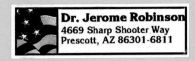
D0742669

OXFORD MEDICAL PUBLICATIONS

AN ACCOUNT OF THE FOXGLOVE
AND ITS MEDICAL USES
1785-1985

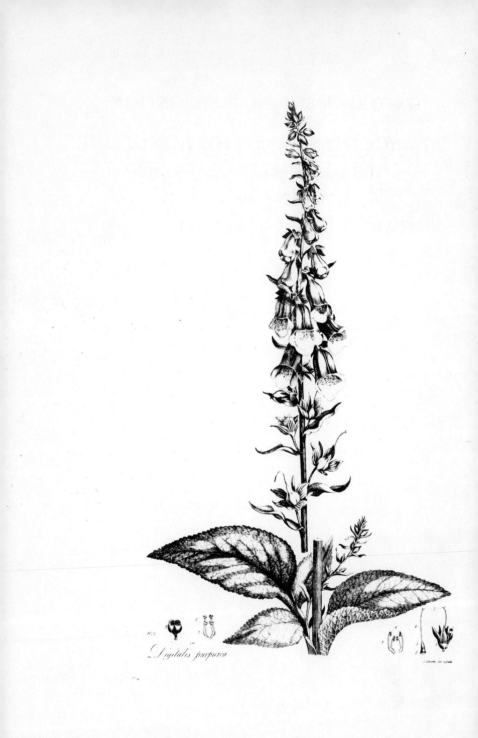

Digitalis purpurea

AN
ACCOUNT OF THE
FOXGLOVE
AND ITS MEDICAL USES
1785-1985

J. K. ARONSON MA DPhil MB FRCP

Clinical Reader in Clinical Pharmacology (Wellcome Lecturer),
University of Oxford
Honorary Consultant in Clinical Pharmacology to the
Oxfordshire Health Authority

London   New York   Tokyo
OXFORD UNIVERSITY PRESS
1985

Oxford University Press, Walton Street, Oxford OX2 6DP
Oxford New York Toronto
Delhi Bombay Calcutta Madras Karachi
Kuala Lumpur Singapore Hong Kong Tokyo
Nairobi Dar es Salaam Cape Town
Melbourne Auckland
and associated companies in
Beirut Berlin Ibadan Nicosia

Oxford is a trade mark of Oxford University Press

British Library Cataloguing in Publication Data
Aronson, J. K.
An account of the foxglove and its medical
uses 1785-1985.—(Oxford medical publications)
1. Digitalis—History
I. Title
615'.32381   RM666.D5
ISBN 0-19-261501-7

Library of Congress Cataloging in Publication Data
Aronson, J. K.
An account of the foxglove and its medical
uses, 1785-1985
Includes a facsimile of W. Withering's original
monograph, Account of the foxglove, and some of its
medical uses.
Bibliography: p.
Includes index.
1. Digitalis—Therapeutic use—History.   2. Digitalis—
Therapeutic use—Case studies—Early works to 1800.
3. Edema—Case studies—Early works to 1800.
4. Withering, William, 1741-1799. Account of the
foxglove, and some of its medical uses. 1985.
I. Withering, William, 1741-1799. Account of the
foxglove, and some of its medical uses. 1985.
II. Title.
RM666.D5A74 1985   615'.32381   85-13829
ISBN 0-19-261501-7

Set by Joshua Associates Limited, Oxford
Printed in Great Britain by
J. W. Arrowsmith Ltd, Bristol

With love, to Renée, who bore my absence from home more
often and
with greater patience than I had reason to expect.

PREFACE

I have written this book to celebrate the 200th anniversary of the publication in 1785 of William Withering's monograph *An Account of the Foxglove and some of its Medical Uses: with Practical Remarks on Dropsy, and other Diseases*. The book is in two parts: in the first I have tried to understand the past through a knowledge of the present, and in the second I have tried to understand the present through a knowledge of the past.

The first part of the book consists of a facsimile of Withering's original monograph, to which I have added annotations which either comment on his text in the light of what we now know about the diseases Withering described or the actions of the compounds he used, or which simply elucidate the meaning of what he is saying (e.g. the modern names of the medicines he refers to, with a brief explanation of what he expected them to do, or an explanation of some technical term which is itself no longer in current use or which refers to some practice no longer applied). In this way I have tried to enliven the text for the modern reader, limited though I was by the constraints of the space available for marginal comments.

The second part of the book consists of my own account of the history of the use of the digitalis glycosides and related compounds over the last 200 years. In writing this section I have restricted myself mostly to clinical matters, introducing only such pharmacological details as seemed necessary to improve understanding. I have also taken pains not simply to recount a bald history of events, interesting though they are in themselves, but also to describe how *attitudes* to the use of digitalis have changed over the years, and how the history of its use has in turn influenced its subsequent use. I have hoped thereby to learn something about how modern practice has been influenced and about what we can learn about our own practices through a knowledge of the previous habits of others.

PREFACE

Withering's *Account of the Foxglove* is the first English text in which the therapeutic effects of a drug are described in detail and its therapeutic usefulness discussed. I believe that it stands as a model for all subsequent such accounts, given the state of the practice of medicine at the time in which it was written, and it deserves commemoration as such.

Oxford   J. K. A.
January 1985

ACKNOWLEDGEMENTS

I owe thanks to more people than I can possibly mention, and I should therefore like to start by expressing my gratitude to everyone who in some way has helped or encouraged me while preparing this book, and to apologize to those whom I shall not mention by name.

My thanks are due in greatest measure to the members of the Wellcome Unit for the History of Medicine in the Banbury Road. They have made space for me in their library, entertained me in their tea-room, and most important of all borne my questions with patience. I owe most to Irvine Loudon, David Hamilton, and Charles Webster, and particularly the last, since it was he who first encouraged me to pursue my interest in the history of digitalis several years ago, and who reassured me that what I was doing was worth while.

I should never have written this book at all had it not been for David Grahame-Smith, who introduced me to digitalis in the first place, and who has carefully led me down the path of scientific rigour, for which I am most grateful.

Finally, I am grateful to the Royal College of Physicians for having lent its copy of Withering's *Account*, from which this annotated facsimile has been prepared.

CONTENTS

AN ACCOUNT OF THE FOXGLOVE
AND SOME OF ITS MEDICAL USES
BY WILLIAM WITHERING

CONTENTS

AN ACCOUNT OF THE FOXGLOVE
AND ITS MEDICAL USES
BY J. K. ARONSON

PART I
INTRODUCTION

PART II
WILLIAM WITHERING OF BIRMINGHAM

CONTENTS

A N

A C C O U N T

O F T H E

F O X G L O V E,

A N D S O M E O F

Its Medical Ufes, &c.

A N

A C C O U N T

O F T H E

F O X G L O V E,

A N D

Some of its Medical Ufes :

W I T H

PRACTICAL REMARKS ON DROPSY,

AND OTHER DISEASES.

B Y

WILLIAM WITHERING, M. D.

Phyſician to the General Hoſpital at Birmingham.

—— *nonumque prematur in annum.*

HORACE.

BIRMINGHAM: PRINTED BY M. SWINNEY;

F O R

G. G. J. AND J. ROBINSON, PATERNOSTER-ROW, LONDON.

M,DCC,LXXXV.

—**nonumque prematur in annum.** This quotation from the *Ars Poetica* of Horace (line 388) is very appropriate:

> ... *nonumque prematur in annum*
> *Membranis intus positis: delere dicebit*
> *Quod non edideris; nescit vox missa reverti*
>
> [Keep your manuscript on the shelf for nine years:
> You can destroy what you haven't published,
> but you can't take back what you have]

As Withering noted (page vi) he waited ten years after starting to use the foxglove before publishing his *Account*.

P R E F A C E.

AFTER being frequently urged to write upon this fubject, and as often declining to do it, from apprehenfion of my own inability, I am at length compelled to take up the pen, however unqualified I may ftill feel myfelf for the tafk.

The ufe of the Foxglove is getting abroad, and it is better the world fhould derive fome inftruction, however imperfect, from my experience, than that the lives of men fhould be hazarded by its unguarded exhibition, or that a medicine of fo much efficacy fhould be condemned and rejected as dangerous and unmanageable.

It

It is now about ten years fince I firft began to ufe this medicine. Experience and
cautious attention gradually taught me how
to ufe it. For the laft two years I have not
had occafion to alter the modes of management ; but I am ftill far from thinking
them perfect.

far from thinking
them perfect Never-
theless, the analyses of
Withering's own case
reports shown in the
Figures on pp. 271-5
suggest that he was as
successful in his use of
digitalis as any other
practitioner until
recent times. For
example, his rate of
toxicity during 1784-5
can be estimated at
about 20 per cent.
Even with the advent
of sophisticated tech-
niques for measuring
the clinical and
pharmacological
effects of digitalis
modern rates of toxi-
city may not be any
better. Rates as high as
29 per cent for in-
patients and 16 per
cent for out-patients
have been observed
(Aronson 1983a).

Apothecaries In his
obituary of
Withering, J. Crane
(1799) wrote, 'He
never prescribed more
medicines than
appeared to be abso-
lutely necessary, con-
sulting by such
conduct the interest of
the patient rather than
the interest of the
apothecary. Hence he
was not generally

It would have been an eafy tafk to have
given felect cafes, whofe fuccefsful treatment
would have fpoken ftrongly in favour of the
medicine, and perhaps been flattering to my
own reputation. But Truth and Science
would condemn the procedure. I have
therefore mentioned every cafe in which I
have prefcribed the Foxglove, proper or improper, fuccefsful or otherwife. Such a
conduct will lay me open to the cenfure of
thofe who are difpofed to cenfure, but it
will meet the approbation of others, who are
the beft qualified to be judges.

To the Surgeons and Apothecaries, with
whom I am connected in practice, both in
this town and at a diftance, I beg leave to
make

make this public acknowledgment, for the
affiftance they fo readily afforded me, in per-
fecting fome of the cafes, and in communicating the events of others.

The ages of the patients are not always
exact, nor would the labour of making them
fo have been repaid by any ufeful confequences. In a few inftances accuracy in that
refpect was neceffary, and there it has been
attempted ; but in general, an approxima-
tion towards the truth, was fuppofed to be
fufficient.

The cafes related from my own experience, are generally written in the fhorteft
form I could contrive, in order to fave time
and labour. Some of them are given more
in detail, when particular circumftances
made fuch detail neceffary ; but the cafes
communicated by other practitioners, are
given in their own words.

I muft caution the reader, who is not a
practitioner in phyfic, that no general de-
ductions, decifive upon the failure or fuccefs

beloved by the subor-
dinate part of the pro-
fession.'

**The ages of the
patients are not
always exact** This
seems uncharacteristic
of Withering. In fact
he gives the ages of all
but 15 of his patients
(see Fig. 4.1, p. 271),
but it is possible that
he did not always
make a note of a
patient's age at the
time, and trusted to
memory when pre-
paring his text.

**who is not a practi-
tioner in physic**
There was an insati-
able thirst for medical
information among
the knowledgeable
gentry of the eigh-
teenth century, and
Withering would have
expected larger sales
of his monograph
among laymen than
among other physi-
cians. This interest
was motivated by
more than idle
curiosity—medical
consultations and
drugs were expensive,
and self-treatment
was widely practised;
furthermore,
informed lay opinions
seem in turn to have
influenced clinical
practice (Jewson 1974).
I was therefore sur-
prised not to have
found a review of
Withering's *Account*
in contemporary
issues of the *Gentle-
man's Magazine*.

of the medicine, can be drawn from the cafes I now prefent to him. Thefe cafes muft be confidered as the moft hopelefs and deplorable that exift ; for phyficians are feldom confulted in chronic difeafes, till the ufual remedies have failed : and, indeed, for fome years, whilft I was lefs expert in the management of the Digitalis, I feldom prefcribed it, but when the failure of every other method compelled me to do it ; fo that upon the whole, the inftances I am going to adduce, may truly be confidered as cafes loft to the common run of practice, and only fnatched from deftruction, by the efficacy of the Digitalis; and this in fo remarkable a manner, that, if the properties of that plant had not been difcovered, by far the greateft part of thefe patients muft have died.

There are men who will hardly admit of any thing which an author advances in fupport of a favorite medicine, and I allow they may have fome caufe for their hefitation; nor do I expect they will wave their ufual modes of judg-

Margin notes:

physicians are seldom consulted See the note to p. vii.

I seldom prescribed it It is a general principle to reserve new, potentially dangerous drugs for intractable or serious cases, as Withering does here. A good recent example of this approach is the careful way in which anti-digoxin antibody was first used in the treatment of digoxin toxicity (Smith *et al.* 1976) (see note to p. 187).

There are men ... Withering's fears were unjustified. The *Account* was universally acclaimed when it appeared (see pp. 292-7).

PREFACE. ix

judging upon the prefent occafion. I could
wifh therefore that fuch readers would pafs
over what I have faid, and attend only to
the communications from correfpondents,
becaufe they cannot be fuppofed to poffefs
any unjuft predilection in favour of the medicine: but I cannot advife them to this ftep,
for I am certain they would then clofe the
book, with much higher notions of the efficacy of the plant than what they would have
learnt from me. Not that I want faith in
the difcernment or in the veracity of my
correfpondents, for they are men of eftab-
lifhed reputation; but the cafes they have
fent me are, with fome exceptions, too
much felected. They are not upon this account lefs valuable in themfelves, but they
are not the proper premifes from which to
draw permanent conclufions.

I wifh the reader to keep in view, that it
is not my intention merely to introduce a
new diuretic to his acquaintance, but one
which, though not infallible, I believe to be
much more certain than any other in prefent ufe.

b 2   After

communications
from correspon-
dents These are
given on pp. 109-178.

a new diuretic It is
clear throughout that
Withering's concept
of the therapeutic
action of digitalis was
limited to his obser-
vations that it acted as
a diuretic (and, there-
fore, he inferred, on
the kidney, see p. 186),
and that it slowed the
rate of the pulse (see
also note to p. 192). In
fact, although digitalis
does have a direct
action on the kidney,
increasing urine flow,
this diuretic effect is
small in patients with
heart failure relative
to its ability to act as a
diuretic by a direct
effect on the heart,
relieving heart failure,
and thus decreasing
fluid retention.

After all, in fpite of opinion, prejudice, or error, TIME will fix the real value upon this difcovery, and determine whether I have impofed upon myfelf and others, or contributed to the benefit of fcience and mankind.

1st July, 1785 The *Account* was published on Monday, 8 July 1785.

Birmingham, 1ft *July,*
    1 7 8 5.

INTRO-

INTRODUCTION.

THE Foxglove is a plant sufficiently common in this island, and as we have but one species, and that so generally known, I should have thought it superfluous either to figure or describe it; had I not more than once seen the leaves of Mullein* gathered for those of Foxglove. On the continent of Europe too, other species are found, and I have been informed that our species is very rare in some parts of Germany, existing only by means of cultivation, in gardens.

Our plant is the *Digitalis purpurea* † of Linnæus. It belongs to the 2d order of the 14th class, or the DIDYNAMIA ANGIOSPERMIA. The *essential characters* of the genus are, *Cup with 5 divisions. Blossom bell-shaped, bulging. Capsule egg-shaped, 2-celled.*— LINN.

DIGITA'LIS *purpu'rea*. Little leaves of the empalement egg-shaped, sharp. Blossoms blunt; the upper lip entire. LINN.

REFE-

---

* Verbascum of Linnæus.

† The trivial name *purpurea* is not a very happy one, for the blossoms though generally purple, are sometimes of a pure white.

b 3

Mullein *Verbascum*, especially *Verbascum thapsus*, also called lungwort. It was at one time regarded as 'the most present remedy in the world' for lung diseases (Topsell 1607). *Verbascum thapsus* was also sometimes colloquially called foxglove (Britten and Holland 1886).

other species are found Boerhaave described eleven such (James 1745)—*Digitalis purpurea, rubella, alba, Hispanica (purpurea minor), latifolia, lutea (magno flore), lutea (minore flore), orientalis, canariensis, angustifolia,* and *minima*. In modern practice only *D. purpurea* and *D. lanata* are used as natural sources of digitalis glycosides.

Linnaeus Carl Linné (1707-78). Swedish botanist and physician. Professor of Botany at Uppsala from 1742. His *Systema Naturae* . . . was published in 1735.

DIDYNAMIA Referring to plants which have two stamens longer (and, hence, supposedly stronger, Greek δυναμις — 'power') than the rest.

ANGIOSPERMIA Plants having their seeds enclosed in a seed-case.

REFERENCES TO FIGURES The references Withering gives here are given in the bibliography as follows: Rivinus (1690-9); *Flora Danica* (1761-1883); Tournefort (1700); Fuchs (1542) (see also note to p. xiv); Bock (Tragus) (1552); Bauhinus and Cherterus (1650-1); Lonicerus (1551 and 1564) Blackwell (1737 and 1750-73); Dodoens (1554) (see also note to p. xiv); Gerard (1633) (see also note to page xviii); Parkinson (1640) (see also note to p. xvi); Gerard (1597); Morison (1672-99); *Flora Danica* (1761-1883).

CHIVES. POINTAL. In the first two editions of his *Botanical Arrangement* Withering preferred the terms 'chive' and 'pointal' to 'stamen' and 'pistil', perhaps to de-emphasize the sexual functions of the parts, having in mind the large number of women attracted to the study of botany. However, since both 'chive' and 'pointal' could mean either 'stamen' or 'pistil' confusion was bound to arise, and in later editions he adopted the latter terms as being those preferred by contemporary botanists.

REFERENCES TO FIGURES. These are disposed in the order of comparative excellence.

Rivini monopet. 104.
Flora danica, 74, *parts of fructification.*
Tournefort Institutiones. 73, *A, E, L, M.*
Fuchsii Hist. Plant. 893, *copied in*
Tragi stirp. histor. 889.
J. Bauhini histor. Vol. ii. 812. 3, *and*
Lonicera 74, 1.
Blackwell. auct. 16.
Dodonæi pempt. stirp. hist. 169, *reprinted in*
Gerard emacul. 790, 1, *and copied in*
Parkinson Theatr. botanic. 653, 1.
Gerard, first edition, 646, 1.
Histor. Oxon. Morison. V. 8, *row* 1. 1.
Flor. danic. 74, *the reduced figure.*

Blossom. The bellying part on the inside sprinkled with spots like little eyes. *Leaves* wrinkled. LINN.

BLOSSOM. Rather tubular than bell-shaped, bulging on the under side, purple; the narrow tubular part at the base, white. *Upper lip* sometimes slightly cloven.

CHIVES. *Threads* crooked, white. *Tips* yellow.

POINTAL. *Seed-bud* greenish. *Honey-cup* at its base more yellow. *Summit* cloven.

S. VESS. *Capsule* not quite so long as the cup.

ROOT. Knotty and fibrous.

STEM.

STEM. About 4 feet high; obſcurely angular; leafy.

LEAVES. Slightly but irregularly ſerrated, wrinkled; dark green above, paler underneath. *Lower leaves* egg-ſhaped; upper leaves ſpear-ſhaped. *Leaf-ſtalks* fleſhy; bordered.

FLOWERS. Numerous, moſtly growing from one ſide of the ſtem and hanging down one over another. *Floral-leaves* ſitting, taper-pointed. The numerous purple bloſſoms hanging down, mottled within; as wide and nearly half as long as the finger of a common-ſized glove, are ſufficient marks whereby the moſt ignorant may diſtinguiſh this from every other Britiſh plant; and the leaves ought not to be gathered for uſe but when the plant is in bloſſom.

PLACE. Dry, gravelly or ſandy ſoils; particularly on ſloping ground. It is a biennial, and flowers from the middle of *June* to the end of *July*.

I have not obſerved that any of our cattle eat it. The root, the ſtem, the leaves, and the flowers have a bitter herbaceous taſte, but I don't perceive that nauſeous bitter which has been attributed to it.

This plant ranks amongſt the LURIDÆ, one of the Linnæan orders in a natural ſyſtem. It has for congenera, NICOTIANA, ATROPA, HYOSCYAMUS, DATURA, SOLANUM, &c. ſo that from the knowledge we poſſeſs of the virtues of thoſe plants, and reaſoning from botanical analogy, we might be led to gueſs at ſomething of its properties.

I in-

---

the leaves ought not to be gathered for use but when the plant is in blossom See notes to pp. 4 and 111.

muscous Mossy.

LURIDAE Plants of a dirty yellow-brown colour.

reasoning from botanical analogy In fact the active principles of the plants Withering mentions here (nicotine, atropine, hyoscine or scopolamine, stramonium, solanine), while having pharmacological actions in common with each other, have none in common with those of digitalis. Withering here disregards his own advice, given to Lady Catherine Wright in a letter dated 3 March 1785: 'Great care should be taken however in reading, not to mistake hypotheses for facts ... In reading it is my earnest desire that you totally disregard all theories and all reasonings from analogy, until you find yourself well acquainted with all the leading facts and even these facts must only be received with slow consenting academic doubt' (Osler Bequest 1928).

Dr. Stokes of Stour-bridge Dr Jonathan Stokes (1755-1831). Physician, botanist, zoologist, geologist, and chemist. He was a member of the Lunar Society and dedicated his dissertation *de Aere Dephlogisticato* (1782) to Withering. His major work was *A Botanical Materia Medica* (1812).

FUCHSIUS Leonhardt Fuchs (1501-66). German botanist, Tubingen. His *De historia stirpium commentarii insignes maximis impensis et vigiliis eld borati*... was published in 1542. See also pp. 216 and 236.

LEWIS William Lewis (1714-81). Physician and chemist. His *Experimental History of the Materia Medica* was published in 1761.

omalade In the original 'ovis placentae', i.e. an omelette. I cannot, however, find the word 'omalade' in any dictionary.

DODONAEUS Rembert Dodoens (16th C.). Dutch botanist and physician. His *Stirpium historiae pemptades* (1554) was translated in English in 1578 by Henry Lyte as *A niewe Herball or Historie of Plantes*. Withering here refers to the revised edition of 1616. Of the fox-glove Dodoens wrote, '[It] hath ... fayre, long, round, hollow floures fashioned like finger stalles.'

I intended in this place to have traced the history of its effects in diseases from the time of Fuchsius, who first describes it, but I have been anticipated in this intention by my very valuable friend, Dr. Stokes of Stourbridge, who has lately sent me the following

HISTORICAL VIEW of the Properties of Digitalis.

FUCHSIUS in his *hist. stirp.* 1542, is the first author who notices it. From him it receives its name of DIGITALIS, in allusion to the German name of *Fingerhut*, which signifies a finger-stall, from the blossoms resembling the finger of a glove.

SENSIBLE QUALITIES. Leaves bitterish, very nauseous. LEWIS *Mat. med.* i. 342.

SENSIBLE EFFECTS. Some persons, soon after eating of a kind of omalade, into which the leaves of this, with those of several other plants, had entered as an ingredient, found themselves much indisposed, and were presently after attacked with vomitings. DODONAEUS *pempt.* 170.

It is a medicine which is proper only for strong constitutions, as it purges very violently, and excites excessive vomitings. RAY. *hist.* 767.

BOERHAAVE judges it to be of a poisonous nature, *hist. plant.* but Dr. ALSTON ranks it among those indigenous vegetables, " which, though now disregarded, " garded,

RAY John Ray (Wray) (1627-1705). Naturalist and philologist. His *Historia Plantarum* was published in three volumes in 1686, 1688, and 1704 respectively.

BOERHAAVE Hermann Boerhaave (1668-1738). Dutch physician and Professor of Botany, Leyden. He is quoted as having said that an infusion of digitalis 'is not used except by the Country People' and that an ointment of Digitalis 'is not in much esteem ... except among the good Women' (Coade 1755). Digitalis is certainly not mentioned in his *Treatise on the Powers of Medicines* (1740).

" garded, are medicines of great virtue, and fcarce-
" ly inferior to any that the Indies afford." LEWIS
Mat. med. i. *p.* 343.

Six or feven fpoonfuls of the decoction produce
naufea and vomiting, and purge ; not without
fome marks of a deleterious quality. HALLER *hift. n.*
330 from *Aerial Infl. p.* 49, 50.

The following is an abridged ACCOUNT of its EFFECTS upon TURKEYS.

M. SALERNE, a phyfician at Orleans, having heard
that feveral turkey pouts had been killed by being
fed with Foxglove leaves, inftead of mullein, he
gave fome of the fame leaves to a large vigorous
turkey. The bird was fo much affected that he
could not ftand upon his legs, he appeared drunk,
and his excrements became reddifh. Good nourifhment reftored him to health in eight days.

Being then determined to pufh the experiment
further, he chopped fome more leaves, mixed them
with bran, and gave them to a vigorous turkey cock
which weighed feven pounds. This bird foon appeared drooping and melancholy ; his feathers ftared,
his neck became pale and retracted. The leaves
were given him for four days, during which time
he took about half a handful. Thefe leaves had
been gathered about eight days, and the winter was
far advanced. The excrements, which are naturally

Dr. ALSTON (p. xiv)
Charles Alston
(1683-1760). Botanist.
His *Lectures on Materia
Medica* were
published post-
humously in 1770.

HALLER Albrecht
von Haller (1708-77).
Swiss anatomist,
botanist, and physio-
logist, Göttingen. Stu-
dent of Boerhaave. His
*Historia stirpium indi-
genarum Helvetiae
inchoata* was published
in Berne in 1768.

ACCOUNT of its
EFFECTS upon
TURKEYS It is
hardly surprising that
the effects of digitalis
on turkeys have not
been widely studied
since the bizarre
experiment recounted
here. However, what
little information
there is (in addition to
common sense)
suggests that it would
be unwise to extrapo-
late from observed
effects in turkeys to
possible effects in man
(see, for example,
Furukawa *et al.* 1980).

turkey pouts Tur-
key poults , young
turkey-cocks; in the
original 'dindonneaux'
(Salerne 1748).

mullein In this case
common mullein, or
Aaron's rod
('bouillon-blanc').

ally green and well formed, became, from the firft, liquid and reddifh, like thofe of a dyfenteric patient.

The animal refufing to eat any more of this mix-- ture which had done him fo much mifchief, I was obliged to feed him with bran and water only; but notwithftanding this, he continued drooping, and without appetite. At times he was feized with con- vulfions, fo ftrong as to throw him down; in the intervals he walked as if drunk; he did not attempt to perch, he uttered plaintive cries. At length he refufed all nourifhment. On the fifth or fixth day the excrements became as white as chalk; after- terwards yellow, greenifh, and black. On the eigh- teenth day he died, greatly reduced in flefh, for he now weighed only three pounds.

On opening him we found the heart, the lungs, the liver, and gall-bladder fhrunk and dried up; the ftomach was quite empty, but not deprived of its villous coat. *Hift. de l'Academ.* 1748. *p.* 84.

polypod. quercin. Poly-
podium quercinum or
Polypodium vulgare. A
fern, polypody,
commonly found
growing at the feet of
oak trees (*Quercus*),
used as a purgative.

Parkinson John Par-
kinson (1567-1650).
Apothecary and herb-
alist. His *Theatrum
Botanicum*... was
published in 1640.

EPILEPSY. — " It hath beene of later experience
" found alfo to be effeĉtual againft the falling fick-
" neffe, that divers have been cured thereby; for
" after the taking of the *Decoĉt. manipulor. ii. c. poly-*
" *pod. quercin. contus. ʒiv. in cerevifia,* they that have
" been troubled with it twenty-fix years, and have
" fallen once in a weeke, or two or three times in a
" moneth, have not fallen once in fourteen or fif-
" teen moneths, that is until the writing hereof."
Parkinfon, p. 654.
SCROPHULA.—

SCROPHULA.—" The herb bruifed, or the juice
" made up into an ointment, and applied to the
" place, hath been found by late experience to be
" availeable for the King's Evill." PARK. p. 654.

Several hereditary inftances of this difeafe faid
to have been cured by it. AEREAL INFLUENCES, *p*
49, 50, quoted by HALLER, *hift. n.* 330.

A man with *fcrophulous ulcers* in various parts of
the body, and which in the right leg were fo virulent that its amputation was propofed, cured by
fucc. exprefs. cochl. i. bis intra xiv. dies, in $\frac{1}{2}$ *pintæ
cerevifiæ calidæ.*

The leaves remaining after the preffing out of the
juice, were applied every day to the ulcers. *Pract.
efs. p.* 40. quoted by MURRAY *apparat. medicam. i. p.*
491.

A young woman with a *fcrophulous tumour of the
eye,* a remarkable *fwelling of the upper lip, and painful
tumours of the joints of the fingers,* much relieved ;
but the medicine was left off, on account of its violent effects on the conftitution. *Ib. p.* 42 quoted as
above.

A man with a *fcrophulous tumour of the right elbow,*
attended for three years *with excruciating pains,* was
nearly cured by four dofes of the juice taken once
a month. *Ib, p.* 43. as above.

The phyficians and furgeons of the Worcefter Infirmary have employed it in ointments and poul-
tices with remarkable efficacy. *Ib. p.* 44. It was re-
com-

SCROPHULA
Tuberculosis of the
skin, the 'King's Evil',
so called because it
was thought to be
curable by the royal
touch.

cerevisiae calidae
Warm beer

MURRAY John
Andrew Murray
(1740-91). Swedish-
born physician of
Scottish parents. Pro-
fessor of Medicine in
Hanover from 1769.
He studied with Lin-
naeus and his *Appara-
tus medicaminum tam
simplicium quam prae-
paratorum et composi-
torum in praxeos
adjumentum considera-
tus* was published in
six volumes between
1776 and 1792 (the
last posthumously and
edited by L. C.
Althoff)

Dr. Baylies William Baylies (1724-87). Physician and apothecary. He emigrated to Germany, because of financial difficulties, in the late 1760s.

commended to them by Dr. Baylies of Evesham, now of Berlin, as a remedy for this difease. Dr. Wall gave it a tryal, as well externally as internally, but their experiments did not lead them to obferve any other properties in it, than thofe of a highly naufeating medicine and draftic purgative.

Dr. Wall John Wall (1708-76). Physician at Worcester from 1736.

WOUNDS. In confiderable eftimation for the healing all kinds of wounds, *Lobel. adv.* 245.

Lobel Matthias de L'Obel (1538-1616). Flemish naturalist. His *Stirpium adversaria nova* ..., with Peter Pena, was published in 1570.

Principally of ufe in ulcers, which difcharge confiderably, being of little advantage in fuch as are dry. HULSE, in R. hift. 768.

HULSE, in R. hist. Edward Hulse (1638-1711). He was a fellow of Emmanuel College, Cambridge, but was ejected 'for nonconformity' (i.e. religious nonconformism). He later graduated MD at Leyden in 1668 with a disseration *De Hydrope*. He was a friend of John Ray, who quoted his comments on the use of an ointment of digitalis in scrofula in volume 1 of his *Raii Historia*, i.e. the *Historia plantarum* (see note to p. xiv).

DOCTOR BAYLIES, phyfician to his Pruffian Majefty, informed me, when at Berlin, that he employed it with great fuccefs in caries, and obftinate fore legs.

DYSPNOEA *Pituitofa* Sauvages i. 657.—" Boiled " in water, or wine, and drunken doth cut and " confume the thicke toughneffe of groffe, and " flimie flegme, and naughtie humours. The " fame, or boiled with honied water or fugar, doth " fcoure and clenfe the breft, ripeneth and bring- " eth foorth tough and clammie flegme. It open- " eth alfo the ftoppage of the liver fpleene and " milt, and of the inwarde parts." GERARDE hift. " ed. I. p. 647.

caries Used here to refer to any bone, not simply, as nowadays, the teeth.

DYSPNOEA *Pituitosa* Or dyspnoea catarrhalis, breathlessness with cough and viscid sputum (L. *pituita* = phlegm).

" Whenfoever there is need of a rarefying or " extenuating of tough flegme or vifcous humours " troubling the cheft,—the decoction or juice here- " of made up with fugar or honey is availeable, as " alfo to clenfe and purge the body both upwards " and

Sauvages Francois Boissier de Sauvages de la Croix (1706-67). French physician and botanist and Professor of Botany at Montpelier from 1751.

GERARDE John Gerard (1545-1612). Herbalist. His *The herball or general historie of plantes* was published in 1597, and was largely a translation of the *Pemptades* of Dodoens (see note to p. xiv). It was revised and enlarged in 1633 by Thomas Johnson. In the extract quoted here he continues: '[It serves] for the same purpose whereunto Gentian doth tend ...', and of gentian he says elsewhere: 'It is excellent good, as Galen faith, when there is need of attenuating, purging, clensing, and removal of obstructions ...'.

INTRODUCTION. xix

" and downwards fometimes, of tough flegme, and
" clammy humours, notwithftanding that thefe
" qualities are found to bee in it, there are but few
" phyfitions in our times that put it to thefe ufes,
" but it is in a manner wholly neglected."

PARKINSON, p. 654.

Previous to the year 1777, you informed me of
the great fuccefs you had met with in curing dropfies by means of the fol. Digitalis, which you then
confidered as a more certain diuretic than any you
had ever tried. Some time afterwards, Mr. Ruffel,
furgeon, of Worcefter, having heard of the fuccefs which had attended fome cafes in which you
had given it, requefted me to obtain for him any
information you might be inclined to communicate
refpecting its ufe. In confequence of this application, you wrote to me in the following terms.*

Mr. Russel ?

In a letter which I received from you in London,
dated *September* 29, 1778, you write as follows:—
" I wifh it was as cafy to write upon the Digitalis—
" I defpair of pleafing myfelf or inftructing others,
" in a fubject fo difficult. It is much eafier to
" write upon a difeafe than upon a remedy. The
" former is in the hands of nature, and a faithful
" obferver, with an eye of tolerable judgment,
" cannot fail to delineate a likenefs. The latter
" will ever be fubject to the whims, the inaccura-
" cies, and the blunders of mankind."—

In

I despair ...
Withering is alluding
in this passage to the
misuse of digitalis by
others, which had
been one of the
reasons for his writing
the *Account* (see
p. 280). Unfortunately,
things did not much
improve following the
publication of the
Account, when as
much, if not more,
misuse occurred (see
pp. 298-313).

* See the extract from this letter at page 5.

In my notes I find the following memorandum— " *February* 20th, 1779, gave an account of Doctor " Withering's practice, with the precautions ne- " ceffary to its fuccefs, to the Medical Society at " Edinburgh."—In the courfe of that year, the Digitalis was prefcribed in the Edinburgh Infirmary, by Dr. Hope, and in the following year, whilft I was Clerk to Dr. Home, as Clinical Profeffor, I had a favourable opportunity of obferving its fenfible effects.

In one cafe in which it was given properly at firft, the urine began to flow freely on the fecond day. On the third, the fwellings began to fubfide. The dofe was then increafed more than *quadruple* in the twenty-four hours. On the fifth day ficknefs came on, and much purging, but the urine ftill increafed though the pulfe funk to 50. On the 7th day, a *quadruple* dofe of the infufion was ordered to be taken every third hour, fo as to bring on naufea again. The pulfe fell to forty-four, and at length to thirty-five in a minute. The patient gradually funk and died on the fixteenth day; but previous to her death, for two or three days, her pulfe rofe to near one hundred.—It is needlefs to obferve to you, how widely the treatment of this cafe differed from the method which you have found fo fuccefsful.

Dr. Hope John Hope (1725-86). Professor of Botany and Materia Medica, and later of Medicine, in Edinburgh.

Dr. Home Francis Home (1719-1813). Professor of Materia Medica in succession to Hope in 1768. He was ever keen to experiment with new drugs, but digitalis is not mentioned in his *Clinical Experiments, Histories, and Dissections* of 1783 (3rd edition, corrected).

In one case ... Some of the manifestations of digitalis intoxication are described here: nausea and vomiting, diarrhoea, bradycardia (probably with heart block), and terminally some arrhythmia (probably atrial tachycardia or flutter with block).

O F

OF THE PLATE.

THE figure of the Foxglove, facing the Title Page, is copied by the permiffion and under the infpection of Mr. Curtis, from his admirable work, entitled FLORA LONDINENSIS. The accuracy of the drawings, the beauty of the colouring, the full defcriptions, the accurate fpecific diftinctions, and the ufes of the different plants, cannot fail to recommend that work to the patronage of all who are interefted in the encouragement of genius, or the promotion of ufeful knowledge.

EXPLANATION.

Fig. 1. The Empalement.

Fig. 2, 3, 4. Four CHIVES two long and two fhort, TIPS at firft large, turgid, oval, touching at bottom, of a yellowifh colour, and often fpotted ; laftly changing both their form and fituation in a fingular manner.

Fig. 5, 6, 7. SEED-BUD rather conical, of a yellow green colour. *Shaft* fimple. *Summit* cloven.

Fig. 8. *Honeycup* a gland, furrounding the bottom of the Seed-bud.

Fig. 9. SEED-VESSEL, a pointed oval *Capfule*, of two cells and two valves, the lowermoft valve fplitting in two.

Fig. 10. SEEDS numerous, blackifh, fmall, lopped at each end.

AN

The figure of the foxglove Withering's *Account* was originally available in two different editions, priced at four shillings (plate plain) and five shillings (plate coloured). In some editions the plate was a mirror image of the original (Brodman 1945). It is not known which was the first version published. One of the two plates is reproduced as the frontispiece to this volume.

Mr. Curtis
William Curtis (1746-99). Botanist to the Society of Apothecaries and a fellow of the Linnean Society.

FLORA LONDINENSIS
Six fascicles of 72 plates each (1777). It established Curtis's reputation as a botanist.

EXPLANATION
The figure numbers refer to the small insets of detail at the foot of the plate (see the frontispiece). *Empalement*—calyx; *chives*—stamens (see note to p. xii); *seed-bud*—the lower part of the pistil, the rudiment of the seed-vessel; *honey-cup*—that part of the flower designed to secrete and contain the nectar; *seed-vessel*—the pericarp.

other modes of analysis Many tests were developed in the early part of this century for pharmaceutical assay of the cardiac glycoside content of digitalis leaf or powder. These included both chemical methods and biological methods, the latter including such techniques as the measurement of the lethal dose in frogs, cats, or guinea-pigs, and the emetic dose in pigeons (for references see Martindale and Westcott 1935). More recently very sensitive assays have been developed to measure concentrations of the order of a nanogram (10^{-9} grams) per millilitre of plasma (see Aronson 1985).

from analogy See note to p. xiii.

AN

ACCOUNT

OF THE

INTRODUCTION of FOXGLOVE

INTO

MODERN PRACTICE.

A S the more obvious and fenfible properties of plants, fuch as colour, tafte, and fmell, have but little connexion with the difeafes they are adapted to cure; fo their peculiar qualities have no certain dependence upon their external configuration. Their chemical examination by fire, after an immenfe wafte of time and labour, having been found ufelefs, is now abandoned by general confent. Poffibly other modes of analyfis will be found out, which may turn to better account; but we have hitherto made only a very fmall progrefs in the chemiftry of animal and vegetable fubftances. Their virtues muft therefore be learnt, either from obferving their effects upon infects and quadrupeds; from analogy, deduced from the already known powers of fome of their congenera, or from the empirical ufages and experience of the populace.

The firft method has not yet been much attended to; and the fecond can only be perfected in proportion as we approach towards the difcovery of a truly natural fyftem; but the laft, as far as it extends, lies

A   within

their peculiar qualities have no certain dependence upon their external configuration this had not always been thought to be so. By the doctrine of signatures (see Cohen 1955) early herbalists gave some plants names according to their resemblance to parts or diseases of the body, and it was thought that they would be useful to treat maladies of those parts. For example, liverwort, or *Hepatica triloba*, so called because of its lobed leaves, of which Dodoens said that it was a 'souveraigne medicine against the heate . . . of the Lyver' (Lyte 1578). Lungwort (see note to p. xi) was so called because of the white spots on its leaves resembling lesions in the lungs.

within the reach of every one who is open to information, regardlefs of the fource from whence it fprings.

It was a circumftance of this kind which firft fixed my attention on the Foxglove.

In the year 1775, my opinion was afked concerning a family receipt for the cure of the dropfy. I was told that it had long been kept a fecret by an old woman in Shropfhire, who had fometimes made cures after the more regular practitioners had failed. I was informed alfo, that the effects produced were violent vomiting and purging; for the diuretic effects feemed to have been overlooked. This medicine was compofed of twenty or more different herbs; but it was not very difficult for one converfant in thefe fubjects, to perceive, that the active herb could be no other than the Foxglove.

My worthy predeceffor in this place, the very humane and ingenious Dr. Small, had made it a practice to give his advice to the poor during one hour in a day. This practice, which I continued until we had an Hofpital opened for the reception of the fick poor, gave me an opportunity of putting my ideas into execution in a variety of cafes; for the number of poor who thus applied for advice, amounted to between two and three thoufand annually. I foon found the Foxglove to be a very powerful diuretic; but then, and for a confiderable time afterwards, I gave it in dofes very much too large

an old woman in Shropshire She has come to be known as 'Mrs Hutton', but there is no information as to who she was or who showed Withering her recipe.

that the active herb could be no other than the Foxglove The ease with which Withering claims to have identified the active constituent suggests that all the other constituents were known to him to be worthless. If there had been any remaining doubt he might have reasoned from analogy with squill (see next page) which he knew to be of some value in dropsy and which, like digitalis, causes vomiting and purging.

Dr. Small William Small (1734-75). Physician and metallurgical chemist. Fellow of the Lunar Society from 1765. See also pp. 254-7.

large, and urged its continuance too long; for mif-
led by reafoning from the effects of the fquill, which
generally acts beft upon the kidneys when it excites
naufea, I wifhed to produce the fame effect by the
Foxglove. In this mode of prefcribing, when I had
fo many patients to attend to in the fpace of one,
or at moft of two hours, it will not be expected that
I could be very particular, much lefs could I take
notes of all the cafes which occurred. Two or three
of them only, in which the medicine fucceeded, I
find mentioned amongft my papers. It was from
this kind of experience that I ventured to affert, in
the Botanical Arrangement publifhed in the courfe of
the following fpring, that the Digitalis purpurea
" merited more attention than modern practice be-
" ftowed upon it."

I had not, however, yet introduced it into the more
regular mode of prefcription; but a circumftance
happened which accelerated that event. My truly
valuable and refpectable friend, Dr. Afh, informed
me that Dr. Cawley, then principal of Brazen Nofe
College, Oxford, had been cured of a Hydrops Pectoris, by an empirical exhibition of the root of the
Foxglove, after fome of the firft phyficians of the age
had declared they could do no more for him. I was
now determined to purfue my former ideas more
vigoroufly than before, but was too well aware of
the uncertainty which muft attend on the exhibition
of the *root* of a *biennial* plant, and therefore continued to ufe the *leaves.* Thefe I had found to vary
much as to dofe, at different feafons of the year;

A 2   but

squill The squill, or sea-onion (*Scilla* or *Urginea maritima*) contains cardiac glyco-sides (e.g. scillaren, proscillaridin) related to those found in *Digitalis* plants. Proscillaridin is used now-adays in some countries for the same indications as digitalis. The squill was a very ancient remedy, and is mentioned, for example, in Syriac texts (Budge 1913). The frequency with which Withering used it for the treatment of drop-sies can be gauged from the index to the medicines and plants mentioned in his text (see p. 386).

Dr. Ash John Ash (1723-98). Physician in Birmingham and then, from 1787, in London.

Dr. Cawley Ralph Cawley (1711-77). An Oxford graduate (BA 1742) and the Princi-pal of Brazen Nose (now Brasenose) College, Oxford between 1770 and 1777, having matricu-lated there in 1738. The college papers relating to his term of office are largely about tedious domestic matters (Coxhill 1946). He was one of seven sons, and his brother Thomas was, among other things, vice-principal of Brasen Nose College from 1746 to 1748. Another brother, Samuel, also matriculated at the College. The brother mentioned here, Robert Cawley, was an apothecary in London. His letter to Wither-ing is given at p. 109.

if gathered always in one condition Modern studies of the seasonal variation in the content of glycosides in foxgloves have confirmed Withering's view. The total amount of the glycosides digitoxin and gitoxin in *Digitalis purpurea* during the first year's growth reaches a peak at between four and eight months, but even when the total amount of these substances is constant during that time the *ratio* of the two varies, being constant only between six and seven months (Evans and Cowley 1972).

decoction A preparation made by boiling the plant in water.

infusion A preparation made by seeping the plant in hot or cold water (first used by Withering in 1778).

began to use the leaves in *powder* In 1779.

but I expected, if gathered always in one condition of the plant, viz. when it was in its flowering state, and carefully dried, that the dose might be ascertained as exactly as that of any other medicine; nor have I been disappointed in this expectation. The more I saw of the great powers of this plant, the more it seemed necessary to bring the doses of it to the greatest possible accuracy. I suspected that this degree of accuracy was not reconcileable with the use of a *decoction*, as it depended not only upon the care of those who had the preparation of it, but it was easy to conceive from the analogy of another plant of the same natural order, the tobacco, that its active properties might be impaired by long boiling. The decoction was therefore discarded, and the *infusion* substituted in its place. After this I began to use the leaves in *powder*, but I still very often prescribe the infusion.

Further experience convinced me, that the *diuretic* effects of this medicine do not at all depend upon its exciting a nausea or vomiting; but, on the contrary, that though the increased secretion of urine will frequently succeed to, or exist along with these circumstances, yet they are so far from being friendly or necessary, that I have often known the discharge of urine checked, when the doses have been imprudently urged so as to occasion sickness.

If the medicine purges, it is almost certain to fail in its desired effect; but this having been the case, I have seen it afterwards succeed when joined with small

ſmall doſes of opium, ſo as to reſtrain its action on the bowels.

In the ſummer of the year 1776, I ordered a quantity of the leaves to be dried, and as it then became poſſible to aſcertain its doſes, it was gradually adopted by the medical practitioners in the circle of my acquaintance.

In the month of *November* 1777, in conſequence of an application from that very celebrated ſurgeon, Mr. Ruſſel, of Worceſter, I ſent him the following account, which I chooſe to introduce here, as ſhewing the ideas I then entertained of the medicine, and how much I was miſtaken as to its real doſe.—
" I generally order it in decoction. Three drams of
" the dried leaves, collected at the time of the bloſ-
" ſoms expanding, boiled in twelve to eight ounces of
" water. Two ſpoonfuls of this medicine, given eve-
" ry two hours, will ſooner or later excite a nauſea.
" I have ſometimes uſed the green leaves gathered in
" winter, but then I order three times the weight;
" and in one inſtance I uſed three ounces to a pint
" decoction, before the deſired effect took place. I
" conſider the Foxglove thus given, as the moſt cer-
" tain diuretic I know, nor do its diuretic effects
" depend merely upon the nauſea it produces, for
" in caſes where ſquill and ipecac. have been ſo
" given as to keep up a nauſea ſeveral days together,
" and the flow of urine not taken place, I have found
" the Foxglove to ſucceed; and I have, in more than
" one inſtance, given the Foxglove in ſmaller and
A 3 " more

small doses of opium The symptoms described in these last two paragraphs, nausea, vomiting, and purging, are all evidence of digitalis intoxication. The diuretic effect in dropsy *should* be achieved without causing nausea and vomiting. As to the treatment of diarrhoea, opium would certainly relieve that, but that it would thereby produce the 'desired effect' of digitalis is unlikely. It is more likely that in such cases opium was having an independent therapeutic effect, acting as a vasodilator and relieving the pressure on the heart.

more distant doses Once it has built up to therapeutic or toxic amounts in the body digitoxin (the main glycoside in *D. purpurea*) takes a long time to be eliminated (with a half-time of seven days). Thus, small doses repeated at longish intervals may be sufficient to maintain an established effect. Repeating such doses daily would lead to toxicity.

Ascites, Anasarca, and Hydrops Pectoris *Ascites* — accumulation of fluid in the belly; *anasarca* — accumulation of fluid in the subcutaneous tissues, especially in the legs, but, in severe cases, widespread; *hydrops pectoris* —accumulation of fluid in the chest (see also Withering's descriptions on pp. 193-207). All of these may occur in heart failure, but also in other diseases. For example, ascites would have been common in chronic liver disease, for which digitalis would not be expected to be beneficial.

Cinnam. Cinnamon, the bark of the *Canella alba* or *Laurus cinnamonum*, used in aqueous solution as a carminative and to relieve nausea and prevent vomiting.

" more diftant dofes, fo that the flow of urine has " taken place without any fenfible affection of the " ftomach; but in general I give it in the manner " firft mentioned, and order one dofe to be taken " after the ficknefs commences. I then omit all me- " dicines, except thofe of the cordial kind are wanted, " during the fpace of three, four, or five days. By " this time the naufea abates, and the appetite be- " comes better than it was before. Sometimes the " brain is confiderably affected by the medicine, and " indiftinct vifion enfues; but I have never yet " found any permanent bad effects from it."—

" I ufe it in the Afcites, Anafarca, and Hydrops " Pectoris; and fo far as the removal of the water " will contribute to cure the patient, fo far may be " expected from this medicine: but I wifh it not to " be tried in afcites of female patients, believing " that many of thefe cafes are dropfies of the ovaria; " and no fenfible man will ever expect to fee thefe " encyfted fluids removed by any medicine."

" I have often been obliged to evacuate the water " repeatedly in the fame patient, by repeating the " decoction; but then this has been at fuch diftances " of time as to allow of the interference of other " medicines and a proper regimen, fo that the patient " obtains in the end a perfect cure. In thefe cafes " the decoction becomes at length fo very difagree- " able, that a much fmaller quantity will produce the " effect, and I often find it neceffary to alter its " tafte by the addition of Aq. Cinnam. fp. or Aq. " Juniper. compofita." " I al-

" I allow, and indeed enjoin my patients to drink
" very plentifully of fmall liquors through the whole
" courfe of the cure ; and fometimes, where the eva-
" cuations have been very fudden, I have found a
" bandage as neceffary as in the ufe of the trochar."—

Early in the year 1779, a number of dropfical
cafes offered themfelves to my attention, the confequences of the fcarlet fever and fore throat which
had raged fo very generally amongft us in the preceding year.   Some of thefe had been cured by
fquills or other diuretics, and relapfed; in others,
the dropfy did not appear for feveral weeks after the
original difeafe had ceafed: but I am not able to
mention many particulars, having omitted to make
notes. This, however, is the lefs to be regretted,
as the fymptoms in all were very much alike, and
they were all without an exception cured by the Foxglove.

This laft circumftance encouraged me to ufe the
medicine more frequently than I had done heretofore, and the increafe of practice had taught me to
improve the management of it.

In *February* 1779, my friend, Dr. Stokes, communicated to the Medical Society at Edinburgh the re-
fult of my experience of the Foxglove; and, in a letter addreffed to me in *November* following, he fays,
" Dr. Hope, in confequence of my mentioning its
" ufe to my friend, Dr. Broughton, has tried the
" Foxglove in the Infirmary with fuccefs." **Dr.**
Stokes

liquors This could
mean either alcoholic
or non-alcoholic
beverages.

bandage ...
trochar See note to
p. 203.

scarlet fever and
sore
throat Common
preludes to rheumatic
fever which can cause
heart failure both
acutely, as a result of
myocarditis, and later
on, as a result of dis-
ease of the cardiac
valves (e.g. mitral
stenosis). Withering's
treatise on the out-
break of scarlet fever
in Birmingham in
1778 is advertised at
the back of the book
(p. 208).

Dr Broughton
Arthur Broughton (c.
1760-96). Physician
and botanist. He grad-
uated MD in Edin-
burgh in 1779 with a
dissertation entitled
De Vermibus Intesti-
norum. He went to
practise in Bristol in
1779 and then to
Jamaica in 1783. The
orchid *Broughtonia* is
named after him.

Dr. Hamilton Of
the several Hamiltons
(not all related) who
studied or practised
medicine in Edin-
burgh at around this
period this is probably
the somewhat eccen-
tric physician James
Hamilton (so called
'the elder')
(1749-1835).

Dr. Duncan
Andrew Duncan the
elder (1744-1828).
Physician and Pro-
fessor of Medicine at
Edinburgh (1774). He
was the influential
editor of the *Medical
Commentaries*. His son,
Andrew Duncan the
younger, became Pro-
fessor of medicine in
1819, jointly with his
father.

**Dr. Charles Dar-
win** Son of Erasmus
Darwin. See
pp. 281-8.

**Edinburgh Phar-
macopoeia**
See note to p. 173.

Stokes also tells me that Dr. Hamilton cured Dropsies with it in the year 1781.

I am informed by my very worthy friend Dr. Duncan, that Dr. Hamilton, who learnt its use from Dr. Hope, has employed it very frequently in the Hospital at Edinburgh. Dr. Duncan also tells me, that the late very ingenious and accomplished Mr. Charles Darwin, informed him of its being used by his father and myself, in cases of Hydrothorax, and that he has ever since mentioned it in his lectures, and sometimes employed it in his practice.

At length, in the year 1783, it appeared in the new edition of the Edinburgh Pharmacopœia, into which, I am told, it was received in consequence of the recommendation of Dr. Hope. But from which, I am satisfied, it will be again very soon rejected, if it should continue to be exhibited in the unre-strained manner in which it has heretofore been used at Edinburgh, and in the enormous doses in which it is now directed in London.

In the following cases the reader will find other diseases besides dropsies; particularly several cases of consumption. I was induced to try it in these, from being told, that it was much used in the West of England, in the Phthisis Pulmonalis, by the common people. In this disease, however, in my hands, it has done but little service, and yet I am disposed to wish it a further trial, for in a copy of Parkinson's Herbal, which I saw about two years ago, I found

I found the following manuscript note at the article Digitalis, written, I believe, by a Mr. Saunders, who practised for many years with great reputation as a surgeon and apothecary at Stourbridge, in Worcestershire.

Mr. Saunders ?

" Confumptions are cured infallibly by weak de-
" coction of Foxglove leaves in water, or wine and
" water, and drank for conftant drink. Or take of
" the juice of the herb and flowers, clarify it, and
" make a fine fyrup with honey, of which take
" three fpoonfuls thrice in a day, at phyfical hours.
" The ufe of thefe two things of late has done, in
" confumptive cafes, great wonders. But be cautious
" of its ufe, for it is of a vomiting nature. In
" thefe things begin fparingly, and increafe the dofe
" as the patient's ftrength will bear, leaft, inftead of
" a fovereign medicine, you do real damage by this
" infufion or fyrup."

Consumptions
There is no reason why digitalis should be beneficial in tuberculosis, but as recently as 1913 it was recommended in William Osler's textbook *The Principles and Practice of Medicine* as a treatment for fever in tuberculosis. See also item 33, p. 205, and the discussion on the use of digitalis in tuberculosis and fevers on pp. 235-7, 310-12, and 320-4.

The precautions annexed to his encomiums of this medicine, lead one to think that he has fpoken from his own proper experience.

I have lately been told, that a perfon in the neighbourhood of Warwick, poffeffes a famous family receipt for the dropfy, in which the Foxglove is the active medicine; and a lady from the weftern part of Yorkfhire affures me, that the people in her country often cure themfelves of dropfical complaints by drinking Foxglove tea. In confirmation of this, I recollect about two years ago being defired to vifit a travelling

Warwick George Eliot, who was born in Warwickshire, wrote in *Silas Marner* (published 1861) of the use of the foxglove by Silas Marner to cure a cobbler's wife of the dropsy, 'recalling the relief his mother had found from a simple preparation of the foxglove' (Chapter 2). For a more extensive extract see p. 221.

travelling Yorkſhire tradeſman. I found him inceſ-
ſantly vomiting, his viſion indiſtinct, his pulſe forty
in a minute. Upon enquiry it came out, that his
wife had ſtewed a large handful of green Foxglove
leaves in half a pint of water, and given him the
liquor, which he drank at one draught, in order to
cure him of an aſthmatic affection. This good woman knew the medicine of her country, but not
the doſe of it, for her huſband narrowly eſcaped
with his life.

It is probable that this rude mode of exhibiting
the Foxglove has been more general than I am at
preſent aware of; but it is wonderful that no author
ſeems to have been acquainted with its effects as a
diuretic.

asthmatic affection
Cardiac asthma (i.e.
pulmonary oedema
due to left ventricular
failure), not bronchial
asthma which would
be unaffected by digi-
talis.

**more general than I
am at present
aware of** It still
happens today, as evi-
denced by a recent
account of poisoning
by foxglove tea (Dick-
stein and Kunkel
1980).

CASES,

C A S E S,

In which the Digitalis was given by the Direction of the Author.

1775.

IT was in the courfe of this year that I began to ufe the Digitalis in dropfical cafes. The patients were fuch as applied at my houfe for advice gratis. I cannot pretend to charge my memory with particular cafes, or particular effects, and I had not leifure to make notes. Upon the whole, however, it may be concluded, that the medicine was found ufeful, or I fhould not have continued to employ it.

at my house At that time Withering was living at 9 Temple Row, in the centre of Birmingham, and had his consulting rooms there too.

C A S E I.

December 8th. A man about fifty years of age, who had formerly been a builder, but was now much reduced in his circumftances, complained to me of an afthma which firft attacked him about the latter end of autumn. His breath was very fhort, his countenance was funken, his belly large; and, upon examination, a fluctuation in it was very perceptible. His urine for fome time paft had been fmall in quantity. I directed a decoction of Fol. Digital. recent. which made him very fick, the ficknefs recurring at intervals for feveral days, during which time he made a large quantity of water. His breath gradually drew eafier, his belly fubfided, and in about

about ten days he began to eat with a keen appetite. He afterwards took fteel and bitters.

1776.
C A S E   II.

January 14th. A poor man labouring under an afcites and anafarca, was directed to take a decoction of Digitalis every four hours. It purged him fmartly, but did not relieve him. An opiate was now ordered with each dofe of the medicine, which then acted upon the kidneys very freely, and he foon loft all his complaints.

C A S E   III.

March 15th. A poor boy, about nine years of age, was brought for my advice. His countenance was pale, his pulfe quick and feeble, his body greatly emaciated, except his belly, which was very large, and, upon examination, contained a fluid. The cafe had been confidered as arifing from worms. He was directed to take the decoction of Digitalis night and morning. It operated as a diuretic, never made him fick, and he got well without any other medicine.

C A S E   IV.

July 25th. Mrs. H————, of A————, near N————, between forty and fifty years of age, a few weeks ago, after fome previous indifpofition, was attacked by a fevere cold fhivering fit, fucceeded by fever; great pain in her left fide, fhortnefs of breath, perpetual cough, and, after fome days,
copious

steel Medicinal iron, thought to be effective in dropsy. It would have been prepared by dowsing red-hot steel in water. Iron salts, such as iron chloride, were sometimes known as salt, flowers, sugar, or tincture of steel. Flowers of steel, for example, was prepared by heating steel filings with sal ammoniac.

bitters Any bitter medicine, such as quinine, gentian, wormwood, and camomile, used as tonics.

Mrs. H—, of A—, near N— This is the case over which Withering and Erasmus Darwin fell out (see pp. 280-91). Darwin identified this patient in his Commonplace Book as Mrs Hill of Aston [near Newcastle-under-Lyme in Staffordshire].

copious expectoration. On the 4th of *June*, Dr. Darwin,* was called to her. I have not heard what was then done for her, but, between the 15th of *June*, and 25th of *July*, the Doctor, at his different visits, gave her various medicines of the deobstruent, tonic, antispasmodic, diuretic, and evacuant kinds.

On the 25th of *July* I was desired to meet Dr. Darwin at the lady's house. I found her nearly in a state of suffocation; her pulse extremely weak and irregular, her breath very short and laborious, her countenance sunk, her arms of a leaden colour, clammy and cold. She could not lye down in bed, and had neither strength nor appetite, but was extremely thirsty. Her stomach, legs, and thighs were greatly swollen; her urine very small in quantity, not more than a spoonful at a time, and that very seldom. It had been proposed to scarify her legs, but the proposition was not acceded to.

She had experienced no relief from any means that had been used, except from ipecacoanha vomits; the dose of which had been gradually increased from 15 to 40 grains, but such was the insensible state of her stomach for the last few days, that even those very large doses failed to make her sick, and consequently purged her. In this situation of things I knew of nothing likely to avail us, except the Digitalis: but this I hesitated to propose, from an apprehension that little could be expected from any thing; that an unfavourable termination would tend to discredit

Then resident at Lichfield, now at Derby.

Dr. Darwin Erasmus Darwin (see pp. 280-91).

deobstruent Of a medicine, opening the natural passages of the body to relieve obstruction. For example, calomel, potassium acetate.

scarify her legs See notes to pp. 21, 40, 65, 86, and 103.

ipecacoanha Ipecacuanha, the root of *Cephaëlis ipecacuanha*, used as an emetic, diaphoretic, and purgative. It contains the alkaloids emetine and cephaeline, and is still used today to induce vomiting after self-poisoning.

prescribed as
follows: The pre-
scription reads, in free
translation: 'Take four
ounces of Digitalis
purpurea boiled in 1½
pounds of pure foun-
tain water until the
water is reduced to 1
pound, then strain. 1½
ounces of this decoc-
tion of digitalis, mixed
with nutmeg water 2
drachms, and made up
into a draught, should
be taken every two
hours'. Compare this
with Darwin's report
given on pp. 284-6.
(Notes elsewhere
explain the symbols
and abbreviations
used in this and other
prescriptions. For
example, the symbols
are explained in a note
at p. 119.)

Nuc. Moschat.
Nucula moschata, nut-
meg, from *Myristica
moschata* (L. *nucula* —
diminutive of *nux*, a
nut), used as a sto-
machic.

pareira brava An
extract of the root of a
Brazilian shrub, either
the *Cissampelos Pareira*
or the *Chondrodendron
tomentosum*. Used in
kidney disorders.

guiacum shavings
Guiacum is an obso-
lete word for guaia-
cum. Shavings of the
wood of the *Guaiacum
officinale*, also called
lignum vitae, were
reputed to be effective
in syphilis. Other
forms of guaiacum
included the resin, the
acid obtained from
the resin, and alkaline
salts of the acid
('soaps').

difcredit a medicine which promifed to be of great
benefit to mankind, and I might be cenfured for a
prefcription which could not be countenanced by
the experience of any other regular practitioner.
But thefe confiderations foon gave way to the defire
of preferving the life of this valuable woman, and
accordingly I propofed the Digitalis to be tried;
adding, that I fometimes had found it to fucceed
when other, even the moft judicious methods, had
failed. Dr. Darwin very politely, acceded immediately to my propofition, and, as he had never
feen it given, left the preparation and the dofe to
my direction. We therefore prefcribed as follows:

R. Fol. Digital. purp. recent. ʒiv. coque ex
    Aq. fontan. puræ ℔ifs ad ℔i. et cola.
R. Decoct. Digital. ʒifs.
    Aq. Nuc. Mofchat. ʒii. M. fiat. hauft. 2dis
horis fumend.

The patient took five of thefe draughts, which
made her very fick, and acted very powerfully upon the kidneys, for within the firft twenty-four
hours fhe made upwards of eight quarts of water.
The fenfe of fulnefs and oppreffion acrofs her ftomach was greatly diminifhed, her breath was eafed,
her pulfe became more full and more regular, and
the fwellings of her legs fubfided.

26th. Our patient being thus fnatched from im-
pending deftruction, Dr. Darwin propofed to give
her a decoction of pareira brava and guiacum fhav-
ings,

ings, with pills of myrrh and white vitriol; and, if coftive, a pill with calomel and aloes. To thefe propofitions I gave a ready affent.

30th. This day Dr. Darwin faw her, and directed a continuation of the medicines laft prefcribed.

Auguft 1ft. I found the patient perfectly free from every appearance of dropfy, her breath quite eafy, her appetite much improved, but ftill very weak. Having fome fufpicion of a difeafed liver, I directed pills of foap, rhubarb, tartar of vitriol, and calomel to be taken twice a day, with a neutral faline draught.

9th. We vifited our patient together, and repeated the draughts directed on the 26th of *June*, with the addition of tincture of bark, and alfo ordered pills of aloes, guiacum, and fal martis to be taken if coftive.

September 10th. From this time the management of the cafe fell entirely under my direction, and perceiving fymptoms of effufion going forwards, I defired that a folution of merc. fubl. corr. might be given twice a day.

19th. The increafe of the dropfical fymptoms now made it neceffary to repeat the Digitalis. The dried leaves were ufed in infufion, and the water was prefently evacuated, as before.

It

myrrh A resinous exudate from the bark of the *Comuniphora (Balsamodendron) myrrha*, also called stacte and ergasma. Used as an antiseptic and vulnerary, to promote menstruation, and as a tonic in fevers.

white vitriol Zinc sulphate.

calomel Mercurous chloride, used as a purgative and diuretic.

pills of soap Medicinal soap was made of two parts oil of almonds to one part caustic alkali (sodium or potassium hydroxide). It was used to dissolve gallstones and urinary stones, in gout and rheumatism, and as an excipient in pills.

rhubarb *Rheum palmatum*, used as a purgative. The active ingredients are anthraquinones.

tartar of vitriol Potassium sulphate.

tincture of bark Peruvian bark, i.e. cinchona or quinine, used as a febrifuge.

sal martis Ferrous sulphate.

merc. subl. corr. Corrosive sublimate of mercury, mercuric chloride.

It is now almoſt nine years ſince the **Digitalis was**
firſt preſcribed for this lady, and notwithſtanding I
have tried every preventive method I could deviſe,
the dropſy ſtill continues to recur at times ; but is
never allowed to increaſe ſo as to cauſe much dif-
treſs, for ſhe occaſionally takes the infuſion and re-
lieves herſelf whenever ſhe chooſes. Since the firſt
exhibition of that medicine, very ſmall doſes have
been always found ſufficient to promote the flow of
urine.

I have been more particular in the narrative of
this caſe, partly becauſe Dr. Darwin has related it rather imperfectly in the notes to his ſon's poſthumous
publication, truſting, I imagine, to memory, and
partly becauſe it was a caſe which gave riſe to a very general uſe of the medicine in that part of Shrop-
ſhire.

**his son's post-
humous publica-
tion** Charles
Darwin's *Experiments
establishing a criterion
between mucaginous and
purulent matter and an
account of the retrograde
motions of the absorbent
vessels of animal bodies
in some diseases* (1780)
(see pp. 280-8).

**very intemperate
living** Probably alco-
holic cirrhosis causing
ascites (he later
became jaundiced),
but an alcoholic car-
diomyopathy with
heart failure could
have contributed.

C A S E V.

December 10th. Mr. L——, Æt. 35. Aſcites
and anaſarca, the conſequence of very intemperate
living. After trying ſquill and other medicines to
no purpoſe, I directed a decoction of the Fol. Digital. recent. ſix drams to a pint; an eighth part to
be taken every fourth hour. This made him ſick,
and produced a copious flow of urine, but not enough
to remove all the dropſical ſymptoms. After a fortnight a ſtronger decoction was ordered, and, upon
a third trial, as the winter advanced, it became
neceſſary to uſe four ounces to the pint decoction;
and thus he got free from all his complaints.

In

In *October* 1777, in confequence of having purfued his intemperate mode of living, his dropfy returned, accompanied by evident marks of difeafed
vifcera. A decoction of two drams of Fol. Digital.
ficcat. to a pint, once more removed the dropfy. He
took a wine glafs full thrice a day.

In *January* 1778, I was defired to vifit him again.
I found he had gone on in his ufual intemperate life,
his countenance jaundiced, and the dropfy coming
on apace. After giving fome deobftruent medicines, I again directed the Digitalis, which again
emptied the water; but he did not furvive many
weeks.

1777.

C A S E VI.

February —. Mrs. M———, Æt. 45. Afcites
and anafarca, but not much otherwife difeafed, and
well enough to walk about the houfe, and fee after
her family affairs. I thought this a fair cafe for a
trial of the Digitalis, and therefore directed a decoction of the frefh leaves, the ftock of dried ones
being exhaufted. About a week afterwards, calling
to fee my patient, I was informed that fhe was dead;
that the third day after my firft vifit fhe fuddenly
fell down, and expired. Upon enquiry I found
fhe had not taken any of the medicine; for the
fnow had lain fo deep upon the ground, that the
apothecary had not been able to procure it. Had

B   the

I thought this a fair case Contrast this approach with Withering's caution in the more seriously ill Mrs H (Case IV, p. 12).

she had not taken any of the medicine Nowadays non-compliance with a doctor's prescription is a not uncommon phenomenon. In the case of digoxin it has been estimated at around 30-40 per cent (Sheiner *et al*. 1974; Johnston *et al*. 1978). However, in Withering's time medicines were very expensive, and any patient who went to the trouble of buying a drug would almost certainly have taken it. In this case the drug was not obtainable.

the medicine been given in a cafe feemingly fo favourable as this, and had the patient died under its
ufe, is it not probable that the death would have
been attributed to it?

is it not probable
See note to p. 14.

C A S E   VII.

February 11th. Mr. E——, of W——, Æt. 61.
Hydrothorax, afcites and anafarca, confequences of
hard drinking.   He had been attended for fome
time by a phyfician in his neighbourhood, who had
treated his cafe with the ufual remedies, but without affording him any relief; nor could I expect to
fucceed better by any other medicine than the Digitalis.   The dried leaves were not to be had; and
the green ones at this feafon being very uncertain in
their ftrength, I ordered four ounces of the roots
in a pint decoction, and directed three fpoonfuls to
be given every fourth hour, until it either excited
naufea, or a free difcharge of urine; both thefe
effects took place nearly at the fame time: he made
a large quantity of water, the fwellings fubfided
very confiderably, and his breath became eafy. Eight
days afterwards he began upon a courfe of bitters
and deobftruents.   The dropfical fymptoms foon
increafed again, but he had fuffered fo much from
the feverity of the ficknefs before, that he was neither willing to take, nor I to give the fame medicine
again.

leaves ... roots See
Withering's com-
ments on the use of
the different parts of
the plant and the
notes thereto
(pp. 179-83).

Perhaps this patient might have been faved, if I
had been well acquainted with the management and
real

real dofes of the medicine, which was certainly in this inftance made very much too ftrong; and notwithftanding the caution to ftop the further exhibition when certain effects fhould take place, it feems the quantity previoufly fwallowed was fufficient to diftrefs him exceedingly.

C A S E VIII.

March 11th. Mrs. H———, Æt. 32. A few days after a tedious labour, had her legs and thighs fwelled to a very great degree; pale and femi-tranfparent,* with pain in both groins. After a purge of calomel and rhubarb, ung. merc. was ordered to be rubbed upon the groins, and the following decoction was directed:

R. Fol. Digital. purp. recent. ʒii.
    Aq. puræ. ℔i. coque ad ℔ifs et colatur. adde.
    Aq. cinn. fp. ʒiv. M. capiat. cyath. vinos.
parv. bis quotidie.

The decoction prefently increafed the fecretion of urine, and abated the diftenfion of the legs: in a fortnight the fwelling was gone; but fome days after leaving her bed, her legs fwelled again about the ancles, which was removed by another bottle of the decoction on the 21ft of *April.*

---

* This difeafe has lately been well defcribed by Mr. White, of Manchefter.

CASE

legs and thighs swelled 'White leg' or *phlegmasia alba dolens*, due to blockage by blood clot of the pelvic veins after childbirth. One would not expect digitalis to help in such a case, and the recovery seen in this patient, and in other similar cases described by Withering (see Cases XXVI, XXXI, and XCVII) was almost certainly spontaneous, since it is in accordance with the natural history of the disease that, in the absence of complications, resolution occurs within two to three weeks.

iss This means 'i semisse', i.e. 1½.

M. *Misce*, i.e. mix.

cyath. vinos. parv. A small wineglassful.

Mr. White Charles White (1728–1813). Surgeon. He is described in de Quincy's *Autobiography* (Masson 1889-90) as 'the most eminent surgeon by much in the North of England'. His *Inquiry into the Nature and Cause of that Swelling in one or both of the Lower Extremities which sometimes happens to Lying-in Women* was published in 1784.

C A S E IX.

March 29th. Mr. G———, Æt. 47. Very much deformed; asthma of several years continuance, but now dropsical to a great degree. Took several medicines without relief, and then tried the Digitalis, but with no better success.

C A S E X.

April 10th. G—G———, Æt. 70. Asthma and anasarca. Took a decoction of the fresh leaves of the Digitalis, which produced violent sickness, but no immediate evacuation of water. After the sickness had ceased altogether, the urine began to flow copiously, and he was cured.

C A S E XI.

July 10th. Mr. M—— of T——, Æt. 54. A very hard drinker; had been affected since *November* last with ascites and anasarca, for which he had taken several medicines without benefit. A decoction of the recent leaves of the Digitalis was then directed, an ounce and half to a pint, one eighth of which I ordered to be given every fourth hour. A few doses brought on great nausea, indistinct vision, and a great flow of urine, so as presently to empty him of all the dropsical water. Indeed the evacuation was so rapid and so complete, that it became necessary to apply a bandage round the belly, and to support him with cordials.

indistinct vision
Visual symptoms sometimes occur in digitalis intoxication (see note to p. 184) and are related in severity to the dose (Lely and van Enter 1970). Blurred vision, however, is very uncommon, and suggests severe toxicity with retrobulbar neuritis.

In

In fomething more than a year and a half, his dropfy returned, but the Digitalis did not then fucceed to our wifhes. In *Auguft*, 1779, he was tapped, and lived afterwards only about five weeks.

For more particulars, fee the extract of a letter from Mr. Lyon.

C A S E   XII.

September 12th.   Mifs C—— of T——, Æt. 48. An ovarium dropfy, and anafarcous legs and thighs. For three months in the beginning of this year fhe had been under the care of Dr. Darwin, who at different times had given her blue vitriol, elaterium, and calomel; decoction of pareira brava, and guiacum wood, with tincture of cantharides; oxymel of fquills, decoction of parfley roots, &c. Finding no relief, fhe difcontinued the ufe of medicines, until the urgency of her fymptoms induced her to afk my advice about the end of *Auguft*. She was greatly emaciated, and had almoft a total lofs of appetite. I firft tried fmall dofes of Merc. fublim. corr. in folution, with decoction of burdock roots, and blifters to the thighs. No advantage attending the ufe of this plan, I directed a decoction of Fol. Digit. a dram and half to a pint; one ounce to be taken twice a day. It prefently reduced the anafarcous fwellings, but made no alteration in the diftenfion of the abdomen.

B 3   C A S E

---

a letter from Mr. Lyon Given at p. 142.

blue vitriol Copper sulphate, also called vitriol of copper or vitriol of Venus. Used as a tonic and emetic, and externally as an astringent (e.g. in ulcers or haemorrhoids).

elaterium This word was used as a general term for a purgative, but here probably means English elaterium, a powerful purgative drug (beta-elaterin) obtained from the squirting cucumber (*Ecballium agreste* or *Momordica elaterium*).

cantharides The dried beetle *Lytta (Cantharis) vesiccatoria* ('Spanish fly') containing cantharidin. It was used as a blister, as a diuretic, and to stimulate the urinary tract.

parsley *Apium* or *Carum petroselinum*. The roots were used as a diuretic and aperient.

burdock *Arctium lappa*, used as a diuretic, aperient, and sudorific.

blisters Substances (e.g. acetic acid, cantharides) applied to the skin to cause blisters, via which fluid might drain (cf. notes to pp. 40, 65, 86, and 203).

made no alteration Digitalis, as Withering noted (p. 6), has no effect on 'ovarium dropsy', i.e. ovarian cyst.

C A S E   XIII.

October 9th. Mrs. B———, Æt. 40. An ovarium dropfy. Took a decoction of Digitalis without effect. Her life was preferved for fome years by repeated tapping.

1778.

C A S E   XIV.

February 8th. Mr. R——— of K———. Had formerly fuffered much from gout, and lived very intemperately. Jaundiced countenance; afcites; legs and thighs greatly fwollen; appetite none; extremely weak; confined to his bed. Had taken many medicines from his apothecary without advantage. I ordered him decoction of Digitalis, and a cordial; but he furvived only a few days.

C A S E   XV.

March 13th. Mr. M———, Æt. 54. A thorax greatly deformed; afthma through the winter, fucceeded by dropfy in belly and legs. Pulfe very fmall; face leaden coloured; cough almoft continual. Decoction of feneka was directed, and fmall dofes of Dover's powder at night.

17th. Gum-ammoniac and fquill, with elixir paregor. at night.—26th, Squill and decoction of feneka.—30th, His complaints ftill increafing, decoction

seneka Or senega. Rattle-snake root, *Polygala senega*, used as a febrifuge and as an antidote to rattle-snake bite.

Dover's powder
Ipecacuanha root, opium, and potassium sulphate, used as a sudorific. Thomas Dover (1660–1742) was a physician in Bristol and the sea-captain of the *Duke*. The original powder, as decribed in his *The Ancient Physician's legacy to his Country* (1732), contained opium, ipecacuanha, liquorice, saltpetre, and vitriolated tartar (potassium sulphate).

Gum-ammoniac
The juice of an umbelliferous plant (*Dorema ammoniacum*), used as an expectorant, often with squill.

elixir paregor.
Paregoric elixir, a tincture of opium, which was either camphorated (English paregoric) or ammoniated (Scottish pare-

coction of Digitalis was then directed, which relieved him in a few days; but his complaints returned again, and he died in the month of *June*.

goric), and flavoured with aniseed and benzoic acid, used as an analgesic (Greek παραγορεειν, to assuage).

C A S E XVI.

August 18th. Mr. B——, Æt. 33. Pulmonary confumption and dropfy. The Digitalis, and that failing, other diuretics were ufed, in hopes of gaining fome relief from the diftrefs occafioned by the dropfical fymptoms; but none of them were effectual. He was then attended by another phyfician, and died in about two months.

C A S E XVII.

September 21ft. Mrs. M—— W—— G——, Æt. 50. An ovarium dropfy. She took half a pint of Infuf. Digitalis, which made her fick, but did not increafe the quantity of urine. She was afterwards relieved by tapping.

C A S E XVIII.

October 28th. R—— W——, Æt. 33. Afcites and univerfal anafarca; countenance quite pale and bloated; appetite none, and the little food he forces down is generally rejected.

R. Fol. Digit. purp. ficcat. ʒiii.
Aq. bull. ℔i. digere per horas duas, et colat. adde aq. junip. comp. ʒiii.

He

He was directed to take one ounce of this infusion every two hours until it should make him sick. This was on Wednesday. The fifth dose made him vomit. On Thursday afternoon he vomited again very freely, without having taken any more of the medicine. On Friday and Saturday he made more water than he had done for a week before, and the swellings of his face and body were considerably abated. He was directed to omit all medicine so long as the urine continued to flow freely, and also to keep an account of the quantity he made in twenty-four hours.

These were his reports:

October 31st.	Saturday,	5 half pints.
November 1st.	Sunday,	6
2d.	Monday,	8
3d.	Tuesday,	8
4th.	Wednesday,	7
5th.	Thursday,	8

On Wednesday he began to purge, and the purging still continues, but his appetite is better than he has known it for a long time. No swelling remains but about his ancles, extending at night half way up his legs.

Omit all medicines at present.

7th.	Saturday,	$7\frac{1}{2}$ half pints.
8th.	Sunday,	8
9th.	Monday,	$6\frac{3}{4}$
10th.	Tuesday,	$6\frac{1}{2}$
11th.	Wednesday,	6
12th.	Thursday,	$6\frac{1}{4}$

On

These were his reports The extent of this man's anasarca can be gauged by the extent of his diuresis—a total of $41\frac{1}{2}$ pints, or 23.6 litres, i.e. approximately 56 pounds weight, lost over a period of two weeks.

On Tuesday the 17th, some swelling still remained about his ancles, but he was in every other respect perfectly well.

He took a few more doses of the infusion, and no other medicine.

C A S E XIX.

December 8th. W—— B——, Æt. 60. A hard drinker. Diseased viscera; ascites and anasarca. An infusion of Digitalis was directed, but it had no other effect than to make him sick.

1 7 7 9.

In the beginning of this year we had many dropsies in children, who had suffered from the Scarlatina Anginosa; they all yielded very readily to the Digitalis, but in some the medicine purged, and then it did not prove diuretic, nor did it remove the dropsy until opium was joined with it, so as to prevent it purging. ——I did not keep notes of these cases, but I do not recollect a single instance in which the Digitalis failed to effect a cure.

C A S E XX.

January 1st. Mr. H————. Hydrops Pectoris; legs and thighs prodigiously anasarcous; a very distressing sense of fulness and tightness across his stomach; urine in small quantity; pulse intermitting; breath very short.

He

diseased viscera A phrase which recurs several times in these case reports and which suggests enlargement of the liver and spleen. The liver would have been enlarged in this case because of alcoholic cirrhosis, and the spleen because of hepatic portal venous hypertension. The ascites and anasarca in such a case would be due to, among other things, lowered production of albumin by the liver. Digitalis would be ineffective in such a case. (The term 'cirrhosis' was not invented until Laennec's observations at the beginning of the nineteenth century.)

Scarlatina Anginosa Scarlet fever (see note to p. 7). There had been an outbreak of scarlet fever in Birmingham in 1778, which Withering chronicled (see the advertisement for his book on p. 208 and the bibliography on p. 265).

pulse intermitting Probably due to atrial fibrillation, but perhaps due to multiple ventricular extrasystoles.

He had taken various medicines, and been blistered, but without relief. His complaints continuing to increase, I directed an infusion of Digitalis, which made him very sick; acted powerfully as a diuretic, and removed all his symptoms.

About three months afterwards he was out upon a journey, and, after taking cold, was suddenly seized with difficulty of breathing, and violent palpitation of his heart: he sent for me, and I ordered the infusion as before, which very soon removed his complaints. He is now active and well; but, whenever he takes cold, finds some return of difficult breathing, which he soon removes by a dose or two of the infusion.

palpitation of his heart Withering's first mention of the heart (see notes to pp. 81 and 192). Note here, as elsewhere (cf. note to p. 43), Withering's use of intermittent dosing, in contrast to the modern habit of continual dosing (see pp. 227-30).

(called asthma) Withering did not recognize that heart failure was the link between hydrothorax (i.e. pleural effusion) and cardiac asthma (i.e. intermittent dyspnoea due to left ventricular failure).

she became so languid Withering overdid the diuresis—the patient lost too much fluid and suffered the symptoms of dehydration.

Mr. Ward ?

C A S E XXI.

January 5th. Mrs. M——, Æt. 69. Hydrothorax, (called asthma) ascites and anasarca. I directed an infusion of Fol. Digital. siccat. three drams to a pint; a small wine glass to be taken every third or fourth hour. It made her violently sick, acted powerfully as a diuretic, set her breath perfectly at liberty, and carried off the swelling of her legs; when she was nearly emptied, she became so languid, that I thought it necessary to order cordials, and a large blister to her back. Mr. Ward, who attended as her apothecary, tells me she had some return of her asthma in *June* and *October* following, which was each time removed by the same medicine.

CASE

C A S E XXII.

January 11th. Mr. H———, Æt. 59. Afcites and general anafarca. A large corpulent man, and a hard drinker: he had repeatedly fuffered under complaints of this kind, but had been always relieved by the judicious affiftance of Dr. Afh. In the prefent inftance, however, not finding relief as ufual from the prefcriptions of my worthy friend, he fent for me; after examining into his fituation, and informing myfelf what had been done to relieve him, I was fatisfied that the Digitalis was the only medicine from which I had any thing to hope. It was therefore directed; but another patient requiring my affiftance at a diftance from town, I defired he would not begin the medicine before I returned, which would be early on the third day; for I was well aware of the difficulties before me, and that he would inevitably fink under too rapid an evacuation of the water. On my return I was informed, that the preceding evening, as he fat on his chair, his head funk upon his breaft, and he died.

This cafe, as well as cafe VI. is mentioned with a view to demonftrate to younger practitioners, how fudden and unexpected the deaths of dropfical patients fometimes happen, and how cautious we fhould be in affigning caufes for effects.

C A S E XXIII.

Auguſt 31ft. Mr. C———, Æt. 57. Difeafed vifcera, jaundice, afcites and anafarca. After trying

how cautious we should be Again Withering tries to defuse criticism in cases where the use of the foxglove might be rapidly succeeded by death apparently caused by the treatment. Note that he seems not to have been criticized for having failed to do anything in this case.

CASE XXIII See also Case XLIX, p. 45.

jallap A drug obtained from the tuberous roots of *Exogonium purga (Ipomoea purga)*, first brought from Jalapa in Mexico, used as a purgative, diuretic, and anthelminthic.

chrystals of tartar Potassium tartrate.

sal succini Literally salt of amber. Succinic acid.

eleterium A misprint for 'elaterium' (see note to p. 21).

CASE XXIV See also Case LXXVI, p. 60.

emetic tartar Potassio-antimonious tartrate, a particularly powerful emetic.

His father died The family history of left ventricular failure is consistent with at least two different possibilities: familial hyperlipoproteinaemia (associated with a high incidence of coronary artery disease) or hypertension. Both might lead to left ventricular failure, but the former is more likely.

ing calomel, faline draughts, jallap purges, chryftals of tartar, pills of gum ammoniac, fquills, and foap, fal fuccini, eleterium, &c. infufion of Digitalis was directed, which removed all his urgent fymptoms, and he recovered a pretty good ftate of health.

C A S E XXIV.

September 11th. I was defired to vifit Mr. L——, Æt. 63; a middle fized man; rather thin; not habitually intemperate; found him in bed, where he had been for three days. He was in a ftate of furious infanity, and had been gradually lofing his reafon for ten days before, but was not outrageous the firft week: his apothecary had given him ten grains of emetic tartar, a dram of ipecacoanha, and an ounce of tincture of jallap, in the fpace of a few hours, which fcarcely made him fick, and only occafioned a ftool or two; upon enquiring into the ufual ftate of his health, I was told that he had been troubled with fome difficulty of breathing for thirty years paft, but for the nine laft years this complaint had increafed, fo that he was often obliged to fit up the greater part of the night; and, for the laft year, the fenfe of fuffocation was fo great, when he lay down, that he often fat up for a week together. His father died of an afthma before he was fifty. A few years ago, at an election, where he drank more than ufual, his head was affected as now, but in a flighter degree, and his afthmatic fymptoms vanifhed; and now, notwithftanding he has been feveral

days

days in bed, he feels not the leaſt difficulty in breathing.

Apprehending that the infanity might be owing to the ſame cauſe which had heretofore occaſioned the aſthma, and that this cauſe was water; I ordered a decoction of the Fol. ſiccat Digital. three drams to half a pint; three ſpoonfuls to be taken every third hour: the fourth doſe made him ſick; the medicine was then ſtopped; the ſickneſs continued at intervals, more or leſs, for four days, during which time he made a great quantity of water, and gradually became more rational. On the fifth day his appetite began to return, and the ſickneſs ceaſed, but the flow of urine ſtill continued.

A week afterwards I ſaw him again, and examined him particularly; his head was then perfectly rational, apetite very good, breath quite eaſy, permitting him to lie down in bed without inconvenience, makes plenty of water, coughs a little, and expectorates freely. He took no other medicine, except a little rhubarb when coſtive.

C A S E XXV.

September 15th. Mr. J. R——, Æt. 50. Subject to an aſthmatical complaint for more than twenty years, but was this year much worſe than uſual, and ſymptoms of dropſy appeared. In *July* he took G. ammon. ſquill and ſeneka, with infuſ. amarum and foſſil alkaly. In *Auguſt*, infuſum amar. with

amarum (L. *amarum* — bitter). Amarine, or benzoline, an alkaloid obtained from the action of ammonia on bitter almonds. It is an isomer of hydroxy-benzamine.

fossil alkaly Sodium carbonate.

vin. chalyb. 'Steel wine', a weak solution of iron, prepared by adding steel filings to wine.

styr. Storax, a fragrant gum-resin obtained from *Styrax officinalis*, used for catarrhal complaints. Another form of storax was prepared from *Liquidamber orientale*, but it had little medical use.

with vin. chalyb. and at bed-time pil. ftyr. and fquill. His complaints increafing, the fquill was pufhed as far as could be borne, but without any good effect. *September* 15th, an infufion of Digitalis was directed, but he died the next morning.

C A S E XXVI.

September 18th. Mrs. R——, Æt. 30. After a fevere child-bearing, found both her legs and thighs fwelled to the utmoft ftretch of the fkin. They looked pale, and almoft tranfparent. The cafe being fimilar to that related at No. VIII. I determined upon a fimilar method of treatment; but as this patient had an inflammatory fore throat alfo, I wifhed to get that removed firft, and in three or four days it was done. I then directed an infufion of Digitalis, which foon increafed the urinary fecretion, and reduced the fwellings, without any difturbance of her ftomach.

A few days after quitting her bed and coming down ftairs, fome degree of fwelling in her legs returned, which was removed by calomel, an opening electuary, and the application of rollers.

C A S E XXVII.

October 7th. Mr. F——, a little man, with a fpine and thorax greatly deformed; for more than a year paft had complained of difficult refpiration, and a fenfe of fulnefs about his ftomach; thefe complaints increafing, his abdomen gradually enlarged, and

and a fluctuation in it became perceptible. He had no anasarca, no appearance of diseased viscera, and no great paucity of urine. Purges and diuretics of different kinds affording him no relief, my assistance was desired. After trying squill medicines without effect, he was ordered to take Pulv. fol. Digital. in small doses. These producing no sensible effect, the doses were gradually increased until nausea was excited; but there was no alteration in the quantity of urine, and consequently no relief to his complaints. I then advised tapping, but he would not hear of it; however, the distress occasioned by the increasing fulness of his belly at length compelled him to submit to the operation on the 20th of *November*. It was necessary to draw off the water again upon the following days:

> *December* the 8th.
> — — 27th.
> 1780. *February* the 4th.
> — — 23d.
> *March* the 9th.

During the intervals, no method I could think of was omitted to prevent the return of the disease, but nothing seemed to avail. In the operation of *February* 23d, his strength was so much reduced, that the water was not entirely removed; and on the 9th of March, before his belly was half emptied, notwithstanding the most judicious application of bandage, his debility was so great, that it was judged prudent to stop. After being placed in bed, the faintness and sickness continued; severe rigors

ensued,

Pulv. fol. Digital.
This is the first time that Withering mentions the use of *powdered* foxglove leaf as such (see p. 4). All of his previous references to the dried leaf (Fol. Digit. purp. siccat.,), would have been to an infusion prepared from the dried leaf, even where he did not specify it as such, e.g. in Case XVIII.

enfued, and violent vomiting; thefe vomitings continued through the night, and in the intervals he lay in a ftate nearly approaching to fyncope. The next day I found him with nearly the fame fymptoms, but remarked that the quantity of fluid he had thrown up was very much more than what he had taken, and that his abdomen was confiderably fallen; in the courfe of two or three days more, he difcharged the whole of the effufed fluid; his ftrength and appetite gradually returned, and he was in all refpects much better than he had been before the laft operation.

Some time afterwards, his belly began to fill again, and he again applied to me; upon an accurate examination, I judged the quantity of fluid might then be about four or five quarts. Nature had pointed out the true method of cure in this cafe; I therefore ordered him to bed, and directed ipecacoanha vomits to be given night and morning: in two or three days the whole of the water was removed by vomiting, for he never purged, nor was the quantity of his urine increafed; his appetite and ftrength gradually returned; he never had any further relapfe, and is now an active healthy man. I muft leave the reader to make his own reflections on this fingular cafe.

this singular case
This is a case of ascites (with clear fluid, if we may so interpret the term 'water'), which seems to have resolved either spontaneously or as a direct result of vomiting. It certainly did not respond to either squill or digitalis. I cannot reach a diagnosis in this case, and others to whom I have shown the case have been equally puzzled.

C A S E

1 7 8 0.

C A S E XXVIII.

January 11th. Captain V——, Æt. 42. Had
suffered much from residing in hot climates, and
drinking very freely, particularly rum in large quantity, He had tried many physicians before I saw
him, but nothing relieved him. I found him
greatly emaciated, his countenance of a brownish
yellow; no appetite, extremely low, distressing
fulness across his stomach; legs and thighs greatly
swollen; pulse quick, and very feeble; urine in
small quantity. As he had evidently only a few
days to live, I ordered him nothing but a solution
of sal diureticus in cinnamon water, slightly acidu-
lated with syrup of lemons. This medicine effect-
ing no change, and his symptoms becoming daily
more distressing, I directed an infusion of Digitalis.
A few doses occasioned a copious flow of urine,
without sickness or any other disturbance. The medicine was discontinued; and the next day the urine
continuing to be secreted very plentifully, he lost
his most distressing complaints, was in great spirits,
and ate a pretty good dinner. In the evening, as
he was conversing chearfully with some friends, he
stooped forwards, fell from his chair, and died in-
stantly. Had he been in bed, I think there is reason to believe this fatal syncope, if such it was,
would not have happened.

sal diureticus
Potassium acetate,
used as a diuretic and
deobstruent.

C   C A S E

C A S E   XXIX.

February 6th.   Mr. H——, Æt. 63.   A corpulent man; had fuffered much from gout, which for the laft year or two had formed very imperfectly. He had now fymptoms of water in his cheft, his belly and his legs.   An infufion of Digitalis removed thefe complaints, and after being confined for the greater part of the winter, he was well enough to get abroad again.   In the courfe of a month the dropfical fymptoms returned, and were again removed by the fame medicine.   Bitters and tonics were now occafionally prefcribed, but his debility gradually increafed, and he died fome time afterwards; but the dropfy never returned.

C A S E   XXX.

February 17th.   Mr. D——, Æt. 50.   Afcites and anafarca, with fymptoms of phthifis.   He had been a very hard drinker.   The infufum Digitalis removed his dropfical fymptoms, and he was fufficiently recovered to take a journey; but as the fpring advanced, the confumptive fymptoms increafed, and he died foon afterwards, perfectly emaciated.

C A S E   XXXI.

March 5th.   I was defired to vifit Mrs. H——, a very delicate woman, who after a fevere lying-in, had her legs and thighs fwollen to a very great degree;

gree; pale and femi-tranfparent. I found her extremely faint, her pulfe very fmall and flow; vomiting violently, and frequently purging. She was attended by a gentleman who had feen me give the Digitalis in a fimilar cafe of fwelled legs after a lying-in (fee Cafe XXVI.) about fix months before. He had not confidered that this patient was delicate, the other robuft; nor had he attended to ftop the exhibition of the medicine when its effects began to take place. The great diftrefs of her fituation was evidently owing to the imprudent and unlimited ufe of the Digitalis. I was very apprehenfive for her fafety; ordered her cordials and volatiles; a free fupply of wine, chamomile tea with brandy for common drink, and blifters. The next day the fituation of things was much the fame, but with all this difturbance no increafed fecretion of urine. The fame methods were continued; an opiate ordered at night, and liniment. volatile upon flannel applied to the groins, as fhe now complained of great pain in thofe parts. The third day the naufea was lefs urgent, the vomitings lefs frequent, the pulfe not fo flow. Camphorated fpirit, with cauftic volatile alkaly, was applied to the ftomach, emulfion given for common drink, and the fame medicines repeated. From this time, the intervals became gradually longer between the fits of vomiting, the flow of urine increafed, the fwellings fubfided, the appetite returned, and fhe recovered perfectly.

C 2 CASE

this patient was delicate, the other robust Appreciating the need to adjust doses according to body weight. The vomiting, diarrhoea, and bradycardia which occurred in this patient were all signs of digitalis intoxication, and the subsequent course typical of the long duration of action of digitoxin (see note to p. 6).

chamomile tea Tea prepared from the flowers of the common camomile, *Anthemis nobilis*, or the wild camomile, *Matricaria chamomilla*, and used as a stomachic.

liniment. volatile Ammonia in olive oil, used as a liniment for rheumatic pains, bruises, and numbness.

Camphorated spirit Camphor (from *Laurus camphora*) dissolved in rectified spirit (i.e. 89% v/v alcohol), used in fevers, epilepsy, and mania, and as an antiseptic.

caustic volatile alkaly Ammonia, used as rubefacient and irritant of mucous membranes. Internally for asphyxia, paralysis, syncope, and hysteria.

emulsion A milky liquor obtained by seeping seeds or kernels (e.g. of almonds) in water.

C A S E XXXII.

March 16th. Mr. D——, Æt. 70. A paralytic stroke had for some weeks past impaired the use of his left side, and he complained much of his breath, and of a straitness across his stomach; at length, an anasarca and ascites appearing, I had no doubt as to the cause of the former symptoms; but, upon account of his advanced age, and the paralytic affection, I hesitated to give the Digitalis, and therefore tried the other usual modes of practice, until at length his breath would not permit him to lie down in bed, and his other symptoms increased so rapidly as to threaten a speedy dissolution. In this dilemma I ventured to prescribe an infusion of the Fol. siccat. Digital. which presently excited a copious flow of urine, and made him very sick; a strong infusion of chamomile flowers, with brandy, relieved the sickness, but the diuretic effects of the Digitalis continuing, his dropsy was removed, and his breathing became easy. The palsy remained nearly in the same state. He lived until *August* 1782, and without any return of the dropsy.

I hesitated to give the Digitalis A stroke is not a contraindication to the use of digitalis. Indeed, digitalis inhibits the secretion of cerebrospinal fluid, an action which might be beneficial in cases where intracranial pressure was increased (e.g. the next case). However, this action of digitalis is clinically detectable only at very high doses, and consequently the risk of toxicity would be high if it were to be used for this purpose.

C A S E XXXIII.

March 18th. Miss S——, Æt. 5. Hydrocephalus internus. As the case did not yield to calomel, when matters were nearly advanced to extremities, it occurred to me to try the Infusum Digitalis; a few doses of which were given, but had no sensible effect.

Hydrocephalus internus A child aged five would need larger doses, weight for weight, than an adult. Thus, if Withering corrected the dose for weight alone here he would have used a relatively

CASE

C A S E XXXIV.

March 19th. A young lady, foon after the birth of an illegitimate child, became infane. After being near a month under my care, fwellings of her legs, which at firft had been attributed to weaknefs, extended to her thighs and belly; her urine became foul, and fmall in quantity, and the infanity remained nearly the fame. As it had been very difficult to procure evacuations by any means, I ordered half an ounce of Fol. Digital. ficcat. in a pint infufion, and directed two fpoonfuls to be given every two hours: this had the defired effect; the dropfy and the infanity difappeared together, and fhe had afterwards no other medicine but fome aperient pills to take occafionally.

C A S E XXXV.

April 12th. Mr. R——, Æt. 32. For the laft three or four years had had more or lefs of what was confidered as afthma;—it appeared to me Hydrothorax. I directed an infufion of Digitalis, which prefently removed his complaints. In *June* following he had a relapfe, and took two grains of the Pulv. fol. Digit. three times a day, which cured him after taking forty grains, and he has never had a return.

CASE

lower dose than usual. Since very high doses of digitalis are required to reduce the production of cerebrospinal fluid (see previous note) it is not surprising that he failed to produce an effect here.

C A S E   XXXVI.

May 15th. Mrs. H——, Æt. 40. A fpafmodic afthma, attended with fymptoms of effufion.
An infufion of Digitalis relieved her very confiderably, and fhe lived four years afterwards without
any relapfe.

C A S E   XXXVII.

May 26th. R—— B——, Æt. 12. Scrophulous, confumptive, and at length anafarcous. Took
Infuf. Digital. without advantage. Died the *July*
following.

C A S E   XXXVIII.

June 4th. Mrs. S——, of W——, Æt 49.
Afcites and anafarca. Had taken many medicines;
firft from her apothecary, afterwards by the direction of a very judicious and very celebrated phyfician, but nothing retarded the increafe of the
dropfy. I firft faw her along with the phyfician
mentioned above, on the 14th of *May;* we directed an electuary of chryftals of tartar, and Seltzer
water for common drink; this plan failing, as others
had done before, we ordered the Infuf. Digital. which
in a few days nearly removed the dropfy. I then
left her to the care of her phyfician; but her conftitution was too much impaired to admit of reftor-
ation to health, and I underftand fhe died a few
weeks afterwards.

CASE

Seltzer water An effervescent mineral water containing common salt and carbonates of sodium, calcium, and magnesium, used in a variety of conditions, including urinary disorders, fevers, and disorders of the bowel. The water came originally from Seltser in Prussia, but Withering probably concocted its equivalent himself, since his son, William junior, noted in his Memoir of his father (1822) that Withering senior's knowledge of the composition of mineral waters was such that he was able to compound 'in exact imitation the waters of Spa, Pyrmont, and Seltzer'.

C A S E   XXXIX.

June 13th.   Mr. P————, Æt. 35.   A very
hard drinker, was attacked with a fevere hæmoptoe,
which was followed by afcites and anafarca.   He
had every appearance of difeafed vifcera, and his
urine was fmall in quantity.   The powder and the
infufion of Digitalis were given at different times,
but without the defired effect.   Other medicines
were tried, but in vain.   Tapping prolonged his
exiftence a few weeks, and he died early in the
following autumn.

haemoptoe
(hĕm'optŏ'ï) An incorrect form of haemoptysis (expectoration of blood), probably from confusion of -ptysis with -ptosis.

C A S E   XL.

June 27th.   Mr. W————, Æt. 37.   An apparently afthmatic affection, gradually increafing for
three or four years, which not yielding to the ufual
remedies, he took the infufion of Digitalis.   Two
or three dofes made him very fick ; but he thought
his breathing relieved.   After one week he took it
again, and was fo much better as to want no other
medicine.

In the courfe of the following winter he became
hectic, and died confumptive about a year afterwards.

hectic The term 'hectic' is specifically used here to refer to the fever which accompanies tuberculosis.

C A S E   XLI.

July 6th.   Mr. E————, Æt. 57.   Hydrothorax
and anafarca ; his breath fo fhort that he could not
lie

fixed alkaly Sodium or potassium carbonate (see also footnote to p. 95).

dulcified spirit of nitre Ethyl nitrate dissolved in alcohol, used as a febrifuge and diuretic.

quack Quacks flourished so well in the latter half of the eighteenth century that the Government introduced a tax on proprietary medicines, hoping to check their activities. In turn the quacks used the tax stamp as evidence of Government approval of their medicines (Hill 1970). For an entertaining history of quackery see Jameson (1961).

Daphne laureola The laurel. Its bark, containing mezereum, was used to irritate the skin and thus excite a discharge (see notes to pp. 21, 65, 86, and 203). Here, however, it seems to have been taken internally.

vitriolic aether Ether, so-called 'sulphuric aether' because it was prepared from sulphuric acid and alcohol, used for many purposes, including fever and pain, and as a diuretic.

lie down. After a trial of squill, fixed alkaly, and dulcified spirit of nitre, I directed Pulv. Digital. gr. 2, thrice a day. In four days he was able to come down stairs; in three days more no appearance of disease remained; and under the use of aromatics and small doses of opium, he soon recovered his strength.

C A S E   XLII.

July 7th. Mifs H—— of T——, Æt. 39. In the last stage of a phthisis pulmonalis became dropsical. She took the Digitalis without being relieved.

C A S E   XLIII.

July 9th. Mrs. F————, Æt. 70. A chearful, strong, healthy woman; but for a few years back had experienced a degree of difficult breathing when in exercise. In the course of the last year her legs swelled, and she felt great fulness about her stomach. These symptoms continued increasing very fast, notwithstanding several attempts made by a very judicious apothecary to relieve her. The more regular practitioner failing, she had recourse to a quack, who I believe plied her very powerfully with Daphne laureola, or some drastic purge of that kind. I found her greatly reduced in strength, her belly and lower extremities swollen to an amazing size, her urine small in quantity, and her appetite greatly impaired. For the first fortnight of my attendance blisters were applied, solution of fixed alkaly, decoction of seneka with vitriolic æther, chrystals chryftals of tartar, fquill and cordial medicines were fucceffively exhibited, but with no advantage. I then directed Pulv. Fol. Digital. two grains every four hours. After taking eighteen grains, the urine began to increafe. The medicine was then ftopped. The difcharge of urine continued to increafe, and in five or fix days the whole of the dropfical water paffed off, without any difturbance to the ftomach or bowels. As the diftenfion of the belly had been very great, a fwathe was applied, and drawn gradually tighter as the water was evacuated. As no pains were fpared to prevent the return of the dropfy, and as the beft means I could devife proved unequal to my wifhes, both in this and in fome other cafes, I fhall take the liberty to point out the methods I tried at different times in as concife a manner as poffible, for the knowledge of what will not do, may fometimes affift us to difcover what will.

a swathe was applied, and drawn gradually tighter See note to p. 203.

1780.

July 18th. Infufum amarum, fteel, Seltzer water.

September 22d. Neutral faline draughts, with tinct. canthar.

26th. Pills of foap, garlic and millepedes.

30th. The fame pills, with infufum amarum.

October 11th. Pills of aloes, affafetida, and fal martis, in the day-time, and mercury rubbed down, at night.

December 21ft. The accumulation of water now required a repetition of the Digitalis. It was directed in infufion, a dram and half to eight ounces, and an ounce and half given every fourth hour, until

garlic *Allium sativum*, used as a diuretic, expectorant, and sudorific.

millepedes *Oniscus asellus*, the common wood-louse or pill-bug. The expressed juice of 50 or so living lice was used as a diuretic and in jaundice.

until its effects began to appear.   The water was
foon carried off.

30th.   Sal diuretic. twice a day.   To eat preferved
garlic frequently.

1781.

February 1ft.   Pills of calomel, fquill and gum ammoniac.

3d.   Infufion of Digitalis repeated, and after the
water was carried off, Dover's powder was tried
as a fudorific.

March 18th.   Infuf Digital. repeated.

26th.   Pills of fal martis and aromatic fpecies, with
infufum amarum.

May 5th.   Being feverifh; James's powder and
faline draughts.

10th.   Laudanum every night, and an opening
tincture to obviate coftivenefs.

24th.   Infuf. Digitalis, one ounce only every fourth
hour, which foon procured a perfect evacuation
of the water.

Auguft 11th.   Infuf. Digitalis.

October 19th.   An emetic, and fol. Cicut. pulv.
ten grains every fix hours.

November 8th.   A mercurial bolus at bed-time.

16th.   Infuf. Digitalis.

December 23d.   An emetic—Pills of feneka and gum
ammoniac—Vitriolic acid in every thing fhe
drinks.

25th.   Squill united to fmall dofes of opium.

1782.

January 2d.   A troublefome cough—Syrup of garlic and oxymel of fquills.   A blifter to the back.

4th.   Tincture

James's powder A febrifuge, emetic, and expectorant, patented in 1746 by Dr Robert James (1705-66), containing calcium phosphate and antimonious oxide (see also note to p. 167). Recently salts of antimony have been used to treat schistosomiasis.

Laudanum Originally any formulation containing mainly opium. More specifically an alcoholic tincture of opium.

fol. Cicut. pulv. Powdered leaf of hemlock (*Conium maculatum*, of the genus *Cicuta*), used to treat cough and cancers.

mercurial Any compound containing mercury.

Vitriolic acid Concentrated sulphuric acid.

oxymel A drink of vinegar and honey (Gr. οχὺς – 'sharp', μελι – 'honey').

4th.   Tincture of cantharides and paregoric elixir.

28th. Infuf. Digitalis, half an ounce every morning, and one ounce every night, was now fufficient to empty her.

March 26th.   Infuf. Digitalis; and when emptied, vitriol of copper twice a day.

April 1ft.   A cordial mixture for occafional ufe.

Two months afterwards a purging came on, which every now and then returned, inducing great weaknefs—her appetite failed, and fhe died in in *July*.

INTERVALS.

From *July* 9th, 1780, to *December* 21ft, 171 days.
From *December* 21ft to *February* 3d, 1781, 34 days.
From *February* 3d to *March* 18th, 44 days.
From *March* 18th to *May* 24th, 66 days.
From *May* 24th to *Auguft* 11th, 79 days.
From *Auguft* 11th to *November* 16th, 98 days.
From *November* 16th to *January* 28th, 1782, 74 days.
From *January* 28th to *March* 26th, 57 days.

None of the accumulations of water were at all equal to that which exifted when I firft faw her, for finding fo eafy a mode of relief, fhe became impatient under a fmall degree of preffure, and often infifted upon taking her medicine fooner than I thought it neceffary.   After the 26th of *March* the degree of effufion was inconfiderable, and at the time of her death very trifling, being probably carried off by the diarrhœa.

C A S E

vitriol of copper
Copper sulphate. See note to p. 21.

INTERVALS
These are the intervals between successive courses of digitalis, none of which seems to have lasted for more than a few days. One could add at the end 'From March 26th to July, [at least] 98 days'. Note that some of Withering's calculations are wrong—the list should read 166, 45, 44, 68, 80, 98, 74, and 58 days. There is no evidence that Withering ever thought of giving long-term therapy, and indeed his method of dosing, if continued for more than a few days would have led quickly to toxicity—he certainly did not appreciate the concept of giving a large loading dose and following it up with small regular maintenance doses (which for digitoxin should be about one-tenth of the former).

C A S E   XLIV.

July 12th. Mr. H——, of A——, Æt. 60. In the laſt ſtage of a life hurried to a termination by free living, dropſical ſymptoms became the moſt diſtreſſing. He wiſhed to take the Digitalis. It was given, but afforded no relief.

C A S E   XLV.

July 13th. Mr. S——, Æt. 49. Aſthma, or rather hydrothorax, anaſarca, and ſymptoms of a diſeaſed liver. He was directed to take two grains of Pulv. fol. Digital. every two hours, until it produced ſome effect. It ſoon removed the dropſical and aſthmatic affections, and ſteel, with Seltzer water, reſtored him to health.

C A S E   XLVI.

Auguſt 6th. Mr. L——, Æt. 35. Aſcites and anaſarca. Pulv. Digital. grains three, repeated every fourth hour, until he had taken two ſcruples, removed every appearance of dropſy in a few days. He was then directed to take ſolution of merc. ſublimat. and ſoon recovered his health and ſtrength.

C A S E   XLVII.

Auguſt 16th. Mr. G——, of W——, Æt. 86. Aſthma of many years duration, and lately an incipient anaſarca, with a paucity of urine. He had never lived intemperately, was of a chearful diſpoſition, and very ſenſible: for ſome years back had
loſt

He wished to take the Digitalis The wording here suggests that the foxglove's reputation had already spread to the laity. Alternatively, Mr H. of A. may have heard of the use of the foxglove directly through another of Withering's patients, or may even have been the husband of Mrs H. of A. (Case IV).

two scruples One scruple = 20 grains.

merc. sublimat. Sublimate of mercury, i.e. mercuric chloride.

CASE XLVII See also Case CV, p. 71.

loſt all reliſh for animal food, and his only ſupport
had been an ounce or two of bread and cheeſe, or
a ſmall ſlice of ſeed-cake, with three or four pints
of mild ale, in the twenty-four hours. After trying chryſtals of tartar, fixed alkaly, ſquills, &c. I
directed three grains of Pulv. fol. Digital. made
into pills, with G. ammoniac, to be given every ſix
hours; this preſently occaſioned copious diſcharges
of urine, removed his ſwellings, and reſtored him
to his uſual ſtandard of health.

C A S E   XLVIII.

Auguſt 17th. T—— B——, Eſq. of K——,
Æt. 46. Jaundice, dropſy, and great hardneſs in
the region of the liver. Infuſion of Digitalis carried off all the effuſion, and afterwards a courſe of
deobſtruent and tonic medicines removed his other
complaints.

C A S E   XLIX.

Auguſt 23d. Mr. C——, Æt. 58. (The perſon
mentioned at Caſe XXIII.) He had continued free
from dropſy until within the laſt ſix weeks; his appetite was now totally gone, his ſtrength extremely
reduced, and the yellow of his jaundice changed to a
blackiſh hue. The Digitalis was now tried in vain,
and he died ſhortly afterwards.

CASE XLIX This patient had spent a year in remission after his first course of treatment. His response to digitalis in the first place suggests that his liver disease may have been secondary to long-standing congestion due to heart failure (so-called 'cardiac cirrhosis').

C A S E   L.

Auguſt 24th. Mrs. W————, Æt. 39. Anaſarcous legs and ſymptoms of hydrothorax, conſequent
to

to a tertian ague. Three grains of Pulv. Digitalis, given every fourth hour, occafioned a very copious flow of urine, and fhe got well without any other medicine.

C A S E   LI.

Auguft 28th. Mr. J—— H——, Æt. 27. In confequence of very free living, had an afcites and fwelled legs. I ordered him to take two grains of Fol. Digital. pulv. every two hours, until it pro-duced fome effect; a few dofes caufed a plentiful fecretion of urine, but no ficknefs, or purging: in fix days the fwellings difappeared, and he has fince remained in good health.

C A S E   LII.

September 27th. Mr. S——, Æt. 45. Had been long in an ill ftate of health, from what had been fuppofed an irregular gout, was greatly emaciated, had a fallow complexion, no appetite, coftive bow-els, quick and feeble pulfe. The caufe of his com-plaints was involved in obfcurity; but I fufpected the poifon of lead, and was ftrengthened in this fufpicion, upon finding his wife had likewife ill health, and, at times, fevere attacks of colic; but the anfwers to my enquiries feemed to prove my fufpicions fruitlefs, and, amongft other things, I was told the pump was of wood. He had lately fuf-fered extremely from difficult breathing, which I thought owing to anafarcous lungs; there was alfo a flight degree of pale fwelling in his legs. Pulv. fol.

tertian ague A fever recurring every alter-nate day (i.e. every third day, counting, as the Romans did, the first and last days of each cycle). The term 'ague' is used here non-specifically, although it would later be used in speci-fic reference to the fever of malaria. How-ever, malaria-carrying mosquitoes were indigenous to the marshes of Britain in the eighteenth cen-tury. Sydenham had already described ter-tian fever in the seventeenth century and the marshes of Lambeth and West-minster were notor-ious as sources of the mosquito vector (Smith 1956). This case, therefore, could have been one of mal-aria.

poison of lead ... colic That lead poisoning could cause colic was well known before the discovery by Sir George Baker in the 1770s (Baker 1772b, 1785a, 1785b) that Derbyshire colic was due to lead poisoning.

fol. Digital. made into pills, with gum ammoniac
and aromatic fpecies, foon relieved his breathing.
Attempts were then made to affift him in other refpects, but with little good effect, and fome months
afterwards he died, with every appearance of a
worn out conftitution.

About two years after this gentleman's death, I was
talking to a pump-maker, who, in the courfe of con-
verfation, mentioned the corrofion of leaden pumps,
by fome of the water in this town, and inftanced
that at the houfe of Mr. S——, which he had re-
placed with a wooden one about three years before.
The lead, he faid, was eaten away, fo as to be very
thin in fome places, and full of holes in others;—
this accidental information explained the myftery.

The deleterious effects of lead feem to be confiderably modified by the conftitution of the patient;
for in fome families only one or two individuals
fhall fuffer from it, whilft the reft receive it with
impunity.   In the fpring of the year 1776, I was
defired to vifit Mrs. H——, of S—— Park, who
had repeatedly been attacked with painful colics,
and had fuffered much from infuperable coftivenefs;
I fufpected lead to be the caufe of her complaints,
but was unable to trace by what means it was taken.
She was relieved by the ufual methods; but, a few
months afterwards, I was defired to fee her again:
her fufferings were the fame as before, and notwithftanding every precaution to guard againft coftivenefs, fhe was never in perfect health, and feldom
efcaped

efcaped fevere attacks twice or thrice in a year; fhe had alfo frequent pains in her joints. I could not find any traces of fimilar complaints either in Mr. H——, the children, or the fervants. Mrs. H—— was a water drinker, and feldom tafted any fermented liquor. The pump was of wood, as I had been informed upon my firft vifit. Her health continued nearly in the fame ftate for two or three years more, but fhe always found herfelf better if fhe left her own houfe for any length of time. At length it occurred to me, that though the pump was a wooden one, the pifton might work in lead. I therefore ordered the pump rods to be drawn up, and upon examination with a magnifying glafs, found the leather of the pifton covered with an infinite number of very minute fhining particles of lead. Perhaps in this inftance the metal was fo minutely divided by abrafion, as to be mechanically fufpended in the water. The lady was directed to drink the water of a fpring, and never to fwallow that from the pump. The event confirmed my fufpicions, for fhe gradually recovered a good ftate of health, loft the obftinate coftivenefs, and has never to this day had any attack of the colic.

as had been prognosticated Of the cases so far described digitalis had proved almost uniformly ineffective in ascites due to tuberculosis, hepatic cirrhosis, and ovarian cyst (to use the modern terminology). Presumably this case was an example of one of those. Alternatively, Withering may have predicted a poor effect of the drug because of the extreme severity of the illness.

C A S E   LIII.

September 28th. Mrs. J——, Æt. 70. Afcites and very thick anafarcous legs and thighs, total lofs of ftrength and appetite. Infufion of Digitalis was given, but, as had been prognofticated, with no good effect.

C A S E

C A S E LIV.

September 30th. Mr. A——, Æt. 57. A ftrong man; hydrothorax and fwelled legs; in other refpects not unhealthful. He was directed to take two grains of the Pulv. fol. Digit. made into a pill with gum ammoniac. Forty grains thus taken at intervals, effected a cure by increafing the quantity of urine, and he has had no relapfe.

C A S E LV.

November 2d. Mr. P—— of T——, Æt. 42. A very ftrong man, drank a great quantity of ftrong ale, and was much expofed to alterations of heat and cold. About the end of fummer found himfelf fhort winded, and loft his appetite. The dyfpnœa gradually increafed, he got a moft diftreffing fenfe of tightnefs acrofs his ftomach, his urine was little, and high coloured, and his legs began to fwell; his pulfe flender and feeble. From the 20th of *September* I frequently faw him, and obferved a gradual and regular increafe of all his complaints, notwithftanding the ufe of the moft powerful medicines I could prefcribe. He took chryftals of tartar, feneka, gum ammoniac, faline draughts, emetics, tinct. of cantharides, fpirits of nitre dulcified, fquills in all forms, volatile alkaly, calomel, Dover's powder, &c. Blifters and draftic purgatives were tried, interpofing falt of fteel and gentian. I had all along felt a reluctance to prefcribe the Digitalis in this cafe, from a perfuafion that it would not fucceed.

A very strong man ... exposed to alterations of heat and cold ?A black-smith

D   At

The reason of this belief will be mentioned hereafter
This patient fits part of Withering's description, on p. 189, of patients in whom digitalis 'seldom succeeds', i.e. 'in men of great natural strength, of tense fibre …'.

assafetida A resinous gum obtained from the Central Asian plant *Ferula (Narthex) asafoetida*. It was used as an antispasmodic, and for that reason Withering recommended it in 'spasmodic asthma'. In his letter to van Lilyveld (see p. 295) Withering recommended, for the treatment of an established attack, coffee, tar preparations, amber mixture, and solution of assafoetida thus: 'Dissolve two drams of assafoetida in half a pint of water. The dose three or four table spoonfuls, i.e. an ounce and a half, or two ounces'.

Nicotian. *Nicotiana tabacum*, i.e. tobacco.

vomit An obsolete use of the word, meaning 'cause to vomit'.

phthisis pulmonalis Pulmonary tuberculosis. The term 'phthisis' is used here

At length I was compelled to it, and directed one grain to be given every two hours until it should excite nausea. This it did; but, as I expected, it did no more. The reason of this belief will be mentioned hereafter. Five days after this last trial I gave him assafetida in large quantity, flattered by a hope that his extreme sufferings from the state of his respiration, might perhaps arise in part from spasm, but my hopes were in vain. I now thought of using an infusion of tobacco, and prescribed the following:

R. Fol. Nicotian. incif. ʒii.
Aq. bull. ℔fs.
Sp. Vini rectif. ʒi digere per horam.

I directed a spoonful of this to be given every two hours until it should vomit. This medicine had no better effect than the former ones, and he died some days afterwards.

C A S E LVI.

November 6th. Mr. H——, Æt. 47. In the last stage of a phthisis pulmonalis, suffered much from dyspnœa, and anasarca. Squill medicines gave no relief. Digitalis in pills, with gum ammon. purged him, but opium being added, that effect ceased, and he continued to be relieved by them as long as he lived.

C A S E

C A S E LVII.

November 16th. Mrs. F——, Æt. 53. In *August* laſt was ſuddenly ſeized with epileptic fits, which continued to recur at uncertain intervals. Her belly had long been larger than natural, but without any perceptible fluctuation. Her legs and thighs ſwelled very conſiderably the beginning of this month, and now there was evidently water in the abdomen. The medicines hitherto in vain directed againſt the epileptic attacks, were now ſuſpended, and two grains of the Pulv. fol. Digital. directed to be taken every ſix hours. The effects were moſt favourable, and the dropſical ſymptoms were ſoon removed by copious urinary diſcharges.

The attacks of epilepſy ceaſed ſoon afterwards. In *February*, 1781, there was ſome return of the ſwellings, which were ſoon removed, and ſhe now enjoys very good health. Does not the narrative of this caſe throw light upon the nature of the epilepſy which ſometimes attacks women, ſoon after the ceſſation of the menſtrual flux?

1781.

C A S E LVIII.

January 1ſt. Mrs. G——, of H——, Æt. 62. Aſcites and very large hard legs. After trying various medicines, under the direction of a very able phyſician, I ordered her to take one grain of Pulv.

D 2　　　　　　　　　Digital.

rather than 'conſumption' to indicate the preſence of cavitation.

epilepsy ... soon after the cessation of the menstrual flux It is not clear here whether Withering is referring to epilepsy occurring soon after a single menstrual period or after the menopause, but in view of the age of the patient it is likely to have been the latter. It has been said that fits are more likly to occur in epileptic women during the week or so *before* a period, but I can find no evidence that epilepsy is more likely to have its onset soon after the menopause than at any other time.

Digital. every fix hours, but it produced no effect. Other Medicines were then tried to as little purpofe. About the end of *February*, I directed an infufion of the Fol. Digital. but with no better fuccefs. Other methods were thought of, but none proved efficacious, and fhe died a few weeks afterwards.

C A S E   LIX.

January 3d. Mrs. B———, Æt. 53. Afcites, anafarca, and jaundice. After a purge of calomel and jallap, was ordered the Infufion of Digitalis: it acted kindly as a diuretic, and greatly reduced her fwellings. Other medicines were then adminifter-ed, with a view to her other complaints, but to no purpofe, and fhe died about a month afterwards.

C A S E   LX.

January 14th. Mr. B———, of D———. Jaundice and afcites, the confequences of great intemperance. Extremely emaciated; his tongue and fauces covered with apthous crufts, and his appetite gone. He firft took tincture of cantharides with infufum amarum, then vitriolic falts, and various other medicines without relief; Infufum Digitalis was given afterwards, but was equally unfuccefsful.

C A S E   LXI.

February 2d. I was defired by the late learned and ingenious Dr. Groome, to vifit Mifs S———, a young

I directed an infusion Withering clearly did not recognize that the infusion and the powdered leaf should have been equally effective, allowing for some differences in dose (see also Case CIV, p. 71).

aphthous crusts Thrush, i.e. infection with the yeast *Candida albicans*.

vitriolic salts Sulphates.

Dr. Groome ?

young lady in the laſt ſtate of emaciation from a
dropſy. Every probable means to relieve her had
been attempted by Dr. Groome, but to no purpoſe; and ſhe had undergone the operation of the
paracenteſis repeatedly. The Doctor knew, he ſaid,
that I had cured many caſes of dropſy, by the Digitalis, after other more uſual methods had been
attempted without ſucceſs, and he wiſhed this lady
to try that medicine under my direction; after examining the patient, and enquiring into the hiſtory
of the diſeaſe, I was ſatisfied that the dropſy was
encyſted, and that no medicine could avail. The
Digitalis, however, was directed, and ſhe took it,
but without advantage. She had determined not to
be tapped again, and neither perſuaſion, nor diſtreſs
from the diſtenſion, could prevail upon her: I at length
propoſed to make an opening into the ſac, by means of
a cauſtic, which was done under the judicious management of Mr. Wainwright, ſurgeon, at Dudley.
The water was evacuated without any accident, and
the patient afterwards let it out herſelf from time to
time as the preſſure of it became troubleſome, until ſhe died at length perfectly exhauſted.

caustic Sodium or potassium hydroxide.

Mr. Wainwright ?

Query. Is there not a probability that this method, aſſiſted by bandage, might be uſed ſo as to
effect a cure, in the earlier ſtages of ovarium dropſy?

C A S E   LXII.

February 27th. Mrs. O——, of T——, Æt. 52,
with a conſtitution worn out by various complicated
diſorders

diforders, at length became dropfical. The Digitalis was given in fmall dofes, in hopes of temporary
benefit, and it did not fail to fulfil our expectations.

C A S E   LXIII.

March 16th.   Mrs. P——, Æt. 47.   Great debility, pale countenance, lofs of appetite, legs fwelled,
urine in fmall quantity.   A dram of Fol. ficcat. Digital. in a half pint infufion was ordered, and an
ounce of this infufion directed to be taken every
morning.   Myrrh and fteel were given at intervals.
Her urine foon increafed, and the fymptoms of
dropfy difappeared.

C A S E   LXIV.

March 18th.   Mr. W————, in the laft ftage
of a pulmonary confumption became dropfical. The
Digitalis was given, but without any good effect.

C A S E   LXV.

April 6th.   Mr. B————, Æt. 63.   For fome
years back had complained of being afthmatical,
and was not without fufpicion of difeafed vifcera.   The laft winter he had been moftly confined
to his houfe ; became dropfical, loft his appetite,
and his fkin and eyes turned yellow.   By the ufe
of medicines of the deobftruent clafs he became lefs
difcoloured, and the hardnefs about his ftomach
feemed to yield ; but the afcites and anafarcous
fymptoms increafed fo as to opprefs his breathing
exceed-

exceedingly. Alkaline falts, and other diuretics failing of their effects, I ordered him to take an infuf. of Digitalis. It operated fo powerfully that it be came neceffary to fupport him with cordials and blifters, but it freed him from the dropfy, and his breath became quite eafy. He then took foap, rhubarb, tartar of vitriol, and fteel, and gradually attained a good ftate of health, which he ftill continues to enjoy.

C A S E LXVI.

April 8th. Mr. B——, Æt. 60. A corpulent man, with a ftone in his bladder, from which at times his fufferings are extreme. He had been affected with what was fuppofed to be an afthma, for feveral years by fits, but through the laft winter his breath had been much worfe than ufual; univerfal anafarca came on, and foon afterwards an afcites. Now his urine was fmall in quantity and much faturated, the dyfuria was more dreadful than ever; his breath would not allow him to lie in bed, nor would the dyfuria permit him to fleep; in this diftrefsful fituation, after having ufed other medicines to little purpofe, I directed an infufion of Digitalis to be given. When the quantity of urine became more plentiful, the pain from his ftone grew eafier; in a few days the dropfy and afthma difappeared, and he foon regained his ufual ftrength and health. Every year fince, there has been a tendency to a return of thefe complaints, but he has recourfe to the infufion, and immediately removes them.

Every year since
That is a total of at least three or four further bouts, each of which was relieved by a single course of digitalis.

CASE

C A S E   LXVII.

April 24th. Mr. M——, of C——, Æt. 57.
Afthma, anafarca, jaundice, and great hardnefs and
ftraitnefs acrofs the region of the ftomach. After a
free exhibition of neutral draughts, alkaline falt,
&c. the dropfy and difficult breathing remaining the
fame, he took Infufum Digitalis, which removed
thofe complaints. He never loft the hardnefs about
his ftomach, but enjoyed very tolerable health for
three years afterwards, without any return of the
dropfy.

C A S E   LXVIII.

April 25th. Mrs. J——, Æt. 42. Phthifis pulmonalis and anafarcous legs and thighs. She took
the Infufum Digitalis without effect. Myrrh and
fteel, with fixed alkaly, were then ordered, but to
no purpofe.

C A S E   LXIX.

May 1ft. Mafter W————, of St——, Æt. 6.
I found him with every fymptom of hydrocephalus
internus. As it was yet early in the difeafe, in confequence of ideas which will be mentioned hereafter, I directed fix ounces of blood to be immediately taken from the arm; the temporal artery to
be opened the fucceeding day; the head to be fha-
ven, and fix pints of cold water to be poured upon
it every fourth hour, and two fcruples of ftrong mer-
                                            curial

curial ointment to be rubbed into the legs every day. Five days afterwards, finding the febrile fymptoms very much abated, and judging the remaining difeafe to be the effect of effufion, I directed a fcruple of Fol. Digital. ficcat. to be infufed in three ounces of water, and a table fpoonful of the infufion to be given every third or fourth hour, until its action fhould be fomeway fenfible. The effect was, an increafed fecretion of urine; and the patient foon recovered.

C A S E LXX.

May 3d. Mrs. B——, Æt. 59. Afcites and anafarca, with ftrong fymptoms of difeafed vifcera. Infufum Digitalis was at firft prefcribed, and prefently removed the dropfy. She was then put upon faline draughts and calomel. After fome time fhe became feverifh: the fever proved intermittent, and was cured by the bark.

the bark The bark of any variety of the cinchona tree, containing quinine, ground into a powder and used to treat fever in general.

C A S E LXXI.

May 3d. Mr. S——, Æt. 48. A ftrong man, who had lived intemperately. For fome time paft his breath had been very fhort, his legs fwollen towards evening, and his urine fmall in quantity. Eight ounces of the Infuf. Digitalis caufed a confiderable flow of urine; his complaints gradually vanifhed, and did not return.

C A S E

C A S E   LXXII.

May 24th. Jofeph B———, Æt. 50. Afcites, anafarca, and jaundice, from intemperate living. Infufion of Digitalis produced naufea, and lowered the
frequency of the pulfe; but had no other fenfible effects. His diforder continued to increafe, and killed
him about two months afterwards.

C A S E   LXXIII.

June 29th. Mr. B———, Æt. 60. A hard drinker;
afflicted with afthma, jaundice, and dropfy. His
appetite gone; his water foul and in fmall quantity.
Neutral faline mixture, chryftals of tartar, vinum
chalybeat. and other medicines had been prefcribed
to little advantage. Infufion of Fol. Digitalis acted
powerfully as a diuretic, and removed the moft urgent of his complaints, viz. the dropfical and afthmatical fymptoms.

The following winter his breathing grew bad again,
his appetite totally failed, and he died, but without
any return of the afcites.

C A S E   LXXIV.

June 29th. Mr. A———, Æt. 58. Kept a public
houfe and drank very hard. He had fymptoms of
difeafed vifcera, jaundice, afcites, and anafarca. After taking various deobftruents and diuretics, to no
purpofe, he was ordered the Infufion of Digitalis:
a few

**Kept a public
house** It is not sur-
prising that the pre-
valence of hepatic
cirrhosis is increased
among publicans (the
other publicans
Withering treated are
described as Cases
LXXXV, CII, CIII, and
possibly CXXXV).
The current figures
show that death from
cirrhosis is 15.8 times
more common among
publicans than in the
general population.
The figure for bar-
maids and barmen is
6.3 times, and for pro-
prietors and managers
of boarding houses
and hotels 5.1 times.
Only seamen and
fishermen (6.6 to 7.8
times) rival these
figures (Office of
Population Censuses
and Surveys 1978).

a few dofes occafioned a plentiful flow of urine, relieved his breath, and reduced his fwellings; but,
on account of his great weaknefs, it was judged imprudent to urge the medicine to the entire evacuation of the water. He was fo much relieved as to
be able to come down ftairs and to walk about, but
his want of appetite and jaundice continuing, and
his debility increafing, he died in about two
months.

C A S E   LXXV.

July 18th. Mrs. B——, Æt. 46. A little woman, and very much deformed. Afthmatical for
many years. For feveral months paft had been worfe
than ufual; appetite totally gone, legs fwollen,
fenfe of great fulnefs about her ftomach, countenance fallen, lips livid, could not lie down.

The ufual modes of practice failing, the Digitalis
was tried, but with no better fuccefs, and in about a
month fhe died; not without fufpicion of her death
having been accelerated a few days, by her taking
half a grain of opium. This may be a caution to
young practitioners to be careful how they venture
upon even fmall dofes of opium in fuch conftitutions, however much they may be urged by the patient to prefcribe fomething that may procure a little
reft and eafe.

C A S E

**very much de-
formed** The nature
of her deformity is not
clear, but Withering
takes the trouble to
mention it and it may
therefore have been
causally implicated.
This suggests that the
deformity was of the
chest with consequent
emphysema and
chronic bronchitis,
leading to congestive
heart failure ('cor pul-
monale'), and the livid
(i.e. cyanotic) lips
support this diagnosis
(see also Case XCIX,
p. 69). Furthermore,
the therapeutic effects
of digitalis are less
impressive in cor pul-
monale and toxicity is
more likely.

**her death having
been accelerated** In
such a case opium
would be contra-
indicated as being
likely to impair res-
piration.

C A S E   LXXVI.

August 12th.   Mr. L——,   Æt. 65, the perfon
whofe Cafe is recorded at No. XXIV, had a return of his infanity, after near two years perfect
health. He was extremely reduced when I faw him,
and the medicine which cured him before was now
adminiftered without effect, for his weaknefs was
fuch that I did not dare to urge it.

C A S E   LXXVII.

September 10th. Mr. V——, of S——, Æt. 47.
A man of ftrong fibre, and the remains of a florid
complexion. His difeafe an afcites and fwelled legs,
the confequence of a very free courfe of life; he
had been once tapped, and taken much medicine
before I faw him. The Digitalis was now directed:
it lowered his pulfe, but did not prove diuretic. He
returned home, and foon after was tapped again, but
furvived the operation only a few hours.

strong fibre See note
to p. 189.

C A S E   LXXVIII.

September 25th. Mr. O——, of M——, Æt. 63.
Very painful and general fwellings in all his limbs,
which had confined him moftly to his bed fince the
preceding winter; the fwellings were uniform, tenfe,
and refifting, but the fkin not difcoloured. After
trying guiacum and Dover's powder without advantage. I directed Infufion of Digitalis. It acted on
the kidneys, but did not relieve him. It is not
eafy

eafy to fay what the difeafe was, and the patient
living at a diftance, I never learnt the future progrefs or termination of it.

C A S E LXXIX.

September 26th. Mr. D——, Æt. 42, a very
fenfible and judicious furgeon at B——, in Staffordfhire, laboured under afcites and very large
anafarcous legs, together with indubitable fymptoms
of difeafed vifcera. Having tried the ufual diuretics to no purpofe, I directed a fcruple of Fol. Digital. ficcat. in a four ounce infufion, a table fpoonful to be taken twice a day. The fecond bottle
wholly removed his dropfy, which never returned.

C A S E LXXX.

September 27th. Mrs. E——, Æt. 42. A fat
fedentary woman; after a long illnefs, very indif-
tinctly marked; had fymptoms of enlarged liver and
dropfy. In this cafe I was happy in the affiftance
of Dr. Afh.   Digitalis was once exhibited in fmall
dofes, but to no better purpofe than many other
medicines. She fuffered great pain in the abdomen
for feveral weeks, and after her death, the liver,
fpleen, and kidneys were found of a pale colour,
and very greatly enlarged, but the quantity of effufed fluid in the cavity was not more than a pint.

**liver, spleen, and
kidneys were found
of a pale colour**
?Primary amyloidosis,
a disease in which
amyloid, a complex
mucopolysaccharide,
is deposited in the
tissues of the body.

C A S E

C A S E   LXXXI.

October 28th. Mr. B——, Æt. 33. Had drank an immenfe quantity of mild ale, and was now become dropfical. He was a lufty man, of a pale complexion: his belly large, and his legs and thighs fwollen to an enormous fize. I directed the Infufion of Digitalis, which in ten days completely emptied him. He was then put upon the ufe of fteel and bitters, and directed to live temperately, which I believe he did, for I faw him two years afterwards in perfect health.

C A S E   LXXXII.

November 14th. Mr. W——, of T——, Æt. 49. A lufty man, with an afthma and anafarca. He had taken feveral medicines by the direction of a very judicious apothecary, but not getting relief as he had been accuftomed to do in former years, he came under my direction. For the fpace of a month I tried to relieve him by fixed alkaly, feneka, Dovers powder, gum ammoniac, fquill, &c. but without effect. I then directed Infufion of Digitalis, which foon increafed the flow of urine without exciting naufea, and in a few days removed all his complaints.

CASE

1 7 8 2.

C A S E LXXXIII.

January 23d. Mr. Q——, Æt. 74. A ftone in his bladder for many years; dropfical for the laft three months. Had taken at different times foap with fquill and gum ammoniac; foap lees; chryftals of tartar, oil of juniper, feneka, jallap, &c. but the dropfical fymptoms ftill increafed, and the dyfuria from the ftone became very urgent. I now directed a dram of the Fol. Digit. ficcat. in a half pint infufion, half an ounce to be given every fix hours. This prefently relieved the dyfuria, and foon removed the dropfy, without any difturbance to his fyftem.

dysuria from the stone Pain during micturition because of reduced urine flow.

C A S E LXXXIV.

January 27th. Mr. D——, Æt. 86. The debility of age and dropfical legs had long oppreffed him. A few weeks before his death his breathing became very fhort, he could not lie down in bed, and his urine was fmall in quantity. A wine glafs of a weak Infufion of Digitalis, warmed with aromatics, was ordered to be taken twice a day. It afforded a temporary relief, but he did not long furvive.

C A S E LXXXV.

January 28th. Mr. D——, Æt. 35. A publican and a hard drinker. Afcites, anafarca, difeafed
vifcera

vifcera, and flight attacks of hæmoptoe. A dram of Fol. Digital. ficc. in a half pint infufion, of which one ounce was given night and morning, proved diuretic and removed his dropfy. He then took medicines calculated to relieve his other complaints. The dropfy did not return during my attendance upon him, which was three or four weeks. A quack then undertook to cure him with blue vitriol vomits, but as I am informed, he prefently funk under that rough treatment.

C A S E　LXXXVI.

January 29th. Mrs. O——, of D——, Æt. 53. A conftant and diftreffing palpitation of her heart, with great debility. From a degree of anafarca in her legs I was led to fufpect effufion in the Pericardium, and therefore directed Digitalis, but it produced no benefit. She then took various other medicines with the fame want of fuccefs, and about ten months afterwards died fuddenly.

had not lain in bed That is, he had orthopnoea, breathlessness on lying down, due to pulmonary oedema caused by left ventricular failure.

at his age Having lived 81 years at a time when the national life expectancy at birth was 38 to 45 years (Revelle 1972). The average age of the male patients Withering describes in the *Account* was 47 years.

C A S E　LXXXVII.

January 31ft. Mr. T——, of A——, Æt. 81. Great difficulty of breathing, fo that he had not lain in bed for the laft fix weeks, and fome fwelling in his legs. Thefe complaints were fubfequent to a very fevere cold, and he had ftill a troublefome cough. He told me that at his age he did not look for a cure, but fhould be glad of relief, if it could be obtained without taking much medicine. I directed an Infufion of Digitalis. a dram to eight ounces, one

one fpoonful to be taken every morning, and two at night. He only took this quantity; for in four days he could lie down, and foon afterwards quitted his chamber. In a month he had a return of his complaints, and was relieved as before.

C A S E LXXXVIII.

January 31ft. Mrs. J——, of S——, Æt. 67. A lufty woman, of a florid complexion, large belly, and very thick legs. She had been kept alive for fome years by the difcharge from ulcers in her legs; but the fores now put on a very difagreeable livid appearance, her belly grew ftill larger, her breath fhort, her pulfe feeble, and fhe could not take nourifhment. Several medicines having been given in vain, the Digitalis was tried, but with no better effect; and in about a month fhe died.

C A S E LXXXIX.

February 2d. Mr. B——, Æt. 73. An univerfal dropfy. He took various medicines, and Digitalis in fmall dofes, but without any good effect.

C A S E XC.

February 24th. Mafter M——, of W——, Æt. 10. An epilepfy of fome years continuance, which had never been interrupted by any of the various methods tried for his relief. The Digitalis was given for a few days, but as he lived at a diftance, fo that I could not attend to its effects, he only took one

E half

discharge from ulcers in her legs It had for some time been the practice to scarify the legs to release oedematous fluid, and in this case the leg ulcers seem to have served the same purpose. Later on fine copper tubes (Southey's tubes, so called after the English physician Reginald S. Southey, 1835-99) were pushed into oedematous legs to drain them. These tubes were used, or at least recommended in some textbooks, until very recently (Dunlop and Alstead 1966). See also notes to pp. 21, 40, 86, and 203.

half pint infufion, which made no alteration in his complaint.

C A S E XCI.

apoplexy Stroke.

March 6th. Mr. H——, Æt. 62. A very hard drinker, and had twice had attacks of apoplexy. He had now an afcites, was anafarcous, and had every appearance of a difeafed liver. Small dofes of ca-

sal sodae Crystallized sodium carbonate.

lomel, Dover's powder, infufum amarum, and fal fodæ palliated his fymptoms for a while; thefe failing; blifters, fquills, and cordials were given without effect. A weak Infufion of Digitalis, well aromatifed, was then directed to be given in fmall dofes. It rather feemed to check than to increafe the fecretion of urine, and foon produced ficknefs. Failing in its ufual effect, the medicine was no longer continued; but every thing that was tried proved equally inefficacious, and he did not long furvive.

C A S E XCII.

it seemed rather to increase than relieve her symptoms This patient had left ventricular failure which was made worse by digitalis. She may, therefore, have had subvalvular aortic stenosis (nowadays called hypertrophic obstructive cardiomyopathy), in which the increase in contractility of the left ventricle caused by digitalis is deleterious, since it occurs in the face of a fixed obstruction.

May 10th. Mrs. P——, Æt. 40. Spafmodic afthma of many years continuance, which had frequently been relieved by ammoniacum, fquills, &c. but thefe now failing in their wonted effects, an Infuf. of Fol. Digitalis was tried, but it feemed rather to increafe than relieve her fymptoms.

C A S E XCIII.

May 22d. Mr. O——, of B——, Æt. 61. A very large man, and a free liver; after an attack of hemi-

CASES 1782. 67

hemiplegia early in the fpring, from which he only partially recovered, became dropfical. The dropfy occupied both legs and thighs, and the arm of the affected fide. I directed an Infufion of Digitalis in fmall dofes, fo as not to affect his ftomach. The fwellings gradually fubfided, and in the courfe of the fummer he recovered perfectly from the palfy.

CASE XCIV.

July 5th. Mr. C——, of W——, Æt. 28. Had drank very freely both of ale and fpirits; and in confequence had an afcites, very large legs, and great fulnefs about the ftomach. He was ordered to take the Infufion of Digitalis night and morning for a few days, and then to keep his bowels open with chryftals of tartar. The firft half pint of infufion relieved him greatly; after an interval of a fortnight it was repeated, and he got well without any other medicine, only continuing the chryftals of tartar occafionally. I forgot to mention that this gentleman, before I faw him, had been for two months under the care of a very celebrated phyfician, by whofe direction he had taken mercurials, bitters, fquills, alkaline falts, and other things, but without much advantage.

CASE XCV.

March 6th. Mrs. W————, Æt. 36. In the laft ftage of a pulmonary confumption, took the Infuf. Digitalis, but without any advantage.

the dropsy occupied ... the arm of the affected side This man had bilateral dropsy of legs and thighs, consistent with heart failure or, in a 'free liver', hepatic oedema. However, the unilateral oedema in the arm on the side of the stroke was probably due to venous thrombosis consequent upon disuse of the arm and it would, like phlegmasia of the leg, have resolved spontaneously (see note to p. 19).

I forgot to mention Withering's self-satisfaction creeps through, despite himself (see pp. 257-62).

CASE

C A S E XCVI.

August 20th. Mr. P——, Æt. 43. In the year 1781 he had a fevere peripneumony, from which he recovered with difficulty. At the date of this, when he firft confulted me, the fymptoms of hydrothorax were pretty obvious. I directed a purge, and then the Infufum Digitalis, three drams to half a pint, one ounce to be taken every four hours. It made him fick, and occafioned a copious difcharge of urine. His complaints immediately vanifhed, and he remains in perfect health.

C A S E XCVII.

September 24th. Mrs. R——, of B——, Æt. 35, the mother of many children. After her laft lying in, three months ago, had that kind of fwelling in one of her legs which is mentioned at No. VIII. XXVI, and XXXI. A confiderable degree of fwelling ftill remained; the limb was heavy to her feeling, and not devoid of pain. I directed a bolus of five grains of Pulv. Digitalis, and twenty-five of crude quickfilver rubbed down, with conferve of cynofbat. to be taken at bed-time, and afterwards an Infufion of red bark and Fol. Digitalis to be taken twice a day. There was half an ounce of bark and half a dram of the leaves in a pint infufion: the dofe two ounces.

The leg foon began to mend, and two pints of the infufion finifhed the cure.

C A S E

---

peripneumony Inflammation of the lungs, i.e. pneumonia, with or without pleurisy.

His complaints immediately vanished If the hydrothorax was due to pneumonia, as one must suppose, the effect of digitalis is surprising. One cannot easily write it off as a spontaneous remission when such a short space of time had elapsed between the time of onset and the cure of the effusion.

conserve of cynosbat. Rose-hip jam. Cynosbatus is the dogrose, *Rosa canina* (Greek κύον – 'dog', βατος – 'thorn').

red bark Bark from the *Cinchona succirubra* (see also note to p. 57). It contains only a relatively small amount of quinine compared with other *Cinchona* barks.

C A S E   XCVIII.

September 25th. Mr. R———, Æt. 60. Complained to me of a ficknefs after eating, and for
fome weeks paft he had thrown up all his food, foon
after he had fwallowed it.   He had taken various
medicines, but found benefit from none, and had
tried various kinds of diet.   He was now very thin
and weak; but had a good appetite. As feveral
very probable methods had been prefcribed, and as
the ufual fymptoms of organic difeafe were abfent,
I determined to give him a fpoonful of the Infufion
of Digitalis twice a day; made by digefting two
drams of the dried leaves in half a pint of cinnamon
water.   From the time he began to take this medicine he fuffered no return of his complaint, and
foon recovered his flefh and his ftrength.

It fhould be observed, that I had frequently feen
the Digitalis remove ficknefs, though prefcribed for
very different complaints.

C A S E   XCIX.

September 30th. Mrs. A———, Æt. 38. Hydrothorax and anafarca. Her cheft was very confiderably deformed.   One half pint of the Digitalis Infufion entirely cured her.

CASE XCVIII In its description of vomiting immediately after food, without loss of appetite, this case sounds like one of peptic ulcer, perhaps with some degree of pyloric spasm, for which digitalis would have been ineffective. The cinnamon water might have given symptomatic relief.

I had frequently seen the Digitalis remove sickness Congestive cardiac failure may be accompanied by nausea and vomiting, and relief of the former would relieve the latter.

C A S E C.

September 30th. Mr. R——, of W——, Æt. 47.
Hydrothorax and anafarca. An Infufion of Digitalis was directed, and after the expected effects from
that fhould take place, fixty drops of tincture of
cantharides twice a day. As he was coftive, pills
of aloes and fteel were ordered to be taken occafionally.

This plan fucceeded perfectly. About a month
afterwards he had fome rheumatic affections, which
were removed by guiacum.

aloes The inspissated juice of plants of the *Aloe* genus (the *Aloinae*), used as stomachics and cathartics. The main varieties were Socotrine aloes (see note to p. 140) and hepatic aloes.

C A S E CI.

October 2d. Mrs. R——, Æt. 60. Difeafed
vifcera; afcites and anafarca. Had taken various
deobftruent and diuretic medicines to little purpofe.
The Digitalis brought on a naufea and languor, but
had no effect on the kidneys.

C A S E CII.

CASE CII See also Case CXLI, p. 92.

October 12th. Mr. R——, Æt. 41. A publican,
and a hard drinker. His legs and belly greatly
fwollen; appetite gone, countenance yellow, breath
very fhort, and cough troublefome. After a vomit
I gave him calomel, faline draughts, fteel and bitters, &c. He had taken the more ufual diuretics
before I faw him. As the dropfical fymptoms increafed, I changed his medicines for pills made of
foap

foap, containing two grains of Pulv. fol. Digital. in each dofe, and, as he was coftive, two grains of jallap. He took them twice a day, and in a week was free from every appearance of dropfy. The jaundice foon afterwards vanifhed, and tonics reftored him to perfect health.

C A S E CIII.

October 12th. Mr. B——, Æt. 39. Kept a public houfe, drank very freely, and became dropfical; he complained alfo of rheumatic pains. I directed Infufion of Digitalis, half an ounce twice a day. In eight days the fwellings in his legs and the fulnefs about his ftomach difappeared. His rheumatic affections were cured by the ufual methods.

C A S E CIV.

October 22d. Mafter B——, Æt. 3. Afcites and univerfal anafarca. Half a grain of Fol. Digital. ficcat. given every fix hours, produced no effect; probably the medicine was wafted in giving. An infufion of the dried leaf was then tried, a dram to four ounces, two tea fpoonfuls for a dofe; this foon increafed the flow of urine to a very great degree, and he got perfectly well.

C A S E CV.

October 30th. Mr. G——, of W——, Æt. 88. The gentleman mentioned in No. XLVII. His complaints and manner of living the fame as there mentioned.

were cured by the usual methods Probably by using such preparations as *Saponaria officinalis*, antimonials, mercurials, and opium, and local applications. During the nineteenth century digitalis was thought to be effective in cases where fever occurred (see p. 318).

Fol. Digital. siccat. ... produced no effect Probably because not enough had been given. When more digitalis was given as an infusion the therapeutic effect occurred (cf. Case LVIII, pp. 51-2). Of course, it is true that the two different types of preparation are not directly comparable: digitalis would be better absorbed from an infusion than from powdered leaf; on the other hand, the leaf would contain more active ingredients weight for weight than the infusion, and that would probably more than offset the lesser absorption.

mentioned. I ordered an Infusion of the Digitalis, a dram and half to half a pint; one ounce to be taken twice a day; which cured him in a short time.

On *March* the 23d, 1784, he sent for me again. His complaints were the same, but he was much more feeble. On this account I directed a dram of the Fol. Digitalis to be infused for a night in four ounces of spirituous cinnamon water, a spoonful to be taken every night. This had not a sufficient effect; therefore, on the 22d of *April*, I ordered the infusion prescribed two years before, which soon removed his complaints.

He died soon afterwards, fairly worn out, in his ninetieth year.

C A S E   CVI.

November 2d. Mr. S———, of B——h——, Æt. 61. Hydrothorax and swelled legs. Squills were given for a week in very full doses, and other modes of relief attempted; but his breathing became so bad, his countenance so livid, his pulse so feeble, and his extremities so cold, that I was apprehensive upon my second visit that he had not twenty-four hours to live. In this situation I gave him the Infusum Digitalis stronger than usual, viz. two drams to eight ounces. Finding himself relieved by this, he continued to take it, contrary to the directions given, after the diuretic effects had appeared.

The

The ficknefs which followed was truly alarming; it continued at intervals for many days, his pulfe funk down to forty in a minute, every object appeared green to his eyes, and between the exertions of reaching he lay in a ftate approaching to fyncope. The ftrongeft cordials, volatiles, and repeated bliffters barely fupported him. At length, however, he did begin to emerge out of the extreme danger into which his folly had plunged him; and by generous living and tonics, in about two months he came to enjoy a perfect ftate of health.

C A S E CVII.

November 19th. Mafter S———, Æt. 8. Afcites and anafarca. A dram of Fol. Digitalis in a fix ounce infufion, given in dofes of a fpoonful, effected a perfect cure, without producing naufea.

1 7 8 3.

The reader will perhaps remark, that from the middle of *January* to the firft of *May*, not a fingle cafe occurs, and that the amount of cafes is likewife lefs than in the preceding or enfuing years; to prevent erroneous conjectures or conclufions, it may be expedient to mention, that the ill ftate of my own health obliged me to retire from bufinefs for fome time in the fpring of the year, and that I did not perfectly recover until the following fummer.

CASE

At length The description (vomiting, heart block, and abnormal colour vision) suggests severe intoxication with digitalis, and one would have expected it to have worn off only after at least two or three weeks, because of the long half-time of digitoxin.

the ill state of my own health Withering died of tuberculosis in 1799 and had not infrequent bouts of illness attributable to tuberculosis during the several years before.

C A S E   CVIII.

January 15th. Mrs. G——, Æt. 57. A very
fat woman; has been dropfical fince *November* laft;
with fymptoms of difeafed vifcera. Various remedies having been taken without effect, an Infufion
of Digitalis was directed twice a day, with a view
to palliate the more urgent fymptoms. She took it
four days without relief, and as her recovery feemed
impoffible it was urged no farther.

C A S E   CIX.

May 1ft. Mrs. D———, Æt. 72. A thin woman, with very large anafarcous legs and thighs;
no appetite and general debility. After a month's
trial of cordials and diuretics of different kinds, the
furgeon who had fcarified her legs apprehended they
would mortify; fhe had very great pain in them,
they were very red and black by places, and extremely tenfe. It was evident that unlefs the tenfion could be removed, gangrene muft foon enfue.
I therefore gave her Infufum Digitalis, which increafed the fecretión of urine by the following evening, fo that the great tenfion began to abate, and
together with it the pain and inflammation. She
was fo feeble that I dared not to urge the medicine
further, but fhe occafionally took it at intervals until the time of her death, which happened a few
weeks afterwards.

scarified her legs
See note to p. 65.

would mortify
Would become
gangrenous.

CASE

CASE CX.

May 18th. I was defired to prefcribe for Mary Bowen, a poor girl at Hagley. Her difeafe appeared to me to be an ovarium dropfy. In other refpects fhe was in perfect health. I directed the Digitalis to be given, and gradually pufhed fo as to affect her very confiderably. It was done; but the patient ftill carries her big belly, and is otherwife very well.

CASE CXI.

May 25th. Mr. G——, Æt. 28. In the laft ftage of a pulmonary confumption of the fcrophulous kind, took an Infufion of Digitalis, but without any advantage.

CASE CXII.

May 31ft. Mr. H——, Æt 27. In the laft ftage of a phthifis pulmonalis became dropfical. He took half a pint of the Infufum Digitalis in fix days, but without any fenfible effect.

CASE CXIII.

June 3d. Mafter B———, of D——, Æt. 6. With an univerfal anafarca, had an extremely troublefome cough. An opiate was given to quiet the cough at night, and 2 tea fpoonfuls of Infuf. Digit. were ordered every fix hours. The dropfy was prefently removed; but the cough continued, his

flefh

CASE CX Withering gives the name of this patient, and this patient only, of all the patients he treated outside hospital. In contrast he gives *all* the names of those he treated in hospital (p. 101 *et seq*.). Why this should have been is not clear, but it has been suggested to me by Dr Irvine Loudon that he would have regarded his hospital cases as being in the public domain, and would have treated those outside of hospital, who may have been of a higher social class, with more confidentiality. Certainly he takes the trouble to mention here that Mary Bowen was poor, although he does also say the same of other patients whose names he does not reveal (e.g. Cases II, III, and CLVI).

An opiate Good treatment for a dry cough (although here apparently ineffective). the opiate would also be expected to have helped the dropsy (see note to p. 5).

flefh wafted, his ftrength failed, and fome weeks afterwards he died tabid.

tabid Probably this
simple means
emaciated, although
the word could also
mean consumptive
and the boy may have
had tuberculosis.

C A S E   CXIV.

June 19th. Mrs. L——, Æt. 28. A dropfy in
the laft ftage of a phthifis. Infufum Digitalis was
tried to no purpofe.

C A S E   CXV.

June 20th. Mrs. H——, Æt. 46. A very fat,
fhort woman; had fuffered feverely through the laft
winter and fpring from what had been called afthma;
but for fome time paft an univerfal anafarca pre-
vailed, and fhe had not lain down for feveral weeks.
After trying vitriolic acid, tincture of cantharides,
fquills, &c. without advantage, fhe took half a pint
of Infuf. Digitalis in three days. In a week afterwards the dropfical fymptoms difappeared, her
breath became eafy, her appetite returned, and fhe
recovered perfect health. The infufion neither
occafioned ficknefs nor purging.

C A S E   CXVI.

June 24th. Mrs. B——, Æt. 40. A puerperal
fever, and fwelled legs and thighs. The fever not
yielding to the ufual practice, I directed an Infufion
of Fol. Digitalis. It proved diuretic; the fwellings
fubfided, but the fever continued, and a few days
afterwards a diarrhœa coming on, fhe died.

C A S E

C A S E   CXVII.

July 22d. Mr. F——, Æt. 48. A ftrong man, of a florid complexion, in confequence of intemperance became dropfical, with fymptoms of difeafed vifcera, great dyfpnœa, a very troublefome cough, and total lofs of appetite. He took mild mercurials, pills of foap, rhubarb, and tartar of vitriol, with foluble tartar and dulcified fpirits of nitre in barley water. After a reafonable trial of this plan, he took fquill every fix hours, and a folution of affafetida and gum ammoniac, to eafe his breathing: finding no relief, I gave him chryftals of tartar with ginger; but his remaining health and ftrength daily declined, and he was not at all benefited by the medicines. I was averfe to the ufe of Digitalis in this cafe, judging from what I had feen in fimilar inftances of tenfe fibre, that it would not act as a diuretic. I therefore once more directed fquill, with decoction of feneka and fal fodæ; but it was inefficacious. His ftrength being much broken down, I then ordered gum ammoniac, with fmall dofes of opium, and infufum amarum, continuing the fquill at intervals. At length I was urged to give the Digitalis, and confidering the cafe as defperate, I agreed to do it. The event was as I expected; no increafe in the urine took place; and the medicine being ftill continued, his pulfe became flow, and he apparently funk under its fedative effects. He was neither purged nor vomited; and had the Digitalis either been omitted

alto-

tense fibre See note to p. 189.

altogether, or fufpended upon its firft effects upon the pulfe being obferved, he might perhaps have exifted a week longer.

C A S E   CXVIII.

July 26th. Mr. W——, of W——, Æt. 47. Phthifis pulmonalis, jaundice, afcites, and fwelled legs. As it was probable that the only relief I could give in a cafe fo circumftanced, would be by carrying off the effufed fluids. I tried fquill and fixed alkaly; and thefe failing, I ordered the Infufum Digitalis. This had the defired effect, and, I believe, prolonged his life a few weeks.

C A S E   CXIX.

Auguft 15th. Mrs. C———, Æt. 60. Afcites, anafarca, difeafed vifcera, paucity of urine, and total lofs of appetite. Thefe complaints had heretofore exifted repeatedly, and had been removed by deobftruent and diuretic medicines; but in this attack the fymptoms were fuffered to exift a longer time and in a greater degree, before affiftance was fought for. The remedies that ufed to relieve her were now exhibited to no purpofe. Mild mercurials, foap, rhubarb, and fquill were tried; but fhe grew rapidly worfe. Saline draughts with acetum fcilliticum feemed for a few days to check the progrefs of her complaint, but they foon loft their effect, and diarrhœa enfued upon every attempt to increafe the frequency of the dofe. Draughts with Infuf. Digital. were then directed to be taken twice a day.

acetum scilliticum Vinegar of squills, prepared by macerating squills in vinegar, heating gently for 24 hours, and adding proof alcohol to the liquor after removing the sediment.

a day. The effect was a powerful action on the kidneys, and a reduction of the swellings, but without
sickness. A degree of appetite returned, but still
the tendency to diarrhœa existed, and kept her
weak. Tonic medicines were then tried, but without advantage, and in a month it was necessary to
have recourse to the Digitalis again. It was directed in a half pint mixture; an ounce to be taken
thrice in twenty-four hours. On the 2d day, finding her symptoms very much relieved, she took in
the absence of her nurse, nearly a double dose of
the medicine. The consequence was great sickness,
languor continuing for several days, and almost a
total stop to the secretion of urine, from the time the
sickness commenced.

The case now became totally unmanageable in
my hands, and, after a fortnight, I was dismissed,
and another physician called in; but she did not
long survive.

This was not the first, nor the last instance, in which
I have seen too large a dose of the medicine, defeat
the very purpose for which it was directed.

C A S E CXX.

August 22d. Mrs. S——, Æt. 36. Extreme
faintiness; anasarcous legs and thighs; great difficulty of breathing, troublesome cough, frequent
chilly fits succeeded by hot ones; night sweats, and
a tendency to diarrhœa. Apprehensive that the
more

she took ... nearly a double dose This case makes it clear why Withering was so reluctant on other occasions to instruct that treatment be started in his absence.

faintiness This could mean the same as faintness, i.e. weakness. However, elsewhere Withering uses the word 'faintness' and here he could be literally meaning 'a tendency to faint'.

more urgent symptoms were caused by water in the lungs, I directed an Infusion of Digitalis, with an ounce of diacodium to the half pint to prevent it purging, a wine glass full to be taken every night at bed-time, and a mixture with confect. cardiac. and pulv. ipecac. to be given in small doses after every loose stool.

On the fourth day she was better in all respects; had made a large quantity of water and did not purge. In a few days more she lost all her complaints, except the cough, which gradually left her, without any further assistance.

I was agreeably deceived in the event of this case, for I expected after the water was removed, to have had a phthisis to contend with.

C A S E   CXXI.

August 25th. T——W——, Esq; Æt, 50. A free liver, diseased viscera, belly very tense, and much swollen; fluctuation perceptible, but the swelling circumscribed; pulse 132. This gentleman was under the care of my very worthy friend Dr. Ash, who, having tried various modes of cure to no purpose, asked me if I thought the Digitalis would answer in this case. I replied that it would not, for I had never seen it effectual where the swelling appeared very tense and circumscribed. It was tried however, but did not lessen the swelling. I mention this case, to introduce the above remark, and also
to

diacodium An opiate syrup prepared from poppy heads (see note to p. 5).

confect. cardiac. *Confectio cardiaca* or *aromatica*, a sweetened medicine containing cinnamon bark, nutmeg, cloves, cardamom seeds, saffron, sugar, and water, and used as a carminative and stimulant. *Cardiacus* meant 'relating to the stomach' as well as 'relating to the heart' (cf. 'cordial').

a phthisis The symptoms and signs were certainly consistent with a diagnosis of pulmonary tuberculosis. It is therefore a little surprising that Withering tried the foxglove, since it had already proved ineffective in almost all the cases in which he had made a diagnosis of tuberculosis (see Table 4.1, p. 276).

to point out the great effect the Digitalis has upon the action of the heart; for the pulfe came down to 96. He was afterwards tapped, and continued, for-fome time under our joint attendance, but the pulfe never became quicker, nor did the fwelling return.

C A S E   CXXII.

September 7th. Mr. L——, Æt. 43. After feveral fevere attacks of ill formed gout, attended for fome time paft with jaundice and other fymptoms of dif-eafed vifcera, the confequences of intemperate living, was fent to Buxton ; from whence he returned in three weeks with afcites and anafarca. Under this complicated load of difeafe, I prefcribed repeatedly without advantage, and at length gave him the Digi-talis, which carried off the more obvious fymptoms of dropfy ; but the jaundice, lofs of appetite, dif-eafed vifcera, &c. rendered his recovery impoffible.

1784.

C A S E   CXXIII.

February 12th. Mrs. C——, Æt. 54. A ftrong fhort woman of a florid complexion ; complained of great fullnefs acrofs the region of the ftomach ; fhort breath, a troublefome cough, lofs of appetite, pau-city of urine ; and had a brownifh yellow tinge on her fkin and in her eyes. She dated thefe com-plaints from a fall fhe had through a trap door about the beginning of winter. From the beginning of January to this time, fhe had been repeatedly let

F   blood

the action of the heart We must assume this to have been a case of atrial fibrillation, in which the atria do not beat properly and as a consequence the ventri-cles beat too quickly, irregularly, and with unequal volume. Withering clearly associated the pulse with the heart, and elsewhere (p. 192) he notes that digitalis affects the motion of the heart, but nowhere is there evidence that he connects any effect on the heart with its effects as a diuretic (see also note to p. 26).

Buxton A mineral spa in the Peak district of Derbyshire, estab-lished as a rival to Bath by William Cavendish, Fifth Duke of Devonshire, in the late eighteenth cen-tury. The water, of temperature 82°F, was reported to have a large quantity of 'elas-tic vapour', the bubbles of which con-tained azotic gas (i.e. nitrogen), and was particularly recom-mended for chronic gout and rheumatism.

blood, had taken calomel purges with jallap; pills of ſoap, rhubarb and calomel; ſaline julep with acet. ſcillit. nitrous decoction, garlic, mercury rubbed down, infus. amarum purg. &c. After the failure of medicines ſo powerful, and ſeemingly ſo well adapted, and during the uſe of which all the ſymptoms continued to increaſe, it was evident that a favourable event could not be expected. However, I tried the infuſum Digitalis, but it did nothing. I then gave her pills of quickſilver, ſoap and ſquill, with decoction of dandelion, and after ſome time, chryſtals of tartar with ginger. Nothing ſucceeded to our wiſhes, and the increaſe of orthopnœa compelled me occaſionally to relieve her by draſtic purges, but theſe diminiſhed her ſtrength, more in proportion than they relieved her ſymptoms. Tincture of cantharides, ſal diureticus and various other means were occaſionally tried, but with very little effect, and ſhe died towards the end of March.

julep See note to p. 92.

dandelion The vulgar name for the dandelion, first recorded by Gerard in his *Herbal* of 1597 (see note to p. xviii), was piss-a-bed, from its diuretic properties.

CASE CXXIV.

March 31ſt. Miſs W——, Æt. 60. Had been ſubject to peripneumonic affections in the winter. She had now total loſs of appetite, very great debility, difficult breathing; much cough, a conſiderable degree of expectoration, and a paucity of urine. She had been blooded, taken ſoap, aſſaf. and ſquill, afterwards aſſaf. and ammon. with acet. ſcillit.: but all her complaints increaſing, a bliſter was applied to her back, and the Digitalis infuſion directed to be taken every night. The effect was an increaſed

ſecre-

secretion of urine, a confiderable relief to her breath, and fome return of appetite ; but foon afterwards fhe became hectic, fpat purulent matter, and died in a few weeks.

C A S E CXXV.

April 12th. Mrs. H——, of L——, Æt. 61. In *December* laft this Lady, then upon a vifit in London, was attacked with fevere fymptoms of peripneumony. She was treated as an afthmatic patient, but finding no relief, fhe made an effort to return to her home to die. In her way through this place, the latter end of December, I was defired to fee her. By repeated bleedings, blifters, and other ufual methods, fhe was fo far relieved, that fhe wifhed to remain under my care. After a while fhe began to fpit matter and became hectic. With great difficulty fhe was kept alive during the difcharge of the abfcefs, and about the end of March fhe had fwelled legs, and unequivocal fymptoms of dropfy in the cheft. Other diuretics failing, on the 12th of April I was induced to give her the Digitalis in fmall dofes. The relief was great and effectual. After an interval of fifteen days, fome fwellings ftill remaining in the legs, I repeated the medicine, and with fuch good effect, that fhe loft all her complaints, got a keen appetite, recovered her ftrength, and about the end of May undertook a journey of fifty miles to her own home, where fhe ftill remains in perfect health.

abscess A lung abscess, a common sequel to untreated or partly treated pneumonia.

F 2   C A S E

C A S E   CXXVI.

April 17th. Mr. F——, Æt. 59. A very fat
man, and a free liver ; had long been fubject to
what was called afthma, particularly in the winter.
For fome weeks paft his legs fwelled, he had great
fenfe of fullnefs acrofs his ftomach ; a fevere cough ;
total lofs of appetite, thirft great, urine fparing,
his breath fo difficult that he had not lain down in
bed for feveral nights.   Calomel, gum ammoniac,
tincture of cantharides, &c. having been given in
vain, I ordered two grains of pulv. fol. Digitalis
made into pills, with aromatic fpecies and fyrup, to
be given every night.   On the third day his urine
was lefs turbid ; on the fourth confiderably increafed in quantity, and in ten days more he was
free from all complaints, and has fince had no
relapfe.

C A S E   CXXVII.

May 7th. Mifs K——, Æt. 8. After a long
continued ague, became hectic and dropfical.   Her
belly was very large, and fhe had a total lofs of appetite.   Half a grain of fol. Digital. pulv. with 2
gr. of merc. alcalis. were ordered night and morning, and an infufion of bark and rhubarb with fteel
wine to be given in the day time. Her belly began
to fubfide in a few days, and fhe was foon reftored
to health.   Two other children in the family,
affected nearly in the fame way, had died, from the
parents being perfuaded that an ague in the fpring
was

merc. alcalis. *Mercu-*
rius alcalizatus or
hydrargyrus cum creta,
i.e. mercury rubbed
together with chalk,
used in venereal
diseases and 'obstruc-
tions of the viscera'.

was healthful and fhould not be ftopped.—I know not how far the recovery in this cafe may be attributed to the Digitalis, but the child was fo near dying that I dared not truft to any lefs efficacious diuretic.

C A S E   CXXVIII.

June 13th. Mr. C——, Æt. 45. A fat man, had formerly drank hard, but not latterly : laft March began to complain of difficult breathing, fwelled legs, full belly, but without fluctuation, great thirft, no appetite ; urine thick and foul ; compleÂction brownifh yellow. Mercurial medicines, diuretics of different kinds, and bitters, had been trying for the laft three months, but with little advantage.   I directed two grains of the fol. Digital. in powder to be taken every night, and infuf. amar. with tinct. facr. twice a day.   In three days the quantity of his urine increafed, in ten or twelve days all his fymptoms difappeared, and he has had no relapfe.

without fluctuation Tense ascites.

tinct. sacr. *Tinctura sacra*, sacred tincture, a mixture of wine, aloes, and rhubarb or *Canella alba* (wild cinnamon). Also called sacred elixir (cf. *cascara sagrada*, the sacred bark). It was used here to mitigate the bitterness of the amarum.

C A S E   CXXIX.

June 17th. Mr. N——, of W——, Æt. 54. A large man, of a pale complexion ; had been fubject to fevere fits of afthma for fome years, but now worfe than ufual. The intermitting pulfe, the great difturbance from change of pofture, and the fwelled legs induced me to conclude that the exacerbation of his old complaint was occafioned by ferous effufion. I directed pills with a grain and half of the

serous effusion Pleural effusion. Serous could, of course refer to other serous membranes, such as the peritoneum.

pulv. Digital. to be taken every night, and as he was costive, jallap made a part of the compofition. He was alfo directed to take muftardfeed every morning and a folution of affafetida twice in the day. The effect of this plan was perfectly to our wifhes, and in a fhort time he recovered his ufual health. About half a year afterwards he died apoplectic.

mustardseed Seeds of the *Sinapis nigra* or *Sinapis alba*, used to stimulate the appetite and as a diuretic.

C A S E CXXX.

Mary B——. A young unmarried woman. Her difeafe appeared to me a dropfy of the right ovarium. She took an infufion of Digitalis, but, as I expected with no good effect. She is ftill, I am informed nearly in the fame ftate.

C A S E CXXXI.

July 12th. Mrs. A——, of C——, Æt. 56. After a feries of indifpofitions for feveral years, became dropfical ; and had long been confined to her chamber, unable to lie down or to walk. She was fo feeble, her legs fo much fwelled, her breath fo fhort, and the fymptoms of difeafed vifcera fo ftrong, that I dared not to entertain hopes of a cure ; but wifhing to relieve her more urgent fymptoms, directed quickfilver rubbed down and fol. Digital. pulv. to be made into pills : the dofe, containing two grains of the latter, to be given night and morning. She was alfo ordered to take a draught with a dram of æther twice a day, and to have fcapulary iffues. Her breath was fo much relieved, that

scapulary issues Incisions or artificial ulcers made under the shoulder on the back for the purpose of causing a discharge (cf. blisters and scarification, see notes to pp. 21, 40, 65, and 203).

that fhe was able foon afterwards to come down ftairs ; but her conftitution was too much broken to admit of a recovery.

C A S E   CXXXII.

July 16th. Mr. B——, of W——, Æt. 31. After a tertian ague of 12 months continuation, fuffered great indifpofition for 10 months more. He chiefly complained of great ftraitnefs and pain in the hypochondriac region, very fhort breath, fweiled legs, want of appetite. He had been under the care of fome very fenfible practitioners, but his complaints increafed, and he determined to come to Birmingham. I found him fupported upright in his chair, by pillows, every attempt to lean back or ftoop forward giving him the fenfation of inftantaneous fuffocation. He faid he had not been in bed for many weeks. His countenance was funk and pale ; his lips livid ; his belly, thighs and legs very greatly fwollen ; hands and feet cold, the nails almoft black, pulfe 160 tremulous beats in a minute, but the pulfation in the carolid arteries was fuch as to be vifible to the eye, and to fhake his head fo that he could not hold it ftill. His thirft was very great, his urine fmall in quantity, and he was difpofed to purge. I immediately ordered a fpoonful of the infufum Digitalis every fix hours, with a fmall quantity of laudanum, to prevent its running off by ftool, and decoction of leontodon taraxacum to allay his thirft. The next day he began to make water freely, and could

allow

leontodon taraxacum Greek λεον — 'lion', oδϑς — 'tooth', i.e. dens leontis, dens de lion, or dandelion (see note to p. 82). Taraxacum may be a corrupt reading, via Arabic, of the Persian for 'bitter herb'.

allow of being put into bed, but was raifed high
with pillows. Omit the infufion. That night he
parted with fix quarts of water, and the next night
could lie down and flept comfortably. *July* 21ft.
he took a mild mercurial bolus. On the 25th. the
diuretic effects of the Digitalis having nearly ceafed,
he was ordered to take three grains of the pulv.
Digital. night and morning, for five days, and a
draught with half an ounce of vin. chalyb. twice a
day. *Auguft* 15th. He took a purge of calomel and
jallap, and fome fwelling ftill remaining in his legs,
the Digitalis infufion was repeated. The water
having been thus entirely evacuated, he was ordered faline draughts with acetum fcilliticum and
pills of falt of fteel and extract of gentian. About
a month after this, he returned home perfectly well.

C A S E   CXXXIII.

July 28th. Mr. A—— of W——, Æt. 29, became dropfical towards the clofe of a pulmonary
confumption. He was ordered 12 grains of pulv.
fol. cicutæ and 1 of Digitalis twice a day. No remarkable effect took place.

C A S E   CXXXIV.

July 31. Mr. M——, Æt. 37. Hydrothorax.
A fingle grain of fol. Digital. pulv. taken every
night for three weeks cured him. The medicine
never made him fick, but increafed his urine, which
became clear; whereas before it had been high coloured and turbid.

C A S E

C A S E   CXXXV.

Auguſt 6th.   Mr. C——— of B————, Æt. 42.
Aſthma and anaſarca, the conſequence of free living.   He had been for ſome time under the care of
an eminent phyſician of this place, but his complaints proving unuſually obſtinate, he conſulted
me.   I directed an infuſion of Digitalis to be taken
every night, and a mixture with ſquill and tincture
of cantharides twice every day.   In about a week
he became better, and continued daily mending.
He has ſince enjoyed perfect health, having quitted
a line of buſineſs which expoſed him to drink too
much.

C A S E   CXXXVI.

Auguſt 6th. Mr. M——— of C———, Æt. 44. Aſcites
and anaſarca, preceded by ſymptoms of the epileptic
kind.   He was ordered to take two grains of pulv.
Digitalis every morning, and three every night ;
likewiſe a ſaline draught with ſyrup of ſquills, every
day at noon.   His complaints ſoon yielded to this
treatment, but in the month of November following
he relapſed, and again aſked my advice. The Digitalis alone was now preſcribed, which proved as efficacious as in the firſt trial.   He then took bitters
twice a day, and vitriolic acid night and morning,
and now enjoys good health.

Before the Digitalis was preſcribed, he had taken
jallap purges, ſoluble tartar, ſalt of ſteel, vitriol of
copper, &c.

C A S E

C A S E   CXXXVII.

Auguſt 10th.   Mrs. W——, Æt. 55.   An anafarcous leg, and fciatica ; full habit.   After bleeding and a purge, a blifter was applied in the manner recommended by Cotunnius ; and two grains
of fol. Digital. with fifteen of fol. cicutæ were directed to be taken night and morning.   The medicine acted only as a diuretic ; the pain and fwelling
of the limb gradually abated ; and I have not heard
of any return.

I muſt here bear witnefs to the efficacy of Cotunnius's method of bliftering in the fciatica, having
ufed it in a great number of cafes, and generally
with fuccefs.

> **Cotunnius** Domen-
> ico Cotugno
> (1736–1822). Italian
> anatomist. The naso-
> palatine nerve and the
> vestibular aqueduct
> were both described
> by and named after
> him.

C A S E   CXXXVIII.

Auguſt 16th.   Mrs. A—— of S——, Æt. 78.
About the middle of Summer began to complain of
fhort breath, great debility, and lofs of appetite. At
this time there were evident marks of effufion in the
thorax, and fome fwelling in the legs.   The advanced age, the weaknefs, and other circumftances
of this patient, precluded every idea of her recovery;
but fomething was to be attempted.   Squills and
other remedies had been tried ; I therefore directed
pills with two or three grains of the pulv. Digitalis
to be taken every night for fix nights, and a faline
draught with forty drops of acetum fcillit. twice in
the day.   She took but few of the draughts, feldom
                                        more

more than half one at a time, for they purged her,
and fhe difliked them. The pills fhe took regularly,
and with the happieft effect, for fhe could lie down,
her breath was very much relieved, and a degree of
appetite returned. *Sept.* 4th, fome return of her
fymptoms demanded the further ufe of diuretics.
I was afraid to pufh the Digitalis in fo hazardous a
fubject, and therefore directed tinct. amara with tinct.
canthar. and pills of fquill, feneka, falt of tartar and
gum ammoniac. Thefe medicines did not at all
check the progrefs of the difeafe, and on the 26th
it became neceffary to give the Digitalis again. The
pills were therefore repeated as before, and infuf.
amarum with fixed alkaly ordered to be taken twice
a day. The event was as favorable as before ; and
from this time fhe had no confiderable return of
dropfy, but languifhed under various namelefs
fymptoms, until the middle or end of November.

salt of tartar Potassium carbonate (see also note to p. 95).

C A S E   CXXXIX.

Aug. 16th. Mrs. P—— of S——, Æt. 50. For
a particular account of this patient, fee Mr. Yonge's
fecond Cafe.

CASE CXXXIX
See also p. 169.

C A S E   CXL.

Sept. 20th. B—— B——, Efq. A true fpafmodic
afthma of many years continuance. After every
method of relief had failed; both under my management, and alfo under the direction of feveral of the
ableft phyficians of this kingdom; I was induced to
give

give him an infufion of the Digitalis. It was continued until naufea came on, but procured no relief.

C A S E CXLI.

October 5th. Mr. R——, Æt. 43. *(The patient
mentioned at No.* 102.*)* He had purfued his former
mode of life, and had now a return of his complaints, with evident marks of difeafed vifcera. His
belly not very large, but uncommonly tenfe. From
this circumftance I did not expect the Digitalis to
fucceed, and therefore tried for fome time to relieve him by the faline julep, with acet fcillitic.
jallap, mercury, fyrup of fquill, with aq. cinnam. decoction of Dandelion, &c.; but thefe being adminiftered without advantage, I was driven to the
Digitalis. As he was very weak and much emaciated, I only gave two grains night and morning for
five days. As no increafe of urine took place, I
ufed alkaline falt with tinct. cantharides :—This
proving equally unfuccefsful, on the 18th, I directed
two ounces of the infufum Digitalis night and morning. This was continued until naufea took place,
but the kidney fecretion was not increafed. Squill
with opium, deobftruents of different kinds, fubli-
mate folution, fixed alkaly, tobacco infufion, were
now fucceffively tried, but with the fame want of
fuccefs. The fullnefs of his belly made it neceffary
to tap him, and by repeating this operation he
continued alive to the end of the year.

the saline julep A julep was a sweet drink used to carry a medicine, in this case a saline, i.e. a salt of magnesium or of an alkaline metal (potassium, sodium, caesium, lithium, or rubidium).

alkaline salt See previous note.

sublimate solution A solution of corrosive sublimate, i.e. mercuric chloride.

C A S E

C A S E CXLII.

October 19th. Mrs. R——, of B——, Æt. 47. Suppofed Afthma, of eighteen months duration. She had kept her room for four months, and could not lie down without great difturbance; was very thin, and had totally loft all inclination for food. She was directed to take two gr. of pulv. fol. Digital. night and morning for five days, and infufum amarum, at the hours of eleven and five. In the courfe of a week fhe was much relieved, and could remain in bed all night. After a few days interval fhe took the Digitalis for five days more, and was foon after that well enough to come down ftairs and conduct her family affairs.

In *April* 1785, fhe had a flight return, but not fuch as to confine her to her chamber. She experienced the fame relief from the fame medicine, but continuing it for feven days without interruption, it excited naufea.

C A S E CXLIII.

October 28th. Mr. A——, fubject to nephritis calculofa : After an attack of that kind, had ftill a troublefome fenfe of weight about his loins, now and then rifing to pain, and a degree of dyfuria, together with a want of appetite. Thefe fymptoms not readily yielding to the ufual methods of treatment, I directed an infufion of Digitalis. The fourth dofe caufed

nephritis calculosa Renal colic. This man probably had staghorn calculus of one or both kidneys.

caufed a copious flow of urine ; the fixth made him
fick, and he was more or lefs fick at times for three
days ; but felt no more of his complaints.

I don't believe it is at all neceffary to bring on
ficknefs in thefe cafes, but an unexpected abfence
from town prevented me from feeing him time
enough to ftop the exhibition of the medicine.

C A S E   CXLIV.

October 31ft. Mrs. C——, of W——, Æt. 67.
Afthma, and very thick hard legs of long continuance. The laft month or two her breath worfe than
ufual, her belly fwollen, her thighs anafarcous, and
her urine in fmall quantity. After trying garlic,
fquill, and purgatives without advantage, I directed
the Digital. Infuf. After taking about five ounces,
her urine from thick and turbid, changed to clear
and amber coloured, its quantity confiderably increafed, and her breathing eafy. Contrary to my
orders, but impelled by the relief fhe had found,
fhe finifhed the remaining three ounces of the infufion, which made her very fick, and the free flow
of urine immediately ceafed. No medicine was
adminiftered for a fortnight, during which time her
complaints increafed. I then directed an infufion
of tobacco, which affected her head, but did not
increafe her urine. She had recourfe again to the
Digitalis infufion, which once more removed the
fulnefs of the belly, reduced the fwellings of her
thighs, and relieved her breath, but had no effect
upon her legs.

C A S E

thick hard legs
Cardiac oedema can
be quite firm in severe
cases and many of the
cases Withering saw
would have been of
such severity. The fact
that he makes special
mention of it in this
case, in addition to the
lack of response to
digitalis, suggest that
the oedema here may
rather have been due
to lymphoedema. An
alternative diagnosis
would be thickening
of the tissues of the
leg due to repeated
bouts of cellulitis (so-
called 'elephantiasis
nostras') but Wither-
ing would have been
less likely to have con-
fused that with car-
diac oedema.

C A S E CXLV.

Nov. 2d. Mifs B—— of C——, Æt. 22. A very evident fluctuation in the abdomen, which was confiderably diftended, whilft the reft ef her frame was greatly emaciated. The prefence of cough, hectic fever, and other circumftances, made it probable that this apparent afcites was caufed by a purulent, and not a watery effufion. However it was poffible I might be miftaken; the Digitalis was therefore given, but without any advantage.

The further progrefs of the difeafe confirmed my firft opinion, and fhe died confumptive.

a purulent ... effusion That is, due to some infection. Probably here caused by tuberculous peritonitis, which carries a poor prognosis when accompanied by purulent ascites.

C A S E CXLVI.

Nov. 4th. Mr. P—— of M——, Æt. 40. Subject to troublefome nephritic complaints, and after the laft attack did not recover, or void the gravelly concretions as ufual, a fenfe of weight acrofs his loins continuing very troublefome. The ufual medicines failing to relieve him, I ordered four grains of pulv. Digital. to be taken every other night for a week, and fifteen grains of mild fixed vegetable alkaly to be fwallowed twice a day in barley water. He foon loft all his complaints; but we muft not in this cafe too haftily attribute the cure to the Digitalis, as the alkaly has alfo been found a very ufeful medicine in fimilar diforders.

fixed vegetable alkaly Potassium carbonate, also called salt of tartar. A fixed alkali was an alkaline salt of sodium or potassium (as opposed to a volatile alkali, a salt of ammonium). Sodium salts were mineral alkalis, potassium salts vegetable alkalis. Alkalinization of the urine might have increased the solubility of whatever substance was causing the renal stones in this case, and thus, as Withering surmised, brought relief.

CASE

C A S E   CXLVII.

Nov. 4th. Mr. B—— of N——, Æt. 60. Had
been much fubject to gout, but his conftitution being at length unable to form regular fits, he became
dropfical. Pulv. fol. Digital. in dofes of two or three
grains, at bed-time, gave him fome relief, but did
not perfectly empty him. About three months afterwards he had occafion to take it again ; but it
then produced no effect, and he was fo debilitated
that it was not urged further.

**being at length
unable to form
regular fits** 'Fits'
here means attacks (of
gout) (see note to
p. 195). Long-term
gout would have
caused renal damage
due to deposition of
urates in the renal
parenchyma. Digitalis
would not be expected
to have much effect in
renal oedema.

C A S E   CXLVIII.

Nov. 8th. Mr. G——, Æt. 35. In the laft ftage
of a phthifis pulmonalis, was attacked with a moft
urgent and painful difficulty of breathing. Sufpecting this diftrefs might arife from watery effufion in
the cheft, I gave him Digitalis, which relieved him
confiderably ; and during the remainder of his life
his breath never became fo bad again.

C A S E   CXLIX.

Nov. 13th. Mrs. A—— of W——h——, Æt.
68. One of thofe rare cafes in which no urine is
fecreted. It proved as refractory as ufual to remedies, and not having ever fucceeded in the cure of
this difeafe, I determined to try the Digitalis. It
was given in infufion, and, after a few dofes, the
fecretion of a fmall quantity of urine feemed to juf-
tify the attempt. The next day, however, the fecretion

**no urine is
secreted** Acute renal
failure. Digitalis
would not have
helped.

cretion ceafed, nor could it be excited again, tho'
at laft the medicine was pufhed fo as to occafion
ficknefs, which continued at intervals for three
days.

C A S E CL.

Nov. 20th. Mrs. B——, Æt. 28. In the laft
ftage of a pulmonary confumption became dropfical. I directed three grains of the pulv. Digital. to
be taken daily, one in the morning, and two at
night. She took twenty grains without any fenfible effect.

C A S E CLI.

Nov. 23d. Mafter W——, Æt. 7. Suppofed
hydrocephalus internus. A grain of pulv. fol. Digitalis was directed night and morning. After
three days, no fenfible effects taking place, it was
omitted, and the mercurial plan of treatment
adopted. The child lived near five months afterwards. Upon diffection near four ounces of water
were found in the ventricles of the brain.

C A S E CLII.

Nov. 26th. Mrs. W——, Æt. 65. I had attended this lady laft winter in a very fevere peripneumony, from which fhe narrowly efcaped with
her life. When the cold feafon advanced this winter, fhe perceived a difficulty in breathing, which gradually became more and more troublefome. I found

G   her

**near four ounces of
water** The normal
total volume of cere-
brospinal fluid in a
seven-year-old child is
about 80 millilitres of
which only about 20
millilitres would be in
the ventricles. Wither-
ing found four ounces,
i.e. about 120 milli-
litres.

her much harraffed by a cough, which occafioned her to expectorate a little: the leaft motion increafed her dyfpnœa; fhe could not lie down in bed; her legs were confiderably fwelled, her urine fmall in quantity. I directed two grains of pulv. Digitalis made into a pill with gum ammoniac, to be taken every night, and to promote expectoration, a fquill mixture twice in the day. Her urine in five days became clear and copious, and in a fortnight more fhe loft all her complaints, except a cough, for which fhe took the lac ammoniacum.

lac ammoniacum
Gum ammoniac (see note to p. 22).

It is not improbable that the fquill might have fome fhare in this cure.

C A S E   CLIII.

December 7th. Mr. H——, Æt. 42. A large fat man, very fubject to gravelly complaints. After an attack in the ufual manner, continued to feel numbnefs in his lower limbs, and a fenfe of weight acrofs his loins. I directed infufum Digitalis to be given every fix hours. Six ounces made him fick, and he took no more. The next day his urine increafed, a good deal of fand paffed with it, and he loft his difagreeable feels, but the ficknefs did not entirely ceafe before the fourth day from its commencement.

CASE

C A S E CLIV.

CASE CLIV See also p. 166.

December 27th. Mr. B——, of H——, Æt. 55.
Symptoms of hydrothorax, at firft obfcurely, afterwards more diftinctly marked. Many things were
tried, but the fquill alone gave relief. At length
this failed. About the third month of the difeafe,
a grain of pulv. Digital. was ordered to be taken
night and morning. This produced the happieft
effects. In *March* following he had fome flight
fymptoms of relapfe, which were foon removed by
the fame medicine, and he now enjoys good health.
For a more particular narrative fee cafe the firft,
communicated by Mr. Yonge.

C A S E CLV.

December 31ft. Mrs. B——, of E——, Æt. 50.
An ovarium dropfy of long continuance. She took
three grains of pulv. Digital. every night at bed
time, for a fortnight, but without any effect.

C A S E CLVI.

A poor man in this town, after his kidneys had
ceafed to fecrete urine for feveral days, was feized
with hickup, fits of vomiting, and tranfient delirium.
After examination I was fatisfied the difeafe was
the fame as that mentioned at **CXLIX**. A very experienced apothecary having tried various methods to
relieve him, I defpaired of any fuccefs, but determined to try the Digitalis. It was accordingly given

G 2   in

the same as that mentioned at CXLIX It was. The symptoms are those of uraemia, due in this case to acute renal failure.

in infusion. At first it checked the vomitings, but did not occasion any secretion of urine.

1785.

The cases which have occurred to me in the course of this year, are numerous ; but as the events of some of them are not yet sufficiently ascertained, I think it better to withhold them at present.

HOSPITAL

HOSPITAL CASES,

Under the Direction of the Author.

THE four following cafes were drawn out at my requeft by Mr. Cha. Hinchley, late apothecary to the Birmingham Hofpital. They are all the Hofpital cafes for which the Digitalis was prefcribed by me, whilft he continued in that office.

CASE CLVII.

March 15th, 1780. John Butler, Æt. 30. Afthma and fwelled legs. He was directed to take myrrh and fteel every day, and three fpoonfuls of infufum Digitalis every night. On the 8th of April he was difcharged, cured of the fwellings and fomething relieved of his afthmatic affections.

CASE CLVIII.

November 18th, 1780. Henry Warren, Æt. 60. This man had a general anafarca and afcites, and was moreover fo afthmatic, that, neither being able to fit in a chair nor lie in bed, he was obliged conftantly to walk about, or to lean forward againft a window or table. You prefcribed for him thus.

G 3   R. Aq.

R. This symbol, used here and elsewhere in the monograph, stands for the symbol ℞, indicating a prescription. Although it is generally taken to represent the Latin word *recipe* ('take' as an injunction), it may in fact derive from the Egyptian symbol (illustrated here) for Har Wer (Horus the elder), god of medicine, identified with the Greek god Apollo.

℞

aa Ana, of each.

cochlear. Cochleare, a spoonful.

R. Aq. cinn. fpt. ʒiv.
Oxymel. fcillit.
Syr. fcillit. aa. ʒi. m. cap. cochlear. larg. fexta quaque horâ.

This medicine producing no increafed difcharge of urine, on the 25th you ordered the infufion of Digitalis, two fpoonfuls every four hours. After taking this for thirty fix hours, his urine was dif- charged in very great quantity ; his breath became eafy, and the fwellings difappeared in a few days, though he took no more of the medicine. On the 2d of *December* he was ordered myrrh and lac am- moniacum, which he continued until the 23d, when he was difcharged cured, and is now in good health.

CASE CLIX.

November 3d, 1781. Mary Crockett, Æt. 40. Afcites and univerfal anafarca. For one week fhe took fal. diureticus and tincture of cantharides, but without advantage. On the 10th you directed the infufion of Digitalis, a dram and half to half a pint, an ounce to be taken every fourth hour. Before this quantity was quite finifhed, the urine began to be difcharged very copioufly. The medicine was then ftopped as you had directed. On the 15th, being coftive, fhe took a jallap purge, and on the 24th fhe was difcharged cured.

CASE CLX.

March 16th, 1782. Mary Bird, Æt. 61. Great fullnefs about the ftomach ; difeafed liver, and anafarcous

farcous legs and thighs. For the firft week fquill was tried in more forms than one, but without advantage. On the 22d fhe began with the Digitalis, which prefently removed all the fwelling.

She was then put upon the ufe of aperient medicines and tonics, and on the firft of *Auguft* was difcharged perfectly cured.

The three following Cafes were drawn up and communicated to me by Mr. Bayley, who fucceeded Mr. Hinchley as apothecary to the Hofpital at Birmingham:

Mr. Bayley ?

DEAR SIR,   Shiffnal, April 26th, 1785.

        DURING my refidence in the Birmingham General Hofpital, I had frequent opportunities of feeing the great effects of the Digitalis in dropfy. As the exhibition of it was in the following inftances immediately under your own direction, I have drawn them up for your infpection, previous to your publifhing upon that excellent diuretic. Of its efficacy in dropfy I have confiderable evidence in my poffeffion, but confider myfelf not at liberty to fend you any other cafes except thofe you had yourfelf the conduct of. The Digitalis is a very valuable acquifition to medicine; and, I truft, it will ceafe to be dreaded when it is well underftood.

I am, Sir, your obedient,
And very humble fervant,
W. BAYLEY.

CASE

CASE CLXI.

Mary Hollis, aged 62, was admitted an out·patient of the Birmingham General Hofpital *February* 12th, 1784, labouring under all the effects of hydrothorax; her dread of fuffocation during fleep was fo great, that fhe always repofed in an elbow chair. She was directed to take two grains of Digitalis in powder every night and morning, and for a few days found great relief; but, on the eighth day, as fhe had complained of ficknefs, and had been confiderably purged, fhe was ordered to defift taking any more of her powders. On the 14th day fhe was ordered an ounce of the following infufion twice in a day: R. Fol. Digital. purp. ficc. ℥ifs. aq. bullient. ℔fs. digere per femi-horam, colaturæ adde tinct. aromatic ℥i. This infufion did not purge, but fometimes excited naufea, though not fufficient to prevent her from continuing its ufe. She grew gradually better, and on the 6th of *May* was difcharged perfectly cured. The diuretic effects of the Digitalis were in this inftance immediate.

aq. bullient. Boiling water, i.e. a decoction.

tinct. aromatic A solution used as a carminative and identical to a cardiac confection (see note to p. 80) but containing alcohol rather than water.

CASE CLXII.

Edward James, Æt. 21. Admitted *March* 20th, 1784. Complained of great difficulty of breathing, pain in his head, and tightnefs about the ftomach, with a trifling fwelling of his legs. Ordered pil. fcillit. Әi. ter de die. On the third day his legs much more fwelled, his breathing more difficult, and in every refpect worfe; his pulfe very fmall
and

and quick, complained when he turned in bed, of something like water rolling from one fide of the thorax to the other. A remarkable bluenefs about the mouth and eyes, and purged confiderably from the pil. fcill. Ordered to omit the pills and to take ʒi. of infuf. Digitalis every eight hours; the proportion ʒifs. to eight ounces of water and ʒi. of aq. n. m. fp.—7th Day, The infufion had neither purged, nor vomited him: he only complained once or twice of giddinefs. His belly was now very hard, rather black on the right fide the navel, and his legs amazingly fwelled. Ordered a bolus with rhubarb and calomel, to be taken in the morning, and ʒii. julep falin. cum tinct. canthar. gutt. forty ter die. —12th Day, nearly in the fame ftate, except his breathing which was fomewhat more difficult, being now obliged to have his head confiderably raifed. Perfiftat—From this day to the 32d day he became hourly worfe. His belly which at firft was only hard, now evidently contained a large quantity of water, his legs were more fwelled, and a large fphacelated fore appeared upon each outer ancle. Refpiration was fo much obftructed, that he was obliged to fit quite upright to prevent fuffocation. He made very little water, not more than eight ounces in a day and a night, and was much emaciated. Ordered his purging bolus again, and ʒii. of a mixture with fal diuretic. ʒfs. to ʒxii. three times in a day, and a poultice with ale grounds to his legs.

54th day. To this period there was not the leaft probability of his exifting ; his legs and thighs were one

aq. n. m. *Aqua nucula moschata* (see note to p. 14).

sphacelated Gangrenous.

ale grounds The residue of malt, left after brewing.

one continued blubber, his thorax quite flat, and his belly fo large that it meafured within one inch as much as a woman's in this Hofpital the day fhe was tapped, and from whom twenty feven pounds of coagulable lymph were taken. He made about three ounces of water in twenty-four hours: his penis and fcrotum were aftonifhingly fwelled, and no difcharge from the fores upon his legs. Ordered to take a pill with two grains of powdered Fox-glove night and morning. For a few days no fenfible effect, but about the 60th day he complained of being continually giddy, and had fome little pain in his ftomach. He now made much more water, and dared to fleep. His appetite which through the whole of his illnefs had been very bad, was alfo better. 66th day. Breathing very much relieved, the quantity of water he made was three chamber pots full in a day and a night, each pot containing two quarts and four ounces, moderately full. Ordered to continue his pills, and his legs which were very flabby, to be rolled.

69th day. His belly nearly reduced to its natural fize, ftill made a prodigious quantity of water, his appetite very good, habit of body rather lax, and his complexion ruddy. On the 2d of *June*, being ftill rather weak, he was ordered decoct. cort. ʒii. ter de die ; and on the 12th was difcharged from this Hofpital perfectly cured.

W. BAYLEY.

Mr.

coagulable lymph This term was used to mean fibrin. Its use here suggests that the fluid in the belly of the woman with whom this patient is being compared was an exudate (e.g. due to inflammation) rather than a transudate (e.g. due to cardiac failure or liver disease).

Mr. Bayley's refpectful compliments to Doctor Withering: he fends the cafe of Edward James, which he believes is pretty correct. He laments not having it in his power to fend the meafure of his belly, having unfortunately miflaid the tape: he heard from James yefterday, and he is perfectly well.

General Hofpital, Auguft 5, 1784.

C A S E   CLXIII.

On the 26th *February*, 1785, Sarah Ford, aged 42, was admitted an out-patient of the Birmingham General Hofpital: fhe complained of confiderable pain in her cheft, and great difficulty of breathing, her face was much fwelled and her thighs and legs were anafarcous. She had extreme difficulty in making water, and with many painful efforts fhe did not void more than fix ounces in twenty-four hours. She had been in this fituation about fix weeks, during which time fhe had taken ammoniacum, olibanum, and large quantities of fquills, without any other effect than frequent ficknefs. Upon her commencing an Hofpital patient, the following medicine was exhibited. R. gum ammoniac ʒii. pulv. fol. Digital. purp. ɘii. fp. lavand. comp. ut fiat pil. 40. cap. ii. nocte maneque. She continued the ufe of thefe pills for a few days, without any fenfible effect. On the eighth day her breathing was much relieved, her legs and thighs were not fo much fwelled, and in a day and

a night

olibanum An aromatic resin, frankincense (Greek λιβανος, obtained from the *Juniperus lycia*.

lavand. *Lavendula spica*, the common lavender, used in nervous disorders and for general malaise.

a night fhe made five pints of water. By the 12th day her legs and thighs were nearly reduced to their natural fize. She continued to make water in large quantities, and had loft her pain in the thorax. To the 20th of *March*, fhe made rapid advances towards health, when not a fymptom of difeafe remaining, fhe was difcharged.

COMMU-

COMMUNICATIONS

FROM CORRESPONDENTS.

—

London, Norfolk-ftreet,
May 31ft, 1785.

Sir,

I HAD the favour of your letter laft week; and I fhall be very happy if I can give you any intelligence relating to the Foxglove, that can anfwer the purpofe in which you are fo laudably engaged.

It is true that my brother, the late Dr. Cawley, was greatly relieved, and his life, perhaps, prolonged for a year, by a decoction of the Foxglove root; but why it had not a more lafting effect, it is neceffary I fhould tell you that he had all the figns of a diftempered vifcera, long before any watery fwellings appeared; it was manifeft that his dropfy was merely fymptomatic, and he could therefore only from time to time have any relief from medicine. In the year 1776, he returned from London to Oxon. having confulted feveral phyficians at the former place, and Dr. Vivian at the latter, but without any fuccefs; and he was then told of a carpenter at Oxon. that had been cured of a Hydrops pectoris by the Foxglove root, and as he

was

COMMUNICATIONS FROM CORRESPONDENTS Most of these cases, at least some of which Withering seems to have solicited from his acquaintances, demonstrate, to a greater or lesser extent, the safety and efficacy of digitalis, and must be regarded as selected cases (cf. Withering's statement on pp. viii–ix).

your letter last week Withering originally heard of Ralph Cawley's case from John Ash (see p. 3). He clearly wrote to Cawley's brother when preparing his monograph for publication, to ratify the account Ash had given him.

Dr. Vivian Willaim Vivian (1728–1801). Physician and Regius Professor of Medicine at Oxford from 1772.

was a younger, and in other refpeɗs an healthy man, his cure, I believe, remains a perfeɗ one.

I did not attend my brother whilſt he took the medicine, and therefore I ·cannot ſpeak precifely to the operation of it; but I remember, by his letters, that he was dreadfully ſick and ill for ſeveral days before the ſecretion of urine came on, but which it did do to a great degree; relieved his breath, and greatly leſſened the ſwelling in his legs and thighs; but the two inſtances I have lately ſeen in this part of the world, are much ſtronger proofs of the efficacy of it than my brother's caſe.

I am, &c.

ROBERT CAWLEY.

N. B. Whenever I have another opportunity of giving the Foxglove, it ſhall be in ſmall doſes:— In which I ſhould hope it might fuceed, although it might be more ſlowly. If you ſhould try it with ſuccefs, I ſhould be glad to know what mode you made uſe of.

Dr. Cawley's preſcription.

R. Rad. Digital. purpur. ſiccat. et contuf. ℥ii.

Coque ex aq. font. ℔ii. ad ℔i. colat. liquor. adde aq. junip. comp. ℥ii.

Mell. anglic ʒi. m. ſumat cochl. iv. omni noɗe h. ſ. et mane.

Mell. anglic I have not been able to discover precisely what this stands for. Perhaps it is simply *mellina anglica*, i.e. English mead, but *mell*. might also stand for *mellago*, any medicine with the sweetness and consistency of honey (e.g. a *confectio cardiaca*, see note to p. 80).

sumat Let the patient take, i.e. 4 spoonfuls every night.

h. s. *Hora somni*, at bedtime.

I have

—I have elfewhere remarked, that when the Digitalis has been properly given, and the diuretic ef-effects produced, that an accidental over-dofe bringing on ficknefs, has ftopped the fecretion of urine. In the prefent inftance it likewife appears, that violent ficknefs may be excited, and continue for feveral days without being accompanied by a flow of urine; and it is probable that the latter circumftance did not take place, until the feverity of the former abated.   If Dr. Cawley had not had a conftitution very retentive of life, I think he muft have died from the enormous dofes he took; and he probably would have died previous to the augmentation of the urinary difcharge.   For if the root from which his medicine was prepared, was gathered in its active ftate, he did not take at each dofe lefs than *twelve* times the quantity a ftrong man ought to have taken.   Shall we wonder then that patients refufe to repeat fuch a medicine, and that practitioners tremble to prefcribe it?   Were any of the active and powerful medicines in daily ufe to be given in dofes *twelve* times greater than they are, and thefe dofes to be repeated without atttention to the effects, would not the patients die, and the medicines be condemned as dangerous and deleterious?—Yet fuch has been the fate of Foxglove!

if the root from which his medicine was prepared, was gathered in its active state As I have noted elsewhere (see note to p. 4) the quantity of digitalis in foxgloves varies from time to time during the year, and could vary twelvefold. Of all the parts of the plant the root contains the least amount of digitalis, weight for weight.

A Letter

Mr. BODEN ?

A Letter to the Author, from Mr. BODEN, Surgeon, at Brofeley, in Shropfhire.

Dear Sir, Brofeley, 25th May, 1785.

HAVE inclofed the prefcriptions that contained the fol. Digital. which I gave to Thomas Cooke and Thomas Roberts.

Thomas Cooke, Æt. 49, had been ill about two or three weeks. When I faw him he had no appetite, and a conftant thirft : a fullnefs and load in the ftomach : the thighs, legs and hands, much fwell'd, and the face and throat in a morning ; was coftive, and made but little water, which was high coloured ; the pulfe very weak, and his breath exceeding bad. *June* 17th. R. Argent. viv ʒi. conf. cynofbat. Ɔii. fol. Digital. pulv. gr. xv. f. pil. xxiv. capt. ii. omni noᴄte horâ decubitus. He was likewife purged by a bolus of argent. viv. jallap, Digit. elaterium and calomel, which was repeated on the fourth day, to the third time. From *June* 17th to the 29th, the fymptoms were moftly removed, making water freely, and having plenty of ftools ; in a week after he was perfeᴄtly well, and remains fo ever fince. The cure was finifhed by fteel and bitters.

Argent. viv *Argentum vivum* (quicksilver), also called *argentum mobile* or *argentum fusum*, i.e. mercury.

deformed chest See note to p. 59.

Thomas Roberts, Æt. 40, had a deformed cheft, was obliged to be almoft in an ereᴄt pofture when in bed ; the other fymptoms were nearly the fame as Cooke's. *Auguft* 3d. The pills prefcribed *June* 17th

17th for Cooke.——17th. A purging bolus of jalap
and Digitalis, once a week. He continued the medicines till the latter end of *Auguſt*, when he got
very well; but the complaint returned in *Jan.* worſe
than before. He is now much better, but I have great
reaſon to believe the liver to be diſeaſed.

I am, with the greateſt reſpect,

Your very obliged humble ſervant,

DANIEL BODEN.

P. S. The ſecond patient, on his relapſe, took
Digitalis again, combined with other things.

CASE communicated by Mr. CAUSER, Surgeon, at Stourbridge, Worceſterſhire.

Mr. P—— of H—— M——, in the pariſh of
Kingſwinford, aged about 60; had been a ſtrong
healthy, robuſt, corpulent man; worked hard early
in life at edge-tool making, and drank freely of
ſtrong malt liquor; for many years had been ſubject to gout in the extremities; for a few years paſt
had been very aſthmatic, and the gout in the extremities gradually decreaſed. When I firſt ſaw
him, which was *Sept.* 12, 1779, his legs were anaſarcous, his belly much ſwelled, and an evident fluctuation of water. His breathing very bad, an irregular pulſe, and unable to lie down. His eaſieſt

H   poſture

posture was standing with his body leaning over a chair, in which situation he would continue many hours together, labouring for breath, with the sweat trickling down his face very profusely; the urine in very small quantity. Diuretics of every kind I could think of were used with very little or no advantage. Blisters applied to the legs relieved very considerably for a time, but by no means could I increase the urinary discharge. Warm stomachic medicines were given, and at the same time sinapisms applied to the feet, in hopes of enticing gout to the extremities, but without any good effect.— *November* 22d. The swelling considerably increasing, an emetic of acet. scillitic. was given, which acted very violently, and increased the urinary discharge considerably. He continued better and worse, using different kinds of diuretic and expectorating medicines until *September* 1781, when the disease was so much worse, I did not expect he could live many days. The acet. scillitic. was repeated, a table spoonful every half hour, till it acted briskly upwards and downwards; but without increasing the urinary discharge.—On the 17th of *September* I infused ʒiii. of the fol. Digitalis in ℥vi. of boiling water, for four hours; then strained it, and added ℥i. of tinct. aromatica.—On the 18th he began by taking one spoonful, which he was to repeat every half hour, till it made him very sick, unless giddiness, loss of sight, or any other disagreeable effect took place. I had never given the medicine before, and had prepared him to expect the operation to be very severe. I saw him again on the 21st; he

had

had taken the medicine regularly, till the whole quantity was confumed, without perceiving the leaft effect of any kind from it, and continued well till the evening of the following day, when a little ficknefs took place, which increafed, but never fo as to occafion either vomiting or purging, but a furprifing difcharge of urine. The faliva increafed fo as to run out of his mouth, and a watery difcharge from his eyes; thefe difcharges continued, with a continual ficknefs, till the fwelling was totally gone, which happened in three or four days. He afterwards took fteel and bitters; and continued very comfortably, without any return of his dropfy, until the the 7th of *April* 1782, when he was feized with an epidemic cough, which was very frequent with us at that time. His fwellings now returned very rapidly, with the greateft difficulty in breathing, and he died in a few days. Blifters and expectorating medicines were ufed on this laft return.

Extract of a Letter from Mr. CAUSER.

Mrs. S——, the fubject of the following Cafe, was as ill as it is poffible for woman to be and recover; from the inefficacy of the medicines ufed, I am convinced no medicine would have faved her but the Digitalis. I never faw fo bad a cafe recovered; and it fhews, that in the moft reduced ftate of body, the medicine in fmall dofes, will prove fafe and efficacious.

H 2   N. B. The

in the seventh month of her pregnancy There seems to be little risk to the fetus in using therapeutic doses of digitalis during pregnancy, if studies of *digoxin* are to be relied upon (Aronson 1980a). Plasma digoxin concentrations in the newborn are only half of those in the non-pregnant mother (i.e. often subtherapeutic). *Digitoxin* is highly protein-bound, and would pass across the placenta even less well. The secretion of digitalis in the breast milk is so small as to be negligible to the breast-feeding infant (not relevant to this case).

syr. rosar. Syrup (attar) of damask rose petals, used as a mild laxative.

tinct. senn. Senna, from the *Cassia senna*, used as a purgative.

sapon. venet. This might stand for *Saponaria venetia*, i.e. some member of the soapwort family, but I cannot anywhere, even in Withering's *Botany*, find mention of such a variety. The *Saponaria officinalis* was used in the treatment of syphilis, gout, rheumatism, and jaundice. Alternatively, sapon. may simply mean

N. B. The Digitalis, in pills, never occafioned the leaft ficknefs. She took two boxes of them.

C A S E.

January 2d, 1785. Mrs. S——, of W——, near Kidderminfter, aged 38, has been affected with dropfical fwellings of her legs and thighs, about fix weeks, which have gradually grown worfe; has now great difficulty in breathing, which is much increafed on moving; a very irregular, intermittent pulfe, urine in very fmall quantity, and in the feventh month of her pregnancy: a woman of very delicate conftitution, with tender lungs from her infancy, and very fubject to long continued coughs.

R. Pulv. fcillæ gr. iii.
Jalap gr. x. fyr. rofar. folut. tinct. fenn. aa ʒii. aq. menth. v. fimpl. ℥ifs. m. mane fumend.

R. pulv. fcillæ Əi. G. ammoniac. fapon. venet. aa ʒifs. fyr. q. f. f. pilul. 42 cap. iii. nocte maneque.

On the 7th found her worfe, and the fwelling increafed; the urine about ℥x in the twenty-four hours.

R. Fol. ficcat. Digital. ʒiii. coque in. aq. fontan. ℥xii. ad ℥vi. cola et adde. aq. juniper. comp. ʒii. facchar. alb. ℥fs. m. cap. cochlear. i. larg. 4tis horis.

She

She took about three parts of the medicine before any effect took place. The firſt was ſickneſs, ſucceeded by a conſiderable diſcharge of urine. She continued the medicine till the whole was conſumed, which cauſed a good deal of ſickneſs for three or four days.

I ſaw her again on the 12th. The quantity of urine was much increaſed, and the ſwelling diminiſhed. Pulſe and breathing better.

R. Fol. ſicc. Digital. G. aſſafetid. aa ʒi. calomel. pp. gr. x. ſp. lavand. comp. q. ſ. fiat pilul. xxxii. cap. ii. omni noƈte horâ ſomni.

A plentiful diſcharge of urine attended the uſe of theſe pills, and ſhe got perfeƈtly free from her dropſical complaints.

March 15th ſhe was delivered: had a good labour, was treated as is uſual, except in not having her breaſts drawn, not intending ſhe ſhould ſuckle her child, being in ſo reduced a ſtate. Continued going on well till the 18th, when ſhe was ſeized with very violent pains acroſs her loins, at times ſo violent as to make her cry out as much as labour pains. Enema cathartic. Fot. papav. applied to the part.

R. Pulv. ipecacoan. gr. vi. opii. gr. iv. ſyr. q. ſ. fiat pilul. vi. capt. i. 2da quaque horâ durante dolore.

H 3   R. Julep.

some sort of soap (cf. note to p. 141).

sacchar. alb. Saccharinum album, white, or refined, sugar.

G. *Gumma*, gum.

pp. *Pulvis patrum*, Jesuits' bark (literally Fathers' powder), the same as Peruvian bark. The term 'Jesuits' bark' was coined because Jesuit missionaries sent it to Rome in the late seventeenth century. The term was also applied to the bark of the *Iva frutescens* (false or bastard Jesuits' bark).

q. s. *Quantum sufficiat*, sufficient.

not having her breasts drawn Not having lactation stimulated by manual expression of the first milk.

Fot. papav. A fomentation (fotus) of poppies.

durante dolore While the pain persists.

sp. minder. Spirit of Mindererus, a solution of ammonium acetate, used as a febrifuge. Named after the German physician Raimund M. Minder (c. 1580-1621) who was born in Augsburg and graduated from Ingolstadt in 1597.

singul. *Singulorum*, of each.

Balsam. peruv. Peruvian balsam, a black liquid obtained from the *Myroxylon peruiferum*, containing esters of benzoic acid and cinnamic acid, and often dissolved, as here, in mucilage of gum-arabic to render it more palatable.

flor. zinci Flowers of zinc, powdered zinc oxide.

aq. menth. Mint water (see note to p. 135).

Emp. vesicat. *Emplastrum vesicatorium*, a blister plaster.

urgente languore As long as the lassitude is severe.

pice burgund. Burgundy pitch, derived from the Norwegian spruce *Pinus abies*. Applied (here in a plaster to the back) as a stimulant, e.g. in cases of catarrh and whooping cough.

R. Julep. e camphor. fp. minder. aa ℥ii. capt. cochlear. i. larg. poft fingul. pilul.

19th. Breathing fhort, unable to lie down, very irregular low pulfe fcarcely to be felt, fainty, and a univerfal cold fweat: no appetite nor thirft, fpafmodic pains at times acrofs the loins very violent, but not fo frequent as on the preceding day.

R. Gum ammoniac. affafetid. aa ʒi. camphor. gr. xii. fiat pilul. 24. capt. ii. 3tia quaque horâ in cochlear. ii. mixtur. feq.

R. Balfam. peruv. ℈iii. mucilag. G. arab. q. f. flor. zinci g. vi. aq. menth. fimp. ℔fs. m.

Applic. Emp. veficat. femorib. internis.

R. Sp. vol. fœtid. elixir. paregor. balfam. Traumatic. aa ʒiii. capt. cochlear. parv. urgente languore.

20th. Much the fame; makes very little water, and the legs begin to fwell.—Applic. Emp. e pice burgund. lumbis.

23d. The fwelling very much increafed.—Capt. gutt. xv. acet. fcillitic. ter die in two fpoonfuls of the following mixture.

R. Infuf. baccar. juniper. ℥vi. tinct. amar. tinct. ftomachic. aa ℥i. m.

25th.

25th. Much the fame.

28th. The fwelling confiderably increafed, in other refpects very much the fame.

30th. Breathing very bad, with cough and pain acrofs the fternum, unable to lie down, legs, thigh-, and body very much fwelled, urine not more than four or five ounces in the twenty-four hours; hot and feverifh, with thirft.

Applic. Emp. veficat. ftomacho et fterno.

R. G. affafetid. Əii. pulv. jacob. Əi. rad. fcill. recent. gr. xii. extract. thebaic. gr. iv. f. pilul. xvi. cap. iv. omni nocte.

R. Sal. nitr. fal. diuretic. aa ʒii. pulv. e contrayerv. comp. ʒi. facchar. ℥i. emulf. commun. ℔i. aq. cinnam. fimpl. ℥i. m. capt. cochlear. iv. ter die.

April 2d. Much the fame, no increafe of urine.

3d. Breathing much relieved by the blifter, which runs profufely. Repeated the medicines, and continued them till the

12th. The cough very bad, pulfe irregular, fwelling much increafed, urine in very fmall quantity, not at all increafed; great lownefs and fainting. She defired to have fome of the pills which relieved her

---

m. *Mane*, in the morning.

Ə... ʒ... ℥
These symbols, used in the prescriptions throughout the *Account* stand for 'grain', 'drachm', and 'ounce' respectively. In apothecaries' weights 1 grain = 1/7000 lb; 1 drachm (or dram) = 1/8 oz; 1 lb = 16 oz.

jacob. Jacobaea, *Senecio Jacobaea*, ragwort, used in various arthropathies, dysentery, wounds, and bruises.

extract. thebaic. Opium.

Sal. nitr. *Sal ammoniacus nitrosus*, ammonium nitrate, used as a diuretic.

contrayerv. Contrayerva, obtained from the root of plants of the *Dorstenia* species, first brought to Europe in 1581 by Sir Francis Drake and sometimes called *Dorstenia Drakena*. Generally used as an antidote to poison (e.g. snakebite), but also as a diaphoretic and as an antiseptic gargle.

her fo much when with child. I was almoſt afraid to give them, but the inefficacy of the other medicines gave me no hopes of a cure from continuing them, which made me venture to comply with her requeſt.

R. Fol. ſiccat. Digital. G. aſſafetid. aa ʒi. ſp. lavand. comp. q. ſ. f. pilul. xxxii. cap. ii. omni mane; et omni noᶜte cap. pilul. e ſtyrace gr. vi.

17th. Conſiderable increaſe of urine.

21ſt. Swelling a good deal diminiſhed; urine near four pints in twenty-four hours, which is more than double the quantity ſhe drinks.

Applic. Emp. veſicat. femoribus internis.

The Digitalis pills and opiate at bed-time continued. Takes a tea cup of cold chamomile tea every morning.

25th. Swelling much diminiſhed, makes plenty of water, appetite much mended, cough and breathing better. She omitted the medicine for three days; the urine began to diminiſh, the ſwelling and ſhortneſs of breathing worſe. On repeating it for two days, the diſcharge was again augmented, and a diminution of the ſwelling ſucceeded. She has continued the pills ever ſince till the 14th of *May;*

May; the dropfical fymptoms and cough are entirely gone, the water is in fufficient quantity, her ftrength is recovered, and fhe has a good appetite. All fhe now complains of is a weight acrofs her ftomach, which is worfe at times, and fhe thinks, unlefs it can be removed, fhe fhall have a return of her dropfy.

Extract of a Letter from Doctor FOWLER, Phyfician, at Stafford.

I UNDERSTAND you are going to publifh on the Digitalis, which I am glad to hear, for I have long wifhed to fee your ideas in print about it, and I know of no one (from the great attention you have paid to the fubject) qualified to treat on it but yourfelf. There are gentlemen of the faculty who give verbal directions to poor patients, for the preparing and taking of an infufion or decoction of the green plant. Would one fuppofe that fuch gentlemen had ever attended to the nature and operation of a fedative power on the functions, *particularly* the *vital?* Is not fuch a vague and unfcientific mode of proceeding putting a two edged fword into the the hands of the ignorant, and the moft likely method to damn the reputation of any very active and powerful medicine? And is it not more than probable that the *neglect* of adhereing to a *certain* and *regular* preparation of the nicotiana, and the *want* (of what you *emphatically* call) a *practicable* dofe, have been the chief caufes of the once rifing reputation of that

Doctor FOWLER, physician, at Stafford Withering practised at the Staffordshire Infirmary before moving to Birmingham in 1775. Dr Thomas Fowler (1736-1801) succeeded him there. he was best known for having introduced arsenic (Fowler's solution) for the treatment of fevers, and this preparation was included in the *British Pharmacopoeia* in one form or another until about the middle of this century. His *Medical reports of the effects of arsenic, in the cure of agues, remitting fevers, and periodic headachs* ... was published in 1786, and included a letter from Withering on the subject.

who give verbal directions to poor patients That is, who tell the poor how to make their own medicines rather than having them buy, at a high price, the medicines already prepared by experts. Fowler understandably deplores this practice, both because it leads to poor or inadequate treatment, and because it diverts income from reputable physicians and apothecaries.

that noted plant being damned above a century ago? In fhort, the Digitalis is beginning to be ufed in dropfies, (although fome patients are faid to go off fuddenly under its adminiftration) fomewhat in the ftyle of broom afhes; and, in my humble opinion, the public, at this very inftant, ftand in great need of your *precepts, guards,* and *cautions* towards the fafe and fuccefsful ufe of fuch a powerful fedative diuretic; and I have no doubt of your minute attention to thofe particulars, from a regard to the good and welfare of mankind, as well as to your own reputation with refpect to that medicine.

broom *Spartium sco-parium,* used as a diuretic and purgative.

I remember an offcer in the Staffordfhire militia, who died here of a dropfy five years ago. The Digitalis relieved him a number of times in a wonderful manner, fo that in all probability he might have obtained a radical cure, if he would have refrained from hard drinking. I underftood it was firft ordered for him by a medical gentleman, and its fedative effects proved fo mild, and diuretic operation fo powerful, that he ufed to prepare it afterwards for himfelf, and would take it with as little ceremony as he would his tea. It is faid, that he was fo certain of its fuccefsful operation, that he would boaft to his bacchanalian companions, when much fwelled, you fhall fee me in two days time quite another man.

CASES

CASES communicated by Mr. J. FREER, jun. Surgeon, in Birmingham.

CASE I.

Nov. 1780. Mary Terry, aged 60. Had been fubject to afthma for feveral years; after a fevere fit of t her legs began to fwell, and the quantity of urine to diminifh.   In fix weeks fhe was much trouoled with the fwellings in her thighs and abdomen, which decreafed very little when fhe lay down: fhe made not quite a pint of water in the twenty-four hours. I ordered her to take two fpoonfuls of the infufion of Foxglove every three hours.   By the time fhe had taken eight dofes her urine had increafed to the quantity of two quarts in the day and night, but as fhe complained of naufea, and had once vo- mited, I ordered the ufe of the medicine to be fuf- fpended for two days.   The naufea being then re- moved, fhe again had recourfe to it, but at inter- vals of fix hours. The urine continued to difcharge freely, and in three weeks fhe was perfectly cured of her fwellings.

CASE II.

December, 1782. A poor woman, who had been afflicted with an ague during the whole of her preg- nancy, and for two months with dropfical fwellings of the feet, legs, thighs, abdomen, and labia pu- denda; was at the expiration of the feventh month taken

taken in labour. On the day after her delivery the ague returned, with fo much violence as to endanger her life. As foon as the fit left her, I began to give her the red bark in fubftance, which had the defired effect of preventing another paroxyfm. She continued to recover her health for a fortnight, but did not find any diminution in the fwellings; her legs were now fo large as to oblige her to keep conftantly on the bed, and fhe made very little water. I ordered her the infufion of Foxglove three times a day, which, on the third day, produced a very copious difcharge of urine, without any ficknefs; fhe continued the ufe of it for ten days, and was then able to walk. Having loft all her fwellings, and no complaint remaining but weaknefs, the bark and fteel compleated the cure.

Doctor JONES ?

Extract of a Letter from Doctor JONES, Phyfician, in Lichfield.

ANXIOUS to procure authentic accounts from the patients, to whom I gave the Foxglove, I have unavoidably been delayed in anfwering your laft favour. However, I hope the delay will be made up by the efficacy of the plant being confirmed by the enquiry. Long cafes are tedious, and feldom

every case would be a history of dropsy
The differences among the different causes of dropsy were not clearly recognized.

read, and as feldom is it neceffary to defcribe every fymptom; for every cafe would be a hiftory of dropfy. I fhall therefore content myfelf with fpecifying

fying the nature of the difeafe, and when the dropfy is attended with any other affection fhall notice
it.

Two years have fcarcely elapfed fince I firft employed the Digitalis; and the fuccefs I have had
has induced me to ufe it largely and frequently.

C A S E   I.

Ann Willott, 50 years of age, became a patient
of the Difpenfary on the 11th of April 1783. She
then complained of an enlargement of the abdomen, difficulty of breathing, particularly when lying, and coftivenefs. She paffed fmall quantities
of high-coloured urine; and had an evident fluctuation in the belly. Her legs were œdematous.
Chryftals of tartar, fquills, &c. had no effect. The
13th of *June* fhe took two fpoonfuls of a decoction
of Foxglove, containing three drams of the dry
leaves, in eight ounces, three times a day. Her
urine foon increafed, and in a few days fhe paffed
it freely, which continued, and her breath returned.

Dispensary Here meaning a charitable institution where advice and medicines were given either free or for a nominal charge.

C A S E   II.

Mr. ———, 45 years of age, had been long
fubject to dropfical fwellings of the legs, and made
little water. Two fpoonfuls of the fame decoction
twice a day, foon relieved him.

CASE

C A S E   III.

Mrs. ——,aged 70 years. A lady frequently afflicted
with the gout, and an afthmatical cough.   After a
long continuance of the latter, fhe had a great diminution of urine, and confiderable difficulty of
breathing, particularly on motion, or when lying.
Her body was much bound.   There was, however,
no apparent fwelling.   She took three fpoonfuls of
an aperient decoction of forty-five grains in fix
ounces and a half, every other morning. The urine
was plentiful thofe days, and her breathing much
relieved.   In two or three weeks after the ufe of it
fhe was perfectly reftored. The purgative medicine
neither increafed the urine, nor relieved the breathing, till the Foxglove was added.

**the gout in her
stomach** Renal colic,
due to urate stones.

This fpring fhe long laboured with the gout in
her ftomach, which terminated in a fit in her hand.
During the whole of this tedious illnefs, of nearly
three months, fhe paffed little urine, and her breathing was again fhort.

She took the fame preparation of Foxglove without any diuretic effect, and afterwards two and three
grains of the powder twice a day with as little. The
**dulcified spirits of
vitriol** Sulphuric
aether (i.e. ether) plus
aetherial oil (any
essential oil), used as a
stimulant in fevers and
in nervous complaints.
dulcified fpirits of vitriol, however, quickly pro-
moted the urinary fecretion.

CASE

C A S E   IV.

Mr. C——, 46 years of age, had dropfical fwellings of the legs, and paffed little urine. He took
the decoction with three drams, and was foon relieved.

C A S E   V.

Lady ———, took three grains of the dried
leaves twice a day, for fwelled legs, and fcantinefs
of urine, without effect.

C A S E   VI.

Mrs. Slater, aged 36 years. For dropfy of the
belly and legs, and fcantinefs of urine, of feveral
weeks ftanding, took three grains of the powder
twice a day, and was quite reftored in ten days.
She took many medicines without effect.

C A S E   VII.

Mrs. P———, in her 70th year, took three
grains of the powder twice a day, for fcantinefs of
urine, and fwelled legs, without effect.

C A S E   VIII.

Ann Winterleg, in her 26th year, had dropfical
fwellings of the legs, and paffed little urine: fhe
was relieved by two drams, in an eight ounce decoction.

C A S E

C A S E   IX.

William Brown, aged 76. In the laſt ſtage of dropſy of the belly and legs, found a confiderable increaſe of his urine by a decoction of Foxglove, but it was not permanent.

C A S E   X.

Mr.————, — years of age, and of very groſs habit of body, became highly dropſical, and took various medicines, without effect. One ounce of the decoction, with three drams of the dry leaves in eight ounces, twice or three times a day, increaſed his urine prodigiouſly. He was evidently better, but a little attendant nauſea overcame his reſolution, and in the courſe of ſome weeks afterwards he fell a victim to his obſtinacy.

C A S E   XI.

Mrs. Smith, about 50 years of age, after a tedious illneſs of many weeks, had a jaundice, and became dropſical in the legs. Two ſpoonfuls of the decoction, with three drams twice a day, increaſed her urine, and abated the ſwelling.

C A S E   XII.

Widow Chatterton, about 60 years of age. Took the decoction in the ſame way for dropſy of the legs, with little effect.

CASE

C A S E   XIII.

———— Genders, about thirty-four years of age, was delivered of three children, and became dropfical of the abdomen. She paffed little or no urine, had conftant thirft, and no appetite. She took two fpoonfuls of an eight ounce decoction, with three drams twice a day. By the time fhe had finifhed the bottle, (which muft have been on the fourth day,) fhe had evacuated all her water, and could go about. Her appetite increafed with every dofe, and fhe recovered without farther help.

C A S E   XIV.

Mifs M—— M——, in her 20th year. Had been infirm from her cradle, and, after various fufferings, had an aftonifhing œdematous fwelling of one leg and thigh, of many weeks ftanding. She paffed little or no urine, and had all her other complaints. She took 2 fpoonfuls of an eight oz. decoction of two drams, twice a day. Her urine immediately increafed; and, on the third day, the fwelling had entirely fubfided.

C A S E   XV.

Mr. P——, 65 years of age, and of a full habit of body. Had lived freely in his youth, and for many years led rather an inactive life. His health was much impaired feveral months, and he had a confiderable diftention, and evident fluctuation in

I   the

the abdomen, and a very great œdema of the legs and thighs. His breathing was very fhort, and rather laborious, appetite bad, and thirft confiderable. His belly was bound, and he paffed very fmall quantities of high-coloured urine, that depofited a reddifh matter. He had taken medicines fome time, and, I believe, the Digitalis; and had been better.

A blifter was applied to the upper and infide of each thigh; he took two fpoonfuls of the decoction, with three drams of the dry leaves, two or three times a day; and fome opening phyfic occafionally.

He lived at a confiderable diftance, and I did not vifit him a fecond time; but I was well informed, about ten days or a fortnight afterwards, that his urine increafed amazingly upon taking the decoction, and that the water was entirely evacuated.

CASE XVI.

Mrs. G——, aged 50 years. After being long ailing, had a large collection of water in the abdomen and lower extremities. Her urine was high-coloured, in fmall quantities, and had a reddifh fediment. She took the decoction of Digitalis, fquills, &c. without any effect. The chryftals of tartar, however, cured her fpeedily.

CASE

C A S E   XVII.

Mr. ———, about 50 years of age, complained of great tenfion and pain acrofs the abdomen, and of lofs of appetite; his urine, he thought, was lefs than ufual, but the difference was fo trifling he could fpeak with no certainty: his belly feemed to fluctuate. Among other things he tried the Fox-glove leaves dried, twice a day; and, although it appeared to afford him relief, yet the effect was not permanent.

C A S E   XVIII.

Mr. W———, aged between 60 and 70 years; and rather corpulent: was confiderably dropfical, both of the belly and legs, and his urine in fmall quantities. Three grains of the dry leaves, twice a day, evacuated the water in lefs than a fortnight.

C A S E   XIX.

Sarah Taylor, 40 years of age, was admitted into the Difpenfary for dropfy of the abdomen and legs; and was relieved by the Decoctum digitalianum.

C A S E   XX.

Lydia Smith, aged 60. Difpenfary. Laboured many years under an afthma, and became dropfical. She took the decoction without effect.

CASE

C A S E   XXI.

quotidian inter-
mittent A fever
every three days (see
note to p. 46).

John Leadbeater, aged 15 years. Had a quotidian intermittent, which was removed by the humane affiftance of an amiable young lady. His
intermittent was foon attended by a very confiderable afcites; for which he became a patient of the
Difpenfary. He took a decoction of Foxglove night
and morning. His urine increafed immediately,
and he loft all his complaints in four days.

C A S E   XXII.

William Millar, aged 50 years. Admitted into
the Difpenfary for a tertian ague, and general dropfy. The dropfy continuing after the ague was removed, and his urine being ftill paffed in fmall
quantities; he took the powdered leaves, and recovered his health in five days.

C A S E   XXIII.

Ann Wakelin, 10 years of age. Had for feveral weeks a dropfy of the belly after an ague. She
took a decoction of Foxglove, which removed all
complaint by the fourth day.

C A S E   XXIV.

Ann Meachime: a Difpenfary patient. Had an
afcites and fcantinefs of urine. She took the powder

der of Foxglove, and evacuated all her water in
three days.

It may not be improper to obferve, 1ft. That
various diuretics had long been given in many of
thefe cafes before I was confulted. And, 2dly.
That the exhibition of the Foxglove was but feldom
attended with ficknefs.

R E M A R K S.

Thefe Cafes, thus liberally communicated by my
friend, Dr. Jones, are more acceptable, as they
feem to contain a faithful abftract from his notes,
both of the unfuccefsful as well as the fuccefsful
Cafes.

The following Tabular View of them will give us
fome Idea of the efficacy of the Medicine.

Anafarca - - - - 7 Cafes - Cured - - 3
　　　　　　　　　　　　　　Relieved - 1
　　　　　　　　　　　　　　Failed - - 3
Afcites - - - - 5 Cafes - Cured - - 4
　　　　　　　　　　　　　　Relieved - 1
Œdematous leg - - 1 Cafe - Cured - - 1
Afcites and anafarca - 7 Cafes - Cured - - 4
　　　　　　　　　　　　　　Relieved - 2
　　　　　　　　　　　　　　Failed - - 1
Afthma and dropfy - 1 Cafe - Failed - - 1
Hydrothorax and gout 1 Cafe - Cured - - 1
- - - - -, afcites } 2 Cafes - Cured - - 2
　and anafarca - - }

　　　　　　A CASE

Mr. JONES Mr William Jones. His letter to Withering about the use of foxglove in treating cases of insanity and haemoptysis were later published in the *Medical Commentaries* (Jones 1787).

A CASE of Anafarca communicated by Mr. JONES, Surgeon, in Birmingham.

Dear SIR,

HAVING lately experienced the diuretic powers of the Foxglove, in a cafe of anafarca; I do myfelf the pleafure of communicating a fhort hiftory of the treatment to you.

I am, &c.

Birmingham,   W. JONES.
May 17th, 1785.

My patient, Mrs. C———, who is in her 51ft year, had the following fymptoms, viz. alternate fwelling of the legs and abdomen, a little cough, fhortnefs of breath in a morning, thirft, weak pulfe, and her urine, which was fo fmall in quantity as feldom to amount to half a pint in twenty-four hours, depofited a clay-coloured fediment.

April 16th, 1785, I directed the following form:

R. Fol. Digitalis ficcat. ʒii.
   Aq. fontanæ bullient. ℥viii. f. infuf. et cola.
   Sumat cochl. larga iii. o. n. et mane.

cola. *Colata*, strained.

o. n. *Omni nocte*, every night.

On the 17th fhe had taken twice of the infufion, and though by miftake only two tea fpoonfuls for a dofe,

dofe, yet the quantity of urine was increafed to about a pint in the twenty-four hours. She was then directed to take two table fpoonfuls night and morning.   And.

On the 18th, a degree of naufea was produced. A pint and half of urine was made in the laft twenty-four hours. During the time above fpecified fhe had two or three ftools every day.   The infufion was now omitted.

On the 19th the fwelling of the legs was removed. A degree of naufea took place in the morning, and increafed fo much during the day, that fhe vomitted up all her food and medicine.   As fhe was very low, and complained of want of appetite, a cordial julep was directed to be taken occafionally, as well as red port and water, mint tea, &c. She informed me that whatever fhe took generally ftaid about an hour before it came up again, and that the mint tea ftaid longeft on the ftomach. The vomiting decreafed gradually, and ceafed on the 22d. The difcharge of urine remained confiderable during the three following days, but its quantity was not meafured.

mint tea Tea made from different species of *Mentha* was used as a stomachic, antispasmodic, and carminative.

22d. A dofe of neutral faline julep was directed to be taken every fourth hour.

On the 23d fhe complained of thirft, and thought the difcharge of urine not fo copious as on the preceding days, therefore the faline julep was continued ed every fourth hour, with the addition of thirty drops of the following medicine:

R. Aceti fcillitic. ʒvi.
    Tinct. aromat. ʒii.
    Tinct. thebaic. gutt. xx. m.

The bowels have been kept open from the 19th, by the occafional ufe of emollient injections.

emollient injections Lubricating enemas used to soften the stools and to ease their passage.

On the 24th the legs were much fwelled again; fhe complained of languor and a degree of naufea. The difcharge of urine increafed a little fince the 23d. Her pulfe was low and her tongue white. The urine, which had been rendered clear by the infufion of Foxglove, now depofited a whitifh fediment.

On the 25th her appetite began to return, the fwelling of the legs diminifhed, and fhe thought herfelf much relieved. The urine was confiderable in quantity, and clear.

On the 26th fhe was thirfty and languid. The fwelling was removed; the quantity of urine difcharged in the laft twenty-four hours was about a pint. She continued to mend from this time, and is now in good health.

A giddinefs of the head, more or lefs remarkable at times, was obferved to follow the ufe of the Foxglove, and it lafted nine or ten days.

This

This is the fecond time that I have relieved this patient by the infufion of Foxglove.   I ufed the fame proportion of the frefh leaves the firft time as I did of the dried ones the laft.   The violent vomiting which followed the ufe of the infufion made with the dried leaves, did not take place with the frefh, though fhe took near a pint made with the fame proportion of the herb frefh gathered.

R E M A R K S.

T H E above is a very inftructive cafe, as it teaches us how fmall a quantity of the infufion was neceffary to effect every defirable purpofe. At firft fight it may appear from the concluding paragraph, that the green leaves ought to be preferred to the dried ones, as being fo much milder in their operation; but let it be noticed, that the fame quantity of infufion was prepared from the fame weight of the green as of the dried leaves, and confequently, as will appear hereafter, the infufion with the dried leaves was five times the ftrength of that before prepared from the green ones. We need not wonder, therefore, that the effects of the former were fo difagreeable, when the dofe was five times greater than it ought to have been.   But what makes this matter ftill more obvious, is the miftake mentioned at firft, of two tea fpoonfuls only being given for a dofe. Now a tea fpoonful, containing about a fourth or a fifth part of the contents of a table fpoon, the dofe then given, was very nearly the fame as that which had before been taken of the

the dose was five times greater Because the green leaves, as Withering notes later (see p. 181), are four-fifths water.

infufion

infufion of the green leaves, and it produced precifely the fame effects for it increafed the urinary
difcharge, without exciting the violent vomiting.

Doctor JOHN-
STONE Dr Edward
Johnstone (born c.
1760), son of the
better-known Dr
James C. Johnstone.
He graduated from
Edinburgh in 1799
with a dissertation
entitled De Febre Puer-
perali.

Letter from Doctor JOHNSTONE, Phyfician, in Birmingham.

Dear SIR,

          THE following cafes are felected
from many others in which I have given the Digitalis purpurea; and from repeated experience of its
efficacy after other diuretics have failed, I can recommend it as an effectual, and when properly
managed, a fafe medicine.

I am, &c.

Birmingham, May 26.   E. JOHNSTONE.
          1785.

March 8th, 1783, I was called to attend Mr.
G——, a gentleman of a robuft habit, who had led
a regular and temperate life, Æt. 68. He was
affected with great difficulty of refpiration, and cough
particularly troublefome on attempting to lie down,
œdematous fwellings of the legs and thighs, abdomen tenfe and fore on being preffed, pain ftriking
from the pit of the ftomach to the back and fhoul-
ders; almoft conftant naufea, efpecially after taking
food, which he frequently threw up; water thick
and high-coloured, paffed with difficulty and in
                                             fmall

fmall quantity ; body coftive; pulfe natural; face much emaciated, .eyes yellow and depreffed. He had been fubject to cough and difficulty of breathing in the winter for feveral years; and about four years before this time, after being expofed to cold, was fuddenly deprived of his fpeech and the ufe of the right fide, which he recovered as the warm weather came on ; but fince that time had been remarkably coftive, and was in every refpect much debilitated. He firft perceived his legs fwell about a year ago ; by the ufe of medicines and exercife, the fwellings fubfided during the fummer, but returned on the approach of winter, and gradually increafed to the ftate in which I found them, notwithftanding he had ufed different preparations of fquills and a great variety of other diuretic medicines. I ordered the following mixture.

R. Foliorum Digitalis purpur. recent. ℨiii. decoque ex aq. fontan. ℥xii ad ℥vi colaturæ adde Tinctur. aromatic.
Syr. zinzib. aa ℥i. m. capt. cochl. duo larga fecunda quaque hora ad quartam vicem nifi prius naufea fupervenerit.

Syr. zinzib. Syrup of ginger (*Zinziber*), used as an antispasmodic and carminative.

ad quartam vicem nisi prius nausea supervenit To the fourth succession (i.e. four times in all) unless nausea occurs beforehand.

March 9th. He took four dofes of the mixture without being in the leaft fick, and made, during the night upwards of two quarts of natural coloured water.

10th.

10th. Took the remainder of the mixture yefter-day afternoon and evening, and was fick for a fhort time, but made nearly the fame quantity of water as before, the fwellings are confiderably diminifhed, his appetite increafed, but he is ftill coftive.

tere ad extinc-tionem merc. Rub together thoroughly until the mercury disappears. A so-called 'extinction of mercury' (cf. mercurial ointment, p. 207).

R. Argent. viv. balfam peruv. aa ʒfs tere ad ex-tinctionem merc. et adde gum. ammon. Ɔiii aloes focotorin. 3fs rad. fcil. recent. Ɔfs fyr. fimpl. q. f. f. mafs. in pil. xxxii divid. cap. iii. bis in die.

aloes socotorin. Socotrine aloes, prepared from the plant *Aloe Socotrina* (from the island of Socotra in the Indian Ocean at the gulf of Aden) or *Perryi*. See also note to p. 70.

14th. Continues to make water freely. The fwellings of his legs have gradually decreafed ; fore-nefs and tenfion of the abdomen confiderably lefs.

Omittant. pil. cap. miftur. c. decoct. Digitalis. &c. 3tia quaque hora ad 3tiam vicem.

15th. Made a pint and a half of water laft night, without being in the leaft fick, and is in every refpect confiderably better. Repet. Pillul. ut antea.

21ft. Makes water as ufual when in health, and the fwellings are entirely gone.

Rhei spirit. Spirit of rhubarb (see note to p. 15).

R. Infus. amar. ʒv. tinctur. Rhei fpirit. ʒii. fpi-rit vitriol. dulc. ʒii. fyr. zinzib. ʒvi. m. cap. cochl. iii. larg. ter in die.

He foon gained fufficient ftrength to enable him to go a journey, and returned home in much better health

health than he had been from the time he was affected with the paralytic stroke, and excepting some return of his asthmatic complaint in the winter, hath continued so ever since.

C A S E   II.

R—— Howgate, a man much addicted to intemperance, particularly in the use of spirituous liquors, Æt. 60, was admitted into the Hospital near Birmingham, *May* 17, 1783. He complained of difficulty of breathing, attended with cough, particularly troublesome on lying down; drowsiness and frequent dozing, from which he was roused by startings, accompanied with great anxiety and oppression about the breast ; œdematous swellings of the legs; constant desire to make water, which he passed with difficulty, and only by drops ; pulse weak and irregular; body rather costive ; face much emaciated; no appetite for food.—Cap. pil. scil. iii. ter in die.*

May 20th. The pills have had no effect.—Cap. mistur. c. † Decoct. Digital. &c. cochl. ii. larg. 3tia quaque hora, ad 3tiam vicem.

May 21st. Made near two quarts of water in the night, without being in the least sick. He contiued the

sapon. castiliens
Castile soap (Spanish or castle soap). A hard soap made with olive oil and sodium carbonate.

f. mass. *Filix mas*, an extract of the male fern, *Dryopteris filix-mas*, used as a purgative and specifically to treat tapeworm infestations.

---

* R. Rad. scil. recent. sapon. castiliens. pulv. Rhei opt. aa. ℈i. ol. junip. gutt. xvi. syr. balf. q. s. f. mass. in pil. xxiv. divid.

† Prepared in the same manner as in the former case,

the ufe of the mixture three times in the day till the 30th, and made about three pints of water daily, by which means the fwellings were entirely taken away ; and his other complaints fo much relieved, that on the 6th of June he was difmiffed free from complaint, except a flight cough. But returning to his old courfe of life, he hath had frequent attacks of his diforder, which have been always removed by ufing the Digitalis.

Mr. Lyon ?

Extract of a letter from Mr. Lyon, Surgeon, at Tamworth.

—Mr. Moggs was about 54 years of age, his dif-eafe a dropfy of the abdomen, attended with anafarcous fwellings of the limbs, &c. brought on by exceffive drinking. I believe the firft fymptoms of the difeafe appeared the beginning of November, 1776 ; the medicines he took before you faw him, were fquills in different forms, fal diureticus and calomel, but without any good effect ; he begun the Digitalis on the 10th of July 1777 ; a few dofes of it caufed a giddinefs in the head, and almoft de-prived him of fight, with very great naufea, but very little vomiting, after which a confiderable flow of urine enfued, and in a very fhort time, a very little water remained either in the cavity of the abdomen, or the membrana adipofa, but he remained exceffive weak, with a fluttering pulfe at the rate of 150 or frequently 160 in a minute ; he kept pretty free from water for upwards of twelve months ; it then collect-

membrana adiposa The fat of the cells of the so-called 'cellular membrane', part of the subcutaneous and peri-renal fat.

a fluttering pulse The term 'fluttering' should not be taken literally. The condition of atrial flutter

collected, and neither the Digitalis nor any other medicine would carry it off. I tapped him the 2d. of August 1779 in the usual place, and took some gallons of water from him, but he very soon filled again, and as he had a very large rupture, a considerable quantity of the water lodged in the scrotum, and could not be got away by tapping in the usual place. I therefore (on the 28th of the same month) made an incision into the lower part of the scrotum, and drained off all the water that way, but he was so very much reduced, that he died the 8th or 9th of *September* following, which was about two years and two months after he first begun the Digitalis.

I have had several dropsical patients relieved, and some perfectly recovered by the Digitalis, since you attended Mr. Moggs, but as I did not take any notes or make any memorandums of them, cannot give you any of them.

Communications from Dr. STOKES, Physician, in Stourbridge.

Dear SIR,

I ACCEPT with pleasure your invitation to communicate what I know respecting the properties of *Digitalis*; and if an account of what others had discovered before you,* with a detail

---

* See this account in the Introduction.

was not recognized. This was probably a case of atrial fibrillation.

tail of my own experience, fhall be allowed the
merit of at leaft a well meant acknowledgment, for
the early communication you were fo kind to make
me, of the valuable properties you had found in it;
I fhall confider my time as well employed. A knowledge of what has been already done is the beft
ground work of future experiment; on which account I have been the more full on this fubject, in
hopes that given with the cautions which you mean
to lay down in the cure of dropfies, it may prove
alike ufeful in that of other difeafes, one of which
ftands foremoft among the *opprobria* of medicine.

CASE I.

Mrs. M——. Orthopnea, pain, and exceffive
oppreffion at the bottom of the fternum. Pulfe
irregular, with frequent intermiffions. Appetite
very much impaired. Legs anafarcous.

Empl. veficator. pectori dolent.
Infuf. Digital. e ʒiii. ad. aq. &c. ʒviii. cochl. j. o.
   h. donec naufea excitetur vel diurefis fatis copi-
   ofa proveniat.

I ordered it of the above ftrength, and to be repeated often, on account of the great emergency of
the cafe, but the naufea excited by the firft dofe prevented its being given at fuch fhort intervals. A 3d
dofe I found had been given, which was followed by
vomitings. All her complaints gradually abated,
                                                    but

but in about a fortnight recurred, notwithſtanding the uſe of infuſ. amar. &c.

Dec. 2. *Infus. Digit. e.* ʒiſs *ad aq.* &c. ʒviii. *cochl. ii. horis* &c. *u. a.*

u. a. Ut ante, as [preſcribed] before.

Complaints gradually abated, ſwellings of the legs nearly gone down.

About a month afterwards you was deſired to viſit this patient.*

you was Neither a grammatical error nor a misprint. 'Was' was commonly used instead of 'were' during the eighteenth century with the second person singular.

---

* For reaſons aſſigned at p. 100, I did not intend to introduce any caſe, occuring under my own inſpection, in the courſe of the preſent year ; but it may be ſatisfactory to continue the hiſtory of this diſeaſe, as Dr. Stokes's narrative would otherwiſe be incomplete.

1 7 8 5.

C   A   S   E.

Jan. 5th. Mrs. M——, Æt. 48. Hydrothorax and anaſarcous legs, of eight months duration. She had taken jallap, ſquill, ſalt of tartar, and various other medicines. I found her in a very reduced ſtate, and therefore directed only a grain and half of the Pulv. Digital. to be given night and morning. This in a few days encreaſed the ſecretion of urine, removed her difficulty of breathing, and reduced the ſwelling of her legs, without any diſturbance to her ſyſtem.

Three months afterwards, a ſevere attack of gout in her legs and arms, removing to her head, ſhe died.

Dr. Stokes had an opportunity of examining the dead body, and I had the ſatisfaction to learn from him, that there did not appear to have been any return of the dropſy.

K   On

On the examination of the body I noticed, among others, the following appearances.

About $\frac{3}{4}$ oz. of bloody water flowed out, on elevating the upper half of the scull, and a small quantity also was found at the base.

BRAIN. Blood-vessels turgid with blood, and many of those of considerable size distended with air.

A very slight watery effusion between the *Pia Mater* and *Tunica arachnoidea*. About $\frac{3}{4}$ oz. of watery fluid in the *lateral ventricles*.

THORAX. In the left cavity about 4 oz. of bloody serum; in the right but little. Lungs, the hinder parts loaded with blood. Adhesions of each lobe to the pleura. *Pericardium* containing but a very small quantity of fluid. *Heart* containing no coagula of blood. *Valves of the Aorta* of a cartilaginous texture, as if beginning to ossify.

Abdominal Viscera natural, and a profusion of *Fat* under the integuments of the abdomen and thorax, in the former to the thickness of an inch and upwards, and in very considerable quantity on the mesentery, omentum, kidneys, &c.

OBS. The intermitting pulse should seem to have been owing to effusions of water in some of the cavities of the breast, as it disappeared on the removal of the waters.

CASE

C A S E   II.*

Mrs. C—— of K——, Æt. 80. Orthopnœa, with fenfe of oppreffion about the prœcordia. Unable to lie down in bed for fome nights paft. Anafarca of the lower extremities. Urine very fcanty. Complaints of fix weeks ftanding. Had taken *fal. diuret. c. ol. junip.*—*Calom.c. jalap, et gambog.*—*Et ol. junip. c. ol. Terebinth.* without effect.

Feb. 7. Infuf. Digital. e. ʒiii. ad aq. &c. ʒviii. cochl. ii. 4tis horis. Ordered to drink largely of *infus. baccar. junip.* The third dofe produced great naufea which continued ten hours, during which time the urine made was about a quart. The next day her apothecary directed her to begin again with it. The fecond dofe produced vomiting. During the next twenty hours fhe made two quarts of water, about four times as much as fhe drank.

From this time fhe took no more of the *infus. Digital.* but continued the *inf. bacc. junip.* until about *March* 2d, when all the fwellings were gone down, her refpiration perfectly free, and fhe herfelf quite reftored to her former ftate of health. On the 29th fhe had an attack of jaundice which was fome time after removed; fince which fhe has enjoyed a good ftate of health, excepting that for fome little time paft her ancles have been flightly œdematous, which will I truft foon yield to ftrengthening medicines.

junip. Juniper, used as a diuretic. *Ol. junip.* — oil of juniper; *baccar. junip.* — juniper berries.

gambog. Gamboge, a resin obtained from the trees of the *Garcinia* genus, found in Cambodia and elsewhere. It was used as a purgative, often, as here, in combination with other drugs.

ol. Terebinth. Oil of turpentine, used as a laxative and diuretic.

CASE

C A S E III.

Mrs. M—— G——, Æt. 64. Has had fore legs for thefe thirty-four years paft. Orthopnœa. Senfe of oppreffion at the præcordia. Pulfe intermitting. Legs anafarcous. Urine fcanty, high-coloured.

Infus. Digital. c. ʒiſs ad aq. bull. ʒviii. cochl. ii. 4tis horis.

Took fix dofes, when naufea was excited. Urine a quart during the courfe of the night. The flow of urine continued, and complaints relieved. Sal. Mart. c. extr. gent. and afterwards with the addition of extr. cort. for which laft ingredient fhe had a predilection, confirmed the cure.

extr. cort. Although strictly speaking this could mean the extract of any rind or bark it was most often used to mean Peruvian bark.

On the fame day the next year I was called in to her for a fimilar train of fymptoms, excepting that the pulfe was but juft perceptibly irregular.

Infus. Digital. u. a. præfcript.

The directions on the phial not being attended to, *two dofes of it were given after a naufea had been excited*, which, with occafional vomitings, became exceedingly oppreffive. A faline draught, given in Dr. Hulme's method, a draught *fal. c. c. gr. xii. c. conf. card. gr. x.* produced no immediate effect, but the naufea gradually abating, inf. bacc. junip. was ordered; but this appeared to augment it, and

Dr. **Hulme** Nathaniel Hulme (1732-1807). Physician. He graduated from Edinburgh in 1765 with a dissertation entitled *De Scorbuto*.

and a great propensity to sleep coming on, I directed *sal. c. c. conf. card. aa gr. viii. 4tis horis*, which removed the unpleasant symptoms and *myrrh. c. sal. mart.* completed the cure. During the use of the above medicines, the urine was augmented, and the pulmonary complaints removed, even before the nausea left her; and the sores of her legs which were much inflamed before she began with the infus. Digital. in a day's time assumed a much healthier appearance, and on her other complaints going off, they shewed a greater tendency to heal than she had ever observed in them for twenty years before. This instance is a very pleasing confirmation of the experience of Hulse and Dr. Baylies, and of the advantage to be derived from a medicine, which, while it helps to heal the ulcers, removes that from the constitution which often renders the healing of them improper.

In one case in which I ordered it, the infusion, instead of digesting three hours as I had directed, was suffered to stand upon the leaves all night. The consequence was that the first dose produced considerable nausea.

The two following cases, with which I have been favoured by a physician very justly eminent, convince me of the necessity there is that every one who discovers a new medicine, or new virtues in an old one, should, in announcing such discoveries, publish to the world the exact manner in which he exhibits

K 3   bits

sal. c. c. Sal cornu cervi, salt of hartshorn, ammonium carbonate (as incorporated in smelling salts), used in dyspepsia and nervous disorders.

bits fuch medicines, with all the precautions neceffary to obtain the promifed fuccefs.

In thefe (fays my correfpondent) " the infufion
" was given in fmall dofes, repeated every hour or
" two, till a naufea was raifed, when it was omit-
" ted for a day or perhaps two, and then repeated
" in the fame manner."

" An ASCITES emptied by it, but filled again
" very fpeedily, though *its ufe was never difconti-*
" *nued*, and who afterwards found no falutary ef-
" fects from it. Ended fatally."

*its use was never dis-
continued . . . the med-
icine was still given . . .*
the inefficacy of *its*
continued use It is
clear from these
remarks that the
reason for the failure
in these cases was the
accumulation of digi-
talis with consequent
fatal toxicity (see note
to p. 6). Withering
emphasizes the fact by
his use of italics.

" In an ANASARCA it fometimes increafed the
" quantity of urine, and abated the fwelling, but
" which as often returned in as great a degree as
" before, though *the medicine was flill given*, and al-
" ways increafed in quantity fo as to excite naufea.
" Ended fatally."

" I have tried it in many other cafes, but found
" very little difference in the fuccefs attending it."

May we not be allowed to conjecture that the inefficacy of *its continued ufe* is owing to its narcotic property gradually diminifhing the irritability of the
mufcular fibres of the abforbents, or poffibly of the
whole vafcular fyftem, and thus adding to that
weakened action which feems to be the caufe of the
generality of dropfies, which leads us to caution
the medical experimenter againft trying it, at leaft

againft

againſt its continued uſe, even in ſmall doſes, in other
diſeaſes of diminiſhed energy, as continued fever,
palſy, &c.

I remain with the greateſt truth,

Your obliged and affectionate friend,

Stourbridge,   JONATHAN STOKES.
May 17, 1785.

THE three following Hoſpital Caſes, which
  Dr. STOKES had an opportunity of obſerv-
ing, are related as inſtances of bad practice, and tend to demonſtrate how necef-
ſary it is when one phyſician adopts the
medicine of another, that he ſhould alſo
at firſt rigidly adopt his method.

C A S E   I.

Eſther K———, Æt. 33. General anaſarca,
aſcites, and dyſpnœa, of ſeven months duration.

Decoct. e Digit. ʒiv. *c. aq.* ℔i. *coquend. ad* ℔ſs. *cap.*
ʒi. 2*dis. horis.* 1ſt DAY. 4th doſe made her ſick.
2d DAY. The firſt doſe ſhe took to-day produced
vomiting.

3d DAY.

3d Day. *Minuatur dofis ad ℥ fs.* This ftayed upon her ftomach, but produced an almoft conftant ficknefs. Stools more frequent, water fcarce fenfibly increafed; and her fwellings not at all reduced.

4th Day. *Cap. Calomel. gambog. fcill. &c.*

Obs. Sufficient time was not allowed to obferve its effects, neither was the patient enjoined the free ufe of diluents. The difeafe terminated fatally.

C A S E   II.

William T——, Æt. 42. Afcites, with cough and dyfpnœa. Abdomen very much diftended. The reft of his body highly emaciated. Urine thick, high coloured, and in very fmall quantity.

Decoct Digit. (u. in Efther K——,) 4tis horis.

1ft Day of taking it. The 4th dofe produced ficknefs.

2d. Vomiting after the fecond dofe.

10th. Urine increafed to ℔vi.

11th. Flow of urine continues. Abdomen quite flaccid.

12th. Ab-

12th. Abdomen not diminiſhed.

15th. A ſmart purging came on, and the flow of
urine diminiſhed.

23d. Belly much bound. Took a cathart. powder, which was followed by a diminution of the
abdomen.

29th. To take a cathart. powder every 4th morning, continuing the decoɗ. Digit.

32d. Urine exceedingly ſcanty.

35th. *Vin. ſcill,* ℥ſs. *o. m. &c.* This produced
diuretic effeɗs.

44th. Tapped. Terminated fatally.

Obs. Here the medicine was *continued till it ceaſed
to produce diuretic effeɗs;* and theſe effeɗs were not
aided by any ſtrengthening remedies.

C A S E   III.

George R——, Æt. 52. Aſcites, general anaſarca, and dyſpnœa. His legs ſo greatly diſtended
that it was with great difficulty he could draw the
one after the other.

Infuſ.

Infuſ. Digital. ʒiiiſs. ad. aq. ℔ſs. cap. ℥i. altern.
horis donec nauſeam excitaverit. Rep. ʒtiis die-
bus. tempore intermedio cap. ſol. guaic. ℥i. ter in
die ex inf. ſinap.

1ſt DAY of taking it. Became ſickiſh towards
night.

2d DAY. Made a great quantity of water during
the night, and ſpat up a great deal of watery phlegm.
The firſt doſe he took in the morning has produced
a ſickneſs which has continued all day, but he has
never vomited.

3d. DAY. The change in his appearance ſo great
as to make it difficult to conceive him to be the
ſame perſon. Inſtead of a large corpulent man, he
appeared tall, thin, and rather aged. Breathes
freely, and can walk up and down ſtairs without inconvenience.

4th DAY. *Decoȼt. bacc. junip. and cyder for common*
drink.

6th DAY. A ſecond courſe of his medicine produced a flow of urine almoſt as plentiful as the former, though he drank little or nothing at the time.
In a day or two after he walked to ſome diſtance.

12th DAY. *Pot. purgans illico.*

14th DAY. *Pot. purg. c. jalap. ʒſs. 4tis diebus.*
Infuſ. Dig. ʒtiis diebus.

17th DAY.

17th Day. R. *Gamb. gr. iii. calom. gr. ii. camph.*
     gr. i. fyr. fimpl. fiat pil. o. n. fum.
     Infuf. Digit. 3tiis diebus.

21ft Day. Made an out-patient. The fuper-
abundant flow of urine continued for the firft three
days after his laft courfe ; but fince, the flow of faliva has been nearly equal to that of urine.

The fmalls of his legs not quite reduced, and are
fuller at night. He has fhrunk round the middle
from four feet two inches to three feet fix inches ;
and in the calves of his legs, from feventeen inches
to thirteen and a half.*

The smalls of his legs The parts between the ankles and calves.

Obs. The waters were here very fuccefsfully evacuated, but as you remarked to me, on communicating the cafe to you at the time, tonic medicines
fhould have been given, to fecond the ground that
had been gained, inftead of weakening the patient
by draftic purgatives.

* In the three laft recited cafes, the medicine was directed in
dofes quite too ftrong, and repeated too frequently. If Efther
K—— could have furvived the extreme ficknefs, the diuretic
effects would probably have taken place, and, from her time of
life, I fhould have expected a recovery. Wm. T —— feems to
have been a bad cafe, and I think would not have been cured under any management. G. R—— certainly poffeffed a good conftitution, or he muft have fhared the fate of the other two.

A CASE

Mr. SHAW ?

A C A S E from Mr. SHAW, Surgeon, at Stourbridge. — Communicated by Doctor STOKES.

Matth. D——, Æt. 71. Tall and thin. Difeafe a general anafarca, with great difficulty of breathing. The lac ammoniac. fomewhat relieved his breath ; but the fwellings increafed, and his urine was not augmented.   I confidered it as a loft cafe, but having feen the good effects of the Digitalis, as ordered by Dr. Stokes in the cafe of Mrs. G——, I gave him one fpoonful of an infufion of ʒii. to half a pint, twice a day.   His breath became much eafier, his urine increafed confiderably, and the fwellings gradually difappeared; fince which his health has been pretty good, except that about three weeks ago, he had a flight dyfpnœa, with pain in his ftomach, which were foon removed by a repetition of the fame medicine.

Mr. Shaw likewife informs me, that he has removed pains in the ftomach and bowels, by giving a fpoonful of the infufion, ʒifs. to ℥viii. morning and night.

A Letter

A Letter from Mr. V A U X, Surgeon, in Birmingham.

Dear Sir,

I SEND you the two following cafes, wherein the Digitalis had very powerful and fenfible effects, in the cure of the different patients.

C A S E   I.

Mrs. O—— of L—— ftreet, in this town, aged 28, naturally of a thin, fpare habit, and her family inclinable to phthifis, fent for me on the 11th of June, 1779, at which time fhe complained of great pain in her fide, a conftant cough, expectorated much, which funk in water; had colliquative fweats and frequent purging ftools; the lower extremities and belly full of water, and from the great difficulty fhe had in breathing, I concluded there was water in the cheft alfo. The quantity of water made at a time for three weeks before I faw her, never amounted to more than a tea-cup full, frequently not fo much. Finding her in fo alarming a fituation, I gave it as my opinion fhe could receive no benefit from medicine, and requefted her not to take any; but fhe being very defirous of my ordering her fomething, I complied, and fent her a box of gum pills with fquills, and a mixture with falt of tartar: thefe medicines fhe took until the fixteenth, without any good effects : the water in her legs now began to ex-
fude

colliquative sweats Profuse sweats resulting in wasting of the body.

fude through the fkin, and a fmall blifter on one of
her legs broke. Believing fhe could not exift much
longer, unlefs an evacuation of the water could be
procured ; after fully iuforming her of her fituation,
and the uncertainty of her furviving the ufe of the
medicine, I ventured to propofe her taking the Digitalis, which fhe chearfully agreed to. I accordingly fent her a pint mixture, made as under, of
the frefh leaves of the Digitalis. Three drams infufed in one pint of boiling water, when cold ftrain-
ed off, without preffing the leaves, and two ounces
of the ftrong juniper water added to it : of this
mixture fhe was ordered four table fpoonfulls every
third hour, till it either made her fick, purged her,
or had a fenfible effect on the kidneys. This mixture was fent on the feventeenth, and fhe began
taking it at noon on the eighteenth. At one o'clock
the following morning I was called up, and informed fhe was dying. I immediately attended
her, and was agreeably furprifed to find their fright
arofe from her having fainted, in confequence of the
fudden lofs of twelve quarts of water fhe had made
in about two hours. I immediately applied a roller
round her belly, and, as foon as they could be made, 2
others, which were carried from the toes quite up the
thighs. The relief afforded by thefe was immediate ;
but the medicine now began to affect her ftomach fo
much, that fhe kept nothing on it many minutes together. I ordered her to drink freely of beef tea, which
fhe did, but kept it on her ftomach but a very fhort
time. A neutral draught in a ftate of effervefcence was
taken to no good purpofe : She therefore continued
the

the beef tea, and took no other medicine for five days, when her ficknefs went off : her cough abated, but the pain in her fide ftill continuing, I applied a blifter which had the defired effect : her urine after the firft day flowed naturally. Her cure was compleated by the gum pills with fteel and the bitter infufion. It muft be obferved fhe never had any collection of water afterwards.

It affords me great pleafure to inform you that fhe is now living, and has fince had four children ; all of whom, I think I may juftly fay, are indebted to the Digitalis for their exiftence.

There appears in this cafe a ftriking proof of the utility of emetics in fome kinds of confumptions, as it appears to me the dropfy was brought on by the cough, &c. and I believe thefe were cured by the continual vomitings, occafioned by the medicine.

C A S E   II.

Mr. H——, a publican, aged about 48 years, fent for me in *March*, 1778. He complained of a cough, fhortnefs of breathing, which prevented him from laying down in bed ; his belly, thighs and legs very much diftended with water ; the quantity of urine made at a time feldom exceeded a fpoonful. I requefted him to get fome of the Digitalis, and as they had no proper weights in the houfe, I told them to put as much of the frefh leaves as would weigh down a guinea, into half a pint of boiling water ;

to

There appears in this case This paragraph indicates the kind of misinterpretation that might be made of simple observations. Mr Vaux clearly believed firstly that because digitalis is an emetic it was the emetic properties which were important, and secondly that because the dropsy was (as he thought) directly due to the cough digitalis might be useful in treating consumptions.

to let it ftand till cold, then to pour off the clear liquor, and add a glafs of gin to it, and to take three
table fpoonfuls every third hour, until it had fome
fenfible effect upon him.

Before he had taken all the infufion, the quantity of urine made increafed, (he therefore left off
taking it), and it continued to do fo until all the
water was evacuated. His breathing became much
better, his cough abated, though it never quite left
him; he being for fome time before afthmatic.
By taking fome tonic pills he continued quite well
until the next fpring, when he had a return of his
complaint, which was carried off by the fame means.
Two years after, he had a third attack, and this alfo gave way to the medicine. Laft year he died of
a pleurify.

I am, &c.

Moor-Street, 8th May,   J E R. V A U X.
        1785.

P. S. You muft well recollect the cafe of Mrs.
F——.—It was " a general dropfy—every time
" fhe took the medicine its effects were fimilar, viz.
" The difcharge of urine came on gradually at firft,
" increafed afterwards, and the whole of the water
" both in the belly, legs, &c. was perfectly evacuated.
" Although the effects were only temporary, they
" were exceedingly agreeable to the patient, making
" her time much more comfortable."—— (See Cafe
XLIII.)

A Let-

A Letter from Mr. WAINWRIGHT, Surgeon, in Dudley.

Mr. WAINWRIGHT ?
(the same as at p. 53).

Dear SIR,

IT gives me great pleasure to find you intend to publish your observations on the Digitalis purpurea.

Several years are now elapsed since you communicated to me the high opinion you entertained of the diuretic qualities of this noble plant. To ensure success, due attention was recommended to its *preparation*, its *dose*, and its *effects* upon the system.

I always gave the infusion of the dried leaves; the dose the same as in the prescriptions returned. If the medicine operated on the stomach or bowels, it was thought prudent to forbear. When the kidneys began to perform their proper functions, and the urine to be discharged, a continuance of its farther use was unnecessary.

These remarks you made in the case of the first patient for whom you prescribed the Digitalis in our neighbourhood, and I have found them all necessary at this present period. From the *decided* good effects that followed from its use, in those cases where the most powerful remedies had failed, I was soon convinced it was a most valuable addition to the materia medica.

L

The

The want of a certain diuretic, has long been one of the defiderata of medicine. The Digitalis is undoubtedly at the head of that clafs, and will feldom, if properly adminiftered, difappoint the expectation. I can fpeak with the more confidence, having, in an extenfive practice, been a happy witnefs to its good qualities.

For feveral years, I have given the infufion in a variety of cafes, where there was a deficiency in the fecretion of the urine, with the greateft fuccefs. In recent obftructions, I do not recollect many failures. In anafarcous difeafes, and in the anafarca, when combined with the afcites ; in fwellings of the limbs, and in difeafes of the cheft, when there was the greateft reafon to believe an accumulation of ferum, the moft beneficial confequences have followed from its ufe.

serum Any watery fluid.

Had I been earlier acquainted with your intention to publifh an account of the Digitalis, I could have tranfmitted fome cafes, which might have ferved to corroborate thefe affertions : but I am convinced the Digitalis needs not my affiftance to procure a favorable reception. Its own merit will enfure fuccefs, more than a hundred recited cafes.

I could wifh thofe gentlemen who intend to make ufe of this plant, to collect it in a hot dry day, when the petals fall, and the feed-veffels begin to fwell.

The

The leaves kept to the fecond year are weaker, and their diuretic qualities much diminifhed. It will therefore be neceffary to gather the plant frefh every feafon.

Thefe cautions are unneceffary to the accurate botanift, who well knows, that a plant in the fpring, though more fucculent and full of juices, is deftitute of thofe qualities which may be expected when that plant has attained its full vigour, and the feed-veffels begin to be manifeft. But for want of attention to thefe particulars, its virtues may be thought exaggerated, or doubtful, if beneficial confequences do not always flow from its ufe. There are difeafes it cannot cure ; and in feveral of thofe patients in this town, who firft took the Digitalis by your orders, there was the moft pofitive proof of the vifcera being unfound. In thefe defperate cafes it often procured a plentiful flow of urine, and palliated a difeafe which mecine could not remove.

mecine *?Mecina bour-baron*, a bicarbonated chalybeate mineral water from Spain.

At a remote diftance, phyficians are feldom applied to for advice in trifling diforders. Many remedies have been tried without relief, and the difeafe is generally obftinate or confirmed. — It would not be fair to try the merits of the Digitalis in this fcale. It might often fail of promoting the end defired. I flatter myfelf the reputation of this plant will be equal to its merit, and that it will meet with a candid reception.

As

As there is no pleafure equal to relieving the miferies and diftreffes of our fellow-creatures, I hope you will long enjoy that peculiar felicity.

Permit me to return my thankful acknowledgments, for your free communication of a medicine, by which means, through the blefling of providence, I have been enabled to reftore health and happinefs to many miferable objects.

I am, &c.

Yours,

Dudley, April 26th, 1785. J. WAINWRIGHT.

Mr. WARD ?

CASE of Mr. WARD, Surgeon, in Birmingham.—Related by himfelf.

IN *September*, 1782, I was feized with a difficulty of breathing, and oppreffion in my cheft, in confequence of taking cold from being called out in the night. My tongue was foul; my urine fmall in quantity; my breath laborious and diftreffing on the flighteft exercife. I tried the medicines moft generally recommended, fuch as emetics, blifters, lac ammoniacum, oxymel of fquills, &c. but finding little or no relief, I confulted Dr. Withering, who advifed me to try the following prefcription.

R. Fol.

R. Fol. Digital. purp. ficcat. ʒifs.

   Aq. bullientis ℥iv.

   Aq. cinn. fp. ℥fs. digere per horas quatuor, et colaturæ capiat cochlear. i. noɕte maneque.

He alfo defired me to take fifty drops of tinɕure of cantharides three or four times a day.

After taking eight ounces of the infufion, and about twelve drams of the drops, I was perfeɕtly cured, and have had no return fince. The medicine did not occafion ficknefs or vertigo, nor had they any other fenfible effeɕt than in changing the appearance, and increafing the quantity of the urine, and rendering the tongue clean. After the laft dofe or two indeed, I had a little naufea, which was immediately removed by a fmall glafs of brandy.

   Birmingham, 1ft July, 1785.

Communications from Mr. YONGE, Surgeon, in Shiffnall, Shropfhire.

Mr. YONGE ?

Dear SIR,

     I HAVE great fatisfaɕtion in complying with your juft claim, by tranfcribing outlines of the fubfequent cafes, for infertion in your long requefted traɕt on the Digitalis purpurea. The two firft of thefe you will eafily recolleɕt, the cures having been conduɕted immediately under your own management

    L 3

ment

ment, and the whole may add to that weight of evidence which long experience enables you to adduce of the efficacy of that valuable medicine. I have recited the only inftances of its failure which occur to me, but many other, though fuccefsful cafes, wherein its utility might feem dubious, and alfo the accounts received from people whofe accuracy might be fufpected, I fhall not for obvious reafous trouble you with.

I am, dear Sir,

Your obliged friend,

Shiffnall,   WILLIAM YONGE.
May 1, 1785.

C A S E   I.

A Gentleman aged 49, on the night of the 21ft of Auguft, 1784, awaked with a fenfe of fuffocation, which obliged him to rife up fuddenly in bed. I found him complaining of difficult refpiration, particularly on lying down ; the countenance pale, and the pulfe fmaller and quicker than ufual. Some brandy and water having been given, the 'fymptoms gradually abated, fo that he flept in a half recumbent pofture. The following day he expreffed a fenfe of anxiety and weight in the cheft, attended by quicker breathing upon motion of the body. That evening an emetic of ipecacohana was given, and afterwards a draught, with vitriolic æther and

and confect. card. aa ʒi to be repeated as the fymptoms fhould require it.   He continued to be affected with flighter returns of the dyfpnœa at irregular
intervals, until *September* 15th, when upon a more
fevere attack, the emetic was repeated.   He now
recollected fome flight pain in his arms which had
affected him previous to this laft feizure, and was
difpofed to confider his complaint as rheumatic.
Pills with gum ammoniac. gum guaiac. and antimonial powder were directed, with infuf. amar. fimpl.
twice a day.   The bowels were regulated by aperient pills of pulv. jalap. aloes and fal. tartar. and
ʒifs balfam peruv. was given occafionally to alleviate
the paroxyfms of dyfpnœa.

From this period until the beginning of November, little amendment or variation happened,
except that refpiration became more permanently
difficult, and particularly oppreffed upon motion,
nor was it relieved by the expectoration of a mucous difcharge, which now increafed confiderably.
Squills, mufk, ol. fuccini, æther, with other medicines of the fame kind, were now ufed, but without fuccefs.   The effects of opium and venæfection
were tried.   The appetite diminifhed, and his
fleep became fhort and difturbed.   He fometimes
flept lying upon his back, but generally upon his
left fide.   The urine which had hitherto been of
good colour, and fufficient quantity, now became
diminifhed, and lateritious ; and the ancles œdematous.

On

antimonial powder
Antimonious sulphide
plus hartshorn shav-
ings (as a source of
ammonia) heated to a
powder. Used as a
febrifuge, sudorific,
and antispasmodic. It
was introduced as a
substitute for James's
powder (see note to
p. 42).

musk A substance
secreted by the male
musk-deer, used as a
stimulant and anti-
spasmodic.

ol. succini Oil of
amber, obtained from
amber by dry distilla-
tion (cf. spirit of
amber — succinic
acid).

lateritious Brick-
red.

On the 15th of *November* a blifter was laid over the fternum, and ʒifs of oxymel ſcillitic. was given every eight hours.

On the 18th, a more copious difcharge of urine took place ; the fwelling of the feet foon difappeared, and the refpiration became gradually relieved.

On the 30th ʒi tinct. cantharidum twice a day in pyrmont water, with pills of ammoniac, fal tartar, et extract. gentian. were fubftituted, but

On the 7th of *December,* from fome fymptoms of relapfe, the oxymel was ufed as before, and continued to be taken until the 27th, in dofes as large as could be difpenfed with on account of the great naufea which attended its exhibition : The urine was made in the quantity of four or five pints each day, during the whole time ; the quantity then drank being feldom more than three pints. But now the ficknefs being exceedingly depreffing, the ftrength failing, and the diuretic effects beginning to ceafe, the following prefcription was directed.

R. Fol. Digitalis purpur. pulv. ℈fs.
    Spec. Aromatic. ℈i. fp. lav. c. f. pilul. no. x.
capiat i. nocte maneque, et alternis diebus fenfim augeatur dofin.

In three days the effect of this medicine became vifible, and when the dofe of the Digitalis had been increafed

---

pyrmont water
Mineral water, originally from Bad Pyrmont, a spa in Lower Saxony (Westphalia), particularly recommended for anaemia, debility, scrofula, and nervous disorders. It has a high iron content and is similar in composition to the water at Spa in Belgium. However, in this case Yonge may have concocted his own version, and if so may have received instruction from Withering (see note to p. 38).

no. *Numero*, in number.

alternis diebus sensium augeatur
Gradually increasing the dose on alternate days.

increafed to fix grains per day, the flow of urine generally amounted to feven pints every twenty-four hours. Not the leaft ficknefs, nor any other difagreeable fymptom fupervened, though he perfevered in this plan until the end of *January* at which time the dyfpnœa was removed, and he has continued gradually to regain his flefh, ftrength, and appetite, without any relapfe.

C A S E   II.

About the middle of the year 1784 a lady aged 48, returned from London, to her native air in Shropfhire, under fymptoms of complicated difeafe. It was your opinion that the plethoric ftate, confequent to that period, when menftruation firft begins to ceafe, had under various appearances, laid the foundation of that deplorable ftate which now prefented itfelf. The fkin was univerfally of a pale, leaden colour; her perfon much emaciated, and her ftrength fo reduced, as to difable her from walking without fupport. The appetite fluctuating, the digeftion impaired fo much, that folids paffed the inteftines with little appearance of folution : She had generally eight or ten alvine evacuations every day, and without this number, febrile fymptoms, attended with fevere vertiginous affection, and vomiting regularly enfued. The ftools were of a pale afh colour. The urine generally pale, and at firft in due quantity. The region of the ftomach had

alvine Abdominal

had a tenfe feel, without forenefs : the feet and ancles œdematous, her fleep was uncertain : the pulfe varying between 94 and 100, and feeble, except upon the approach of the menftrual periods, which were now only marked by its increafed ftrength, and exacerbation of other febrile fymptoms. Emetics, faline medicines, and gentle aperients were neceffary to alleviate thefe. Six grains of ipecac. operated with fufficient power, and half a grain of calomel would have purged with great violence.

From the time of her arrival till the middle of *Auguft*, mercury had been continued in various forms, and in dofes fuch as the irritable ftate of her ftomach and bowels would admit of. Spirit. nitri dulc. ; fal. tartar. fquill, and cantharides were alternately employed as diuretics, but without fuccefs, to retard the progrefs of an univerfal anafarca. which was then advanced to fuch degree and accompanied by fo great debility, and other dreadful concomitants, as to threaten a fpeedy and fatal cataftrophe.

Spirit. nitri dulc. Sweet spirits of nitre (see note to p. 40).

On the 16th of *Auguft* you firft faw her, and directed thus.

Mercur. cinerei Ashes of mercury, i.e. mercuric oxide, used in syphilis and as a purgative and diaphoretic.

pomeridiana A contraction of *post meridiana*, i.e. in the afternoon.

R. Mercur. cinerei gr. ii.
Fol. Digital. purpur. pulv. ǝi. f. mafs. in pill. no. xvi. dividend.—fumat unam hora meridiaana, iterumque hora quinta pomeridiana quotidie.

Capiat

Capiat lixivii faponac. gutt. L. in hauft. jufcul.
fine fale parati omni noĉte.

On the 20th the flow of urine began to increafe,
and fhe continued the medicine in the fame dofe
until the 20th of *September*, difcharging from fix to
eight pints of water each day for the firft week, and
which quantity gradually diminifhed as fhe became
empty.   During this period fhe complained not of
any ficknefs, except from the lixivium, which was
after the firft dofe reduced to 20 drops ; and her appetite and ftrength increafed daily,   though it was
evident that no bile had yet flowed into the bowels,
nor was the digeftion at all improved.   The anafarcous appearances being then removed, the Digitalis was omitted, and pills, compofed of mercur.
cinereus, aloes, and fal tartari directed twice a day,
with ʒi. of vin. chalybeat. in infuf. amar. fimpl.

Her amendment in other refpects proceeded
flowly, but regularly, from that time until the 9th
of October; when the ftate of plethora again recurring, with its ufual attendant fymptoms, ʒiv. of
blood were taken from the arm; and this was upon
the fame occafion, repeated in the following month,
with manifeft good confequences ; though in both
inftances the colour of the blood, as flowing from
the vein could hardly be called red, and the coagu-
lum was as weak in its cohefion as poffible.   The
ftate of the ftomach and bowels was by this time
greatly improved, in common with other parts of
the

lixivii saponac. A
lixivium was a solu-
tion of alkaline salts
(see notes to pp. 92
and 95). *Lixivium
saponaria*, or *potassae
liquor*, was a solution
of potassium car-
bonate.

**in haust. iuscul.
sine sale** Made into a
draught without
flavouring.

the fyftem; but no intromiffion of bile had yet
happened: the hardnefs about the hypogaftric region, though lefs, continued in a confiderable degree, and you ordered pills of mercury rubbed
down, and juft of iron, to be taken twice a day,
with a decoction of dandelion and fal fodæ.

rust of iron Ferric
oxide.

A cataplafm of linfeed was applied every night
over the ftomach and right fide; and, with little
deviation from this plan, fhe continued to the end
of the year, improving in her general health, but
the hepatic affection yet remaining. It was then
determined to try the effects of electricity, and
gentle fhocks were paffed through the body daily,
and as nearly as could be through the liver, in various directions.

**cataplasm of lin-
seed** A linseed poul-
tice prepared by
sprinkling linseed
flour into boiling
water. It was used as
an emollient.

electricity Electri-
city was thought to
increase the circula-
tion of the bood and
to increase the absor-
bent efficiency of the
lymphatics. John
Wesley (1791) said that
'[electricity] comes the
nearest an universal
medicine, of any yet
known in the world'.

On the fifth day there was reafon to think that
fome gall had been fecreted and poured out, and
this became every day more evident; but it flowed
only in fmall quantity, and irregularly into the
bowels, as appeared from the fæces being partially
tinged by it.

In *February* the lady left this neighbourhood, and
though convalefcent, yet fo nearly well as to pro-
mife us the fatisfaction of feeing her perfectly reftored.

June 29. The bile is now fecreted in pretty good
quantity, her appetite is perfectly good, her ftrength
equal to almoft any degree of exercife, and her
health

health in general better than it has been for fome years.

C A S E   III.

Mr. W——, aged —. In *June*, 1782, was affected with flight difficulty in refpiration, upon taking exercife or lying down in bed. Thefe fymptoms increafed gradually until the end of *July*, when he complained of fenfe of weight and uneafinefs about the præcordia; lofs of appetite; and coftivenefs. The urine was fmall in quantity, and high coloured; his pulfe feeble, and intermitting; he breathed with difficulty when in bed, and flept little. After the exhibition of an emetic, and an opening medicine of rhubarb, fena, and fal tartari, he was directed to take half a dram of fquill pill, pharm. Edinburg. night and morning, with ʒfs fal. fodæ in ℥ifs. infuf. amar. fimpl. twice a day; and thefe medicines were continued during ten days, without any fenfible effect. A blifter was then applied to the fternum, and fix grains of calomel given in the evening. The fymptoms were now increafed very confiderably, in every particular; and the following infufion was fubftituted for the former medicines.

R. Fol. Digital. purpur. ʒiii.
    Cort. limon. ʒii. infund.
    Aq. bullient. ℔i. per hor. 2 et cola. fumat cochl. i. primo mane et repet. omni hora.

Sometime

sena Senna (see note to p. 116).

pharm. Edinburg. As described in the sixth edition of the *Edinburgh Pharmacopoeia* (1774). Digitalis was included in the first three editions (1699, 1722, 1735) but then dropped, perhaps because of Boerhaave's pronouncements (see note to p. xiv). It was reintroduced in the seventh edition (1783) (Cowen 1957).

Cort. limon. Lemon rind, used as a stomachic and in menorrhagia.

infund. *Infunderetur*, poured on.

Sometime in the night confiderable naufea occurred, and the following day he began to make water in great quantity, which he continued to do for three or four days. The pulfe in a few hours became regular, flower, and ftronger, and, in the courfe of a week, all the fymptoms entirely vanifhed, and an electuary of cort. peruvian, fal martis, and fpec. aromatic. confirmed his cure.

In *February*, 1784, this gentleman had a relapfe of his difeafe, from which he again foon recovered by the fame r eans, and is now perfectly well.

C A S E   IV.

G—— A——, a hufbandman, aged 57. Was in the year 1782 affected with a flight, but conftant pain in his breaft, with difficult refpiration. His countenance was yellow; the abdomen fwelled, and hard; his urine high coloured, and in fmall quantity; appetite and fleep little. Complained of frequent naufea, a d of fudden profufe fweatings, which feemed for a fhort time to relieve the dyfpnœa.

After the exhibition of an emetic, fix grains of calomel were given, with a purge of jalap in the morning, and repeated in a few days, with fome appearance of advantage. He was then directed to take fome pills of fquill, foap, and rhubarb, with a draught twice a day, confifting of infuf. amar. fimp. and fal tartari. The fkin foon became clearer and the

electuary A paste consisting of the powdered drug mixed with honey, jam, or syrup. In the case of Peruvian bark, however, gum-arabic would have been used instead of syrup, since it masked the taste of the bark more efficiently.

cort. peruvian Peruvian bark (see note to p. 57).

the pain in his breaſt conſiderably diminiſhed. But every other circumſtance remaining the ſame, and a fluctuation in the belly being now more evident, the infuſion of Digitalis as prefcribed in caſe third, was given in the doſe of one ounce twice a day.

On the 5th day the effects were apparent, and he continued his medicine for a fortnight without nauſea, making four or five pints of water every night, but little in the day, and gradually loſing the ſymptoms of his diſeaſe.

In 1784, this perſon had a relapſe, and was again cured by ſimilar treatment.

C A S E   V.

R—— H——, Aged 43. Towards the end of the year 1783, became affected with ſlight cough and expectoration of purulent matter. In December his ſkin became univerſally of a pale yellow colour. The abdomen was ſwelled and hard ; his appetite little, and he complained of a violent and conſtant palpitation of the heart, which prevented him from ſleeping. The urine pale, and in ſmall quantity. The pulſe exceedingly ſtrong, and rebounding ; beating 114 to 120 ſtrokes every minute. He ſuffered violent pain of his head, and was very feeble and emaciated. After bleeding, and the uſe of gentle aperient medicines, he continued to take the infuſion of Digitalis for ſome days, without any ſenſible effect. Other diuretics were tried to as little purpoſe

violent and constant palpitation of the heart . . . pulse exceedingly strong, and rebounding This description sounds like the 'collapsing' or 'water-hammer' type of pulse first described by Dominic John Corrigan (Corrigan 1832) and hence also known as Corrigan's pulse. It signified aortic regurgitation. As Corrigan reported in his paper, digitalis is not of great value in the treatment of heart failure due to aortic regurgitation. Indeed, Corrigan reported that 'in all, the patients while under its exhibition were always worse'.

pofe. Repeated bleeding had no effect in diminifhing the violent action of the heart. He died in
January following, under complicated fymptoms of
phthifis and afcites.

C A S E   VI.

A man aged 57, who had lived freely in the fummer of 1784, became affected with œdematous
fwelling of his legs, for which he was advifed to
drink Fox Glove Tea. He took a four ounce bafon
of the infufion made ftrong with the green leaves,
every morning for four fucceffive days.

On the 5th he was fuddenly feized with faintnefs
and cold fweatings. I found him with a pale countenance, complaining of weaknefs, and of pain,
with a fenfe of great heat in his ftomach and
bowels. The fwelling of the legs was entirely gone,
he having evacuated urine in very large quantities
for the two preceding days. He was affected with
frequent diarrhœa. The pulfe was very quick and
fmall, and his extremities cold.

A fmall quantity of broth was directed to be given
him every half hour, and blifters were applied
to the ancles, by which his fymptoms became gradually alleviated, and he recovered perfectly in the
fpace of three weeks; except a relapfe of the anafarca, for which the Digitalis was afterwards fuccefsfully employed, in fmall dofes, without any difagreeable confequence.

C A S E

C A S E   VII.

S—— D——, a middle aged fingle woman, was affected in the year eighty-one, with a painful rigidity and flight inflammation of the integuments on the left fide, extending from the ear to the fhoulder. In every other particular fhe was healthy. The ufe of warm fomentations, and opium, with two or three dofes of mercurial phyfic, afforded her eafe and the inflammation difappeared, but was fucceeded by an œdematous fwelling of the part, which very gradually extended along the arm, and downward to the breaft, back, and belly. Friction, electricity and mercurial ointment were amongft the number of applications unfuccefsfully employed to relieve her for the fpace of three months, during which time fhe continued in good general health.

In *November* fhe became afcitic, paffing fmall quantities of urine, and foon afterwards a fudden dyfpnœa gave occafion to fuppofe an effufion of water in the thorax. The Digitalis, fquills, and cantharides were given in very confiderable dofes without effect. She died the latter end of December following.

C A S E   VIII.

W—— C——, a collier aged 58, was attacked in the fpring of 1783 with a tertian ague, which he attributed to cold, by fleeping in a coal

M   pit,

pit, and from which he recovered in a few days, except a fwelling of the lower extremities, which had appeared about that time, and gradually increafed for two or three months. The legs and thighs were greatly enlarged and œdematóus. His belly was fwelled, but no fluctuation perceptible. He made fmall quantities of high coloured water. The appetite bad, and pulfe feeble. He had taken many medicines without relief, and was now fo reduced in ftrength, as to fit up with difficulty. An infufion of the Digitalis was directed for him, in the proportion of one ounce of the frefh leaves to a pint of water, two ounces to be taken three times a day, until the ftomach or bowels became affected. Upon the exhibition of the fixth dofe, naufea fupervened, and continued to opprefs him at intervals for two or three days, during which he paffed large quantities of pale urine. The fwelling, affifted by moderate bandage rapidly diminifhed, and without any repetition of his medicine, at the expiration of fixteen days, he returned to his labour perfectly recovered.

OF THE

PREPARATIONS and DOSES,

OF THE

FOXGLOVE.

EVERY part of the plant has more or lefs of the fame bitter tafte, varying, however, as to ftrength, and changing with the age of the plant and the feafon of the year.

ROOT.—This varies greatly with the age of the plant. When the ftem has fhot up for flowering, which it does the fecond year of its growth, the root becomes dry, nearly taftelefs, and inert.

Some practitioners, who have ufed the root, and been fo happy as to cure their patients without exciting ficknefs, have been pleafed to communicate the circumftance to me as an improvement in the ufe of the plant. I have no doubt of the truth of their remarks, and I thank them. But the cafe of Dr. Cawley puts this matter beyond difpute. The fact is, they have fortunately happened to ufe the root in its approach to its inert ftate, and confequently have not over dofed their patients. I could,

Every part of the plant ... etc. See footnotes to pp. 4 and 111 on the varying amounts of digitalis glycosides to be found in different parts of the plant at different times of the year.

if

if neceffary, bring other proof to fhew that the root is juft as capable as the leaves, of exciting naufea.

STEM.—The ftem has more tafte than the root has, in the feafon the ftem fhoots out, and lefs tafte than the leaves. I do not know that it has been particularly felected for ufe.

LEAVES. — Thefe vary greatly in their efficacy at different feafons of the year, and, perhaps, at different ftages of their growth; but I am not certain that this variation keeps pace with the greater or leffer intenfity of their bitter tafte.

habituated That is, to taking repeated, intermittent courses of foxglove. Constant dosing at the doses used by Withering would have led inevitably to toxicity (see footnote to p. 6).

They have used the leaves in such large proportion This really cannot be the explanation, because of the narrow margin between the therapeutic efficacy of digitalis and its toxic effects. A likelier explanation is that the *total* dose used during a course of treatment would have been varied from season to season, since the patients would have continued taking the drug until it had some effect. During the sea-

Some who have been habituated to the ufe of the recent leaves, tell me, that they anfwer their purpofe at every feafon of the year; and I believe them, notwithftanding I myfelf have found very great variations in this refpect. The folution of this difficulty is obvious. They have ufed the leaves in fuch large proportion, that the dofes have been fufficient, or more than fufficient, even in their moft inefficacious ftate. *The Leaf-ftalks* feem, in their fenfible properties, to partake of an intermediate ftate between the leaves and the ftem.

FLOWERS.—The petals, the chives, and the pointal have nearly the tafte of the leaves, and it has been fuggefted to me, by a very fenfible and judicious friend, that it might be well to fix on the flower for internal ufe. I fee no objection to the propofition; but I have not tried it.

SEEDS.

SEEDS.—Thefe I believe are equally untried.

From this view of the different parts of the plant, it is fufficiently obvious why I ftill continue to prefer the leaves.

Thefe fhould be gathered after the flowering ftem has fhot up, and about the time that the bloffoms are coming forth.

The leaf-ftalk and mid-rib of the leaves fhould be rejected, and the remaining part fhould be dried, either in the fun-fhine, or on a tin pan or pewter difh before a fire.

If well dried, they readily rub down to a beautiful green powder, which weighs fomething lefs than one-fifth of the original weight of the leaves. Care muft be taken that the leaves be not fcorched in drying, and they fhould not be dried more than what is requifite to allow of their being readily reduced to powder.

I give to adults, from one to three grains of this powder twice a day. In the reduced ftate in which phyficians generally find dropfical patients, four grains a day are fufficient. I fometimes give the powder alone ; fometimes unite it with aromatics, and fometimes form it into pills with a fufficient quantity of foap or gum ammoniac.

M 3

If

---

sons when the active content of the leaves was low they would simply have gone on taking them for longer. Because the amount of digitoxin in the body continues to accumulate for up to four or five weeks of regular dosing, a therapeutic or toxic effect would almost inevitably have occurred.

one-fifth of the original weight Withering used this observation in his remarks on the case reported to him by Mr Jones (see p. 137). Withering's comments, on this and the following page, on suitable doses, comparing powdered leaf with infusion, puzzled John Blackall when he later came to use digitalis in the treatment of dropsies, and he commented on them in his book *Observations on the nature and cure of dropsies . . .* (Blackall 1813). However, the differences can be explained on the basis of incomplete extraction of the active principles of the leaves into the aqueous infusion Withering prepared.

If a liquid medicine be preferred, I order a dram of these dried leaves to be infused for four hours in half a pint of boiling water, adding to the strained liquor an ounce of any spirituous water. One ounce of this infusion given twice a day, is a medium dose for an adult patient. If the patient be stronger than usual, or the symptoms very urgent, this dose may be given once in eight hours ; and on the contrary in many instances half an ounce at a time will be quite sufficient. About thirty grains of the powder or eight ounces of the infusion, may generally be taken before the nausea commences.

The ingenuity of man has ever been fond of exerting itself to vary the forms and combinations of medicines. Hence we have spirituous, vinous, and acetous tinctures ; extracts hard and soft, syrups with sugar or honey, &c. but the more we multiply the forms of any medicine, the longer we shall be in ascertaining its real dose. I have no lasting objection however to any of these formulæ except the extract, which, from the nature of its preparation must ever be uncertain in its effects ; and a medicine whose fullest dose in substance does not exceed three grains, cannot be supposed to stand in need of condensation.

It appears from several of the cases, that when the Digitalis is disposed to purge, opium may be joined with it advantageously; and when the bowels are too tardy, jalap may be given at the same time, without

---

One ounce of this infusion Digitalis glycosides are less soluble in water than in organic solvents such as alcohol, and that accounts for the difference between the doses of powdered leaf and the doses of an infusion of the powdered leaf. Here Withering infuses about 60 grains of leaf in about 10 ounces of water, replacing what little would have been lost by evaporation with wine or another alcoholic beverage. If his doses were strictly comparable he would have ended up with a solution containing about 40 grains (i.e. about 66% recovery) in about 10 ounces of water.

extracts hard and soft Extracts were prepared by macerating a vegetable substance in water, alcohol, or ether, and then evaporating to dryness. The hardness or softness of the extract would have depended on the degree to which fluid was removed by evaporation.

without interfering with its diuretic effects ; but I have not found benefit from any other adjunct.

From this view of the dofes in which the Digitalis really ought to be exhibited, and from the evidence of many of the cafes, in which it appears to have been given in quantities fix, eight, ten or even twelve times more than neceffary, we muft admit as an inference either that this medicine is perfectly fafe when given as I advife, or that the medicines in daily ufe are highly dangerous.

the more we multiply the forms of any medicine There is no doubt that different oral formulations of the same drug may have different effects by virtue of different characteristics (of either rate or extent) of absorption of the drug from the gastrointestinal tract. For example, digoxin is absorbed about 67 per cent from a tablet, 80 per cent from an elixir, and 95 per cent from a formulation of elixir encapsulated in a gelatin capsule.

condensation Concentration.

opium may be joined with it advantageously See note to p. 5.

EFFECTS,

EFFECTS, RULES, and CAUTIONS.

THE Foxglove when given in very large and quick-ly-repeated doſes, occaſions ſickneſs, vomiting, purging, giddineſs, confuſed viſion, objects appear-ing green or yellow ; increaſed ſecretion of urine, with frequent motions to part with it, and ſometimes inability to retain it ; ſlow pulſe, even as ſlow as 35 in a minute, cold ſweats, convulſions, ſyncope, death.*

When given in a leſs violent manner, it pro-duces moſt of theſe effects in a lower degree ; and it is curious to obſerve, that the ſickneſs, with a cer-tain doſe of the medicine, does not take place for ma-ny hours after its exhibition has been diſcontinued ; that the flow of urine will often precede, ſometimes accompany, frequently follow the ſickneſs at the diſtance of ſome days, and not unfrequently be checked by it. The ſickneſs thus excited, is ex-tremely different from that occaſioned by any other medicine ; it is peculiarly diſtreſſing to the patient ; it ceaſes, it recurs again as violent as before ; and thus it will continue to recur for three or four days, at diſtant and more diſtant intervals.

Theſe

* I am doubtful whether it does not ſometimes excite a copious flow of ſaliva.—See caſes at pages 115, 154, and 155.

THE Foxglove ... In this paragraph Withering details almost all of the known non-cardiac toxic effects of digitalis. Notable for its absence is anorexia (but see note to next page). His description of the abnormalities of colour vision that can occur in severe intoxication is incomplete, however, since (albeit rarely) patients may complain of seeing objects in other colours, e.g. blue, red, brown, black, and even white. In patients with mild or moderate toxicity, even without symptoms, defects of colour vision can be detected by the use of sensitive tests (Aronson and Ford 1980).

slow pulse Withering is here describing not merely a slowing of the pulse (sinus bradycardia) but complete heart block, which is typically associated with a pulse rate of around 35 per minute.

a copious flow of saliva There is no modern evidence that this is a toxic effect of digitalis, but it was reported as such by others in Withering's time. It may simply have been the excessive salivation which normally accompanies vomiting.

Thefe fufferings of the patient are generally re-
warded by a return of appetite, much greater than
what exifted before the taking of the medicine.

But thefe fufferings are not at all neceffary ;
they are the effects of our inexperience, and would
in fimilar circumftances, more or lefs attend the exhibition of almoft every active and powerful medicine we ufe.

return of appetite
Loss of appetite is a
symptom of both car-
diac failure and digi-
talis toxicity, and
would therefore not
have been remarked
upon as a specific
effect of the latter.
The return of appetite
would have been due
to the relief of the
dropsy.

Perhaps the reader will better underftand how it
ought to be given, from the following detail of my
own improvement, than from precepts peremptori-
ly delivered, and their fource veiled in obfcurity.

At firft I thought it neceffary *to bring on and
continue the ficknefs, in order to enfure the diuretic
effects.*

**At first I thought it
necessary** What
Withering is describ-
ing in the succeeding
paragraphs is the loss
of therapeutic effect of
digitalis which can
occur if toxicity
supervenes.

I foon learnt that the naufea being once excited,
it was unneceffary to repeat the medicine, as it was
certain to recur frequently, at intervals more or lefs
diftant.

Therefore my patients were ordered *to perfift
until the naufea came on, and then to ftop.* But it
foon appeared that the diuretic effects would often
take place firft, and fometimes be checked when the
ficknefs or a purging fupervened.

The

The direction was therefore enlarged thus—*Continue the medicine until the urine flows, or sickness or purging take place.*

I found myself safe under this regulation for two or three years ; but at length cases occurred in which the pulse would be retarded to an alarming degree, without any other preceding effect.

but at length cases occurred It is known (Church *et al*. 1962) that the manifestations of digitalis toxicity differ not only from patient to patient, but also in the same patient at different times, and in the same patient in response to different glycosides.

The directions therefore required an additional attention to the state of the pulse, and it was moreover of consequence not to repeat the doses too quickly, but to allow sufficient time for the effects of each to take place, as it was found very possible to pour in an injurious quantity of the medicine, before any of the signals for forbearance appeared.

Let the medicine therefore be given in the doses, and at the intervals mentioned above:—let it be continued until it either acts on the kidneys, the stomach, the pulse, or the bowels; let it be stopped upon the first appearance of any one of these effects, and I will maintain that the patient will not suffer from its exhibition, nor the practitioner be disappointed in any reasonable expectation.

If it purges, it seldom succeeds well.

enjoined to drink very freely To avoid dehydration due to excessive diuresis (see Case XXI, p. 26).

The patients should be enjoined to drink very freely during its operation. I mean, they should drink whatever they prefer, and in as great quantity

tity as their appetite for drink demands.   This direction is the more neceſſary, as they are very generally prepoſſeſſed with an idea of drying up a dropſy, by abſtinence from liquids, and fear to add to the diſeaſe, by indulging their inclination to drink.

In caſes of aſcites and anaſarca ; when the patients are weak, and the evacuation of the water rapid ; the uſe of proper bandage is indiſpenſably neceſſary to their ſafety.

the use of proper bandage See note to p. 203.

If the water ſhould not be wholly evacuated, it is beſt to allow an interval of ſeveral days before the medicine be repeated, that food and tonics may be adminiſtered ; but truth compels me to ſay, that the uſual tonic medicines have in theſe caſes very often deceived my expectations.

From ſome caſes which have occurred in the courſe of the preſent year, I am diſpoſed to believe that the Digitalis may be given in ſmall doſes, viz. two or three grains a day, ſo as gradually to remove a dropſy, without any other than mild diuretic effects, and without any interruption to its uſe until the cure be compleated.

a remedy to counteract its effects would be a desirable thing Such a remedy has recently become available. If digoxin is chemically conjugated to bovine albumin, and the conjugate injected into sheep or rabbits, they form in their blood antibodies to the digoxin. Specific fragments of these antibodies, if injected into man, can displace digoxin (and other cardiac glycosides) from their binding sites in the tissues and thus rapidly reverse digitalis toxicity (Smith *et al*. 1983).

If inadvertently the doſes of the Foxglove ſhould be preſcribed too largely, exhibited too rapidly, or urged to too great a length ; the knowledge of a remedy to counteract its effects would be a deſirable thing.

thing. Such a remedy may perhaps in time be
difcovered. The ufual cordials and volatiles are
generally rejected from the ftomach ; aromatics and
ftrong bitters are longer retained; brandy will fometimes remove the ficknefs when only flight ; I have
fometimes thought fmall dofes of opium ufeful, but I
am more confident of the advantage from blifters.
Mr. Jones *(Page* 135) in one cafe, found mint tea to
be retained longer than other things.

CON-

CONSTITUTION of PATIENTS.

INDEPENDENT of the degree of difeafe, or of the ftrength or age of the patient, I have had occafion to remark, that there are certain conftitutions favourable, and others unfavourable to the fuccefs of the Digitalis.

From large experience, and attentive obfervation, I am pretty well enabled to decide *a priori* upon this matter, and I wifh to enable others to do the fame: but I feel myfelf hardly equal to the undertaking. The following hints, however, aiding a degree of experience in others, may lead them to accomplifh what I yet can defcribe but imperfectly.

It feldom fucceeds in men of great natural ftrength, of tenfe fibre, of warm fkin, of florid complexion, or in thofe with a tight and cordy pulfe.

If the belly in afcites be tenfe, hard, and circumfcribed, or the limbs in anafarca folid and refifting, we have but little to hope.

On the contrary, if the pulfe be feeble or intermitting, the countenance pale, the lips livid, the fkin cold, the fwollen belly foft and fluctuating, or the

It seldom succeeds This suggestion was later contradicted by William Hamilton in his monograph on the foxglove (Hamilton 1807), thus: 'Of my patients, several were men of very rigid fibre, and great natural body strength; yet the foxglove produced effects upon these equal to what could be expected from it in more enervated habits.'

tense fibre This refers to the tone of the muscles. 'The state of the [muscle] fibres is indicative of various deviations from a healthy standard. When there is a *lax* fibre, debility is supposed to prevail; and, on the opposite extreme of too great *rigidity*, the body is obnoxious to other maladies from the cause.' (*Edinburgh Medical and Physical Dictionary* 1807). Among Withering's patients of 'tense fibre' were those described as Cases LV, LXXVII, and CXVII.

If the belly in ascites be tense ... the limbs in anasarca solid That is, in advanced cases of dropsy, or perhaps in cases of ascites and anasarca not due to cardiac failure.

On the contrary Descriptions of cases associated with atrial fibrillation, or less severe dropsy.

the anafarcous limbs readily pitting under the preffure of the finger, we may expect the diuretic effects to follow in a kindly manner.

In cafes which foil every attempt at relief, I have
been aiming, for fome time paft, to make fuch a
change in the conftitution of the patient, as might
give a chance of fuccefs to the Digitalis.

blood-letting
Which would have
removed some of the
circulating blood
volume, relieving the
pressure on the heart
and leading to
improvement in some
cases.

squills See note to p. 3.

**lowers the tone of
the system** For at
least a century after
Withering it was
thought that digitalis
would be more effec-
tive if the tone of the
vasculature was first
reduced. Hence the
advice to let blood.

By blood-letting, by neutral falts, by chryftals
of tartar, fquills, and occafional purging, I have
fucceeded, though imperfectly. Next to the ufe
of the lancet, I think nothing lowers the tone of
the fyftem more effectually than the fquill, and confequently it will always be proper, in fuch cafes, to
ufe the fquill; for if that fail in its defired effect, it
is one of the beft preparatives to the adoption of the
Digitalis.

A tendency to paralytic affections, or a ftroke of
the palfy having actually taken place, is no objection to the ufe of the Digitalis; neither does a
ftone exifting in the bladder forbid its ufe. Theoretical ideas of fedative effects in the former, and
apprehenfions of its excitement of the urinary organs in the latter cafe, might operate fo as to
make us with-hold relief from the patient; but experience tells me, that fuch apprehenfions are
groundlefs.

INFER-

INFERENCES.

INFERENCES
Apart perhaps from
inference numbers
VII and VIII one can-
not fault Withering
on his observations, in
the context of the
knowledge of his time.

TO prevent any improper influence, which the above recitals of the efficacy of the medicine, aided by the novelty of the fubject, may have upon the minds of the younger part of my readers, in raifing their expectations to too high a pitch, I beg leave to deduce a few inferences, which I apprehend the facts will fairly fupport.

I. That the Digitalis will not univerfally act as a diuretic.

II. That it does do fo more generally than any other medicine.

III. That it will often produce this effect after every other probable method has been fruitlefsly tried.

IV. That if this fails, there is but little chance of any other medicine fucceeding.

V. That in proper dofes, and under the management now pointed out, it is mild in its operation, and gives lefs difturbance to the fyftem, than fquill, or almoft any other active medicine.

VI. That when dropfy is attended by palfy, unfound vifcera, great debility, or other complication of difeafe, neither the Digitalis, nor any other diuretic

the cure of diseases, unconnected with dropsy It is true that digitalis is useful in atrial fibrillation (a condition not recognized by Withering as such), and he may be referring here to the weak, fast, irregular pulse of that condition in patients without dropsy. However, it is more likely that he is referring to other conditions unassociated with the heart, such as hydrocephalus. It is also of interest that his son notes at the end of his collection of his father's miscellaneous tracts (Withering 1822) that 'By the application of *Fol. Digital. Recent.* (fresh Foxglove leaves) renewed night and morning, Dr. Withering was in the habit of removing *Bronchocele.*'

That it has a power over the motion of the heart Withering mentions the heart twice elsewhere in the *Account* (see footnotes to pp. 26 and 81), and on the second occasion he mentions it we can see that he reasoned that it must affect the heart because it affected the pulse. He may also have reasoned from its effects in relieving symptoms of palpitation in some patients.

retic can do more than obtain a truce to the urgency of the fymptoms; unlefs by gaining time, it may afford opportunity for other medicines to combat and fubdue the original difeafe.

VII. That the Digitalis may be ufed with advantage in every fpecies of dropfy, except the encyfted.

VIII. That it may be made fubfervient to the cure of difeafes, unconnected with dropfy.

IX. That it has a power over the motion of the heart, to a degree yet unobferved in any other medicine, and that this power may be converted to falutary ends.

PRACTICAL

P R A C T I C A L

REMARKS ON DROPSY,

AND SOME OTHER DISEASES.

SOME OTHER DISEASES See Table 4.2, p. 000.

T H E following remarks confift partly of matter of fact, and partly of opinion. The former will be permanent; the latter muft vary with the detection of error, or the improvement of knowledge. I hazard them with diffidence, and hope they will be examined with candour; not by a contraft with other opinions, but by an attentive comparifon with the phœnomena of difeafe.

A N A S A R C A.

§ 1. THE anafarca is generally curable when feated in the fub-cutaneous cellular membrane, or in the fubftance of the lungs.

cellular membrane See note to p. 142.

§ 2. When the abdominal vifcera in general are greatly enlarged, which they fometimes are, without effufed fluid in the cavity of the abdomen; the difeafe is incurable. After death, the more folid vifcera are found very large and pale. If the cavity contains water, that water may be removed by diuretics.

N   § 3. In

resistance to pressure is considerable That is, in very severe cases of cardiac failure, or in non-cardiac swelling, due, for example, to lymphatic obstruction.

alteration of posture In mild cases of peripheral oedema the fluid may drain into the circulation if the legs are raised. Thus some patients will comment that their ankle swelling is absent first thing in the morning and worsens as the day progresses.

spissitude Thickness or denseness.

§ 3. In fwollen legs and thighs, where the refiftance to preffure is confiderable, the tendency to tranfparency in the fkin not obvious, and where the alteration of pofture occafions but little alteration in the ftate of diftenfion, the cure cannot be effected by diuretics.

Is this difficulty of cure occafioned by fpiffitude in the effufed fluids, by want of proper communication from cell to cell, or is the difeafe rather caufed by a morbid growth of the folids, than by an accumulation of fluid?

Is not this difeafe in the limbs fimilar to that of the vifcera (§ 2)?

§ 4. Anafarcous fwellings often take place in palfied limbs, in arms as well as legs; fo that the fwelling does not depend merely upon pofition.

is it not probable ...? Not in lymphatic oedema.

§ 5. Is there not caufe to fufpect that many dropfies originate from paralytic affections of the lymphatic aoforbents? And if fo, is it not probable that the Digitalis, which is fo effectual in removing dropfy, may alfo be ufed advantageoufly in fome kinds of palfy?

A S C I T E S,

§ 6. IF exifting alone, (i. e.) without accompanying anafarca, is in children curable; in adults generally incurable by medicines. Tapping may be ufed uſed here with better chance for ſucceſs than in more complicated dropſies. Sometimes cured by vomiting.

ASCITES and ANASARCA.

§ 7. I N C U R A B L E if dependant upon irremediably diſeaſed viſcera, or on a gouty conſtitution, ſo debilitated, that the gouty paroxyſms no longer continue to be formed.

In every other ſituation the diſeaſe yields to diuretics and tonics.

A S C I T E S, A N A S A R C A, and H Y D R O T H O R A X.

§ 8. U N D E R this complication, though the ſymptoms admit of relief, the reſtoration of the conſtitution can hardly be hoped for.

A S T H M A.

§ 9. T H E true ſpaſmodic aſthma, a rare diſeaſe —is not relieved by Digitalis.

§ 10. In the greater part of what are called aſthmatical caſes, the real diſeaſe is anaſarca of the lungs, and is generally to be cured by diuretics. (See § 1.) This is almoſt always combined with ſome ſwelling of the legs.

N 2   § 11. There

Sometimes cured by vomiting For example, the puzzling Case XXVII.

that the gouty paroxysms no longer continue to be formed Withering here refers to the fact that in its chronic (so-called 'burnt-out') state gout does not cause acute attacks of inflammation in the joints and tissues. See also note to p. 96.

THE true spasmodic asthma Withering here distinguishes *cardiac* asthma, which is due to left ventricular failure, from *bronchial* asthma, which is nowadays quite common and which is not, as he rightly says, relieved by digitalis.

combined with some swelling of the legs Pure left ventricular failure does not cause peripheral oedema. Withering is describing combined left and right heart failure.

§ 11. There is another kind of afthma, in which change of pofture does not much affect the patient. I believe it to be caufed by an infarction of the lungs. It is incurable by diuretics; but it is often accompanied with a degree of anafarca, and fo far it admits of relief.

Is not this difeafe fimilar to that in the limbs at (§ 3,) and alfo to that of the abdominal vifcera at (§ 2.)?

infarction of the lungs Pulmonary embolism (usually from a blood clot in the deep veins of the legs), which can result in acute shortness of breath, sometimes with haemoptysis, and acute heart failure. A single mild attack would resolve spontaneously. Repeated attacks of pulmonary embolism can cause chronic heart failure.

ASTHMA and ANASARCA.

§ 12. IF the afthma be of the kind mentioned at (§§ 9 and 11,) diuretics can only remove the accompanying anafarca. But if the affection of the breath depends alfo upon cellular effufion, as it moftly does, the patient may be taught to expect a recovery.

ASTHMA and ASCITES.

§ 13. A RARE combination, but not incurable if the the abdominal vifcera are found. The afthma is here moft probably of the anafarcous kind (§ 10;) and this being feldom confined to the lungs only, the difeafe generally appears in the following form.

ASTHMA,

ASTHMA, ASCITES, and ANASARCA.

§ 14. T H E curability of this combination will depend upon the circumſtances mentioned in the preceding ſection, taking alſo into the account the ſtrength or weakneſs of the patient.

E P I L E P S Y.

§ 15. I N epilepſy dependant upon effuſion, the Digitalis will effect a cure; and in the caſes alluded to, the dropſical ſymptoms were unequivocal. It has not had a ſufficient trial in my hands, to determine what it can do in other kinds of epilepſy,

H Y D A T I D   D R O P S Y.

§ 16. T H I S may be diſtinguiſhed from common aſcites, by the want of evident fluctuation. It is common to both ſexes. It does not admit of a cure either by tapping or by medicine.

H Y D R O C E P H A L U S.

§ 17. T H I S diſeaſe, which has of late ſo much attracted the attention of the medical world, I believe, originates in inflammation; and that the water found in the ventricles of the brain after death, is the conſequence, and not the cauſe of the illneſs.

It has ſeldom happened to me to be called upon in the earlier ſtages of this complaint, and the ſymp-

N 3   toms

epilepsy dependant upon effusion This is probably epilepsy due to hyponatraemia (i.e. a low concentration of sodium in the blood) secondary to severe cardiac failure. Digitalis is not effective in epilepsy.

HYDATID DROPSY An encysted mass due to infection with the *Echinococcus* tapeworms. It does not respond to digitalis.

HYDROCE-PHALUS See notes to pp. 36 and 97.

dentition The
cutting of the teeth.

toms are at firſt ſo ſimilar to thoſe uſually attendant upon dentition and worms, that it is very difficult to pronounce decidedly upon the real nature of the diſeaſe; and it is rather from the failure of the uſual modes of relief, than from any other more decided obſervation, that we at length dare to give it a name.

At firſt, the febrile ſymptoms are ſometimes ſo unſteady, that I have known them miſtaken for the ſymptoms of an intermittent, and the cure attempted by the bark.

In the more advanced ſtages, the diagnoſtics obtrude themſelves upon our notice, and put the ſituation of the patient beyond a doubt. But this does not always happen. The variations of the pulſe, ſo accurately deſcribed by the late Dr. Whytt, do not always enſue. The dilatation of the pupils, the ſquinting, and the averſion to light, do not univerſally exiſt. The ſcreaming upon raiſing the head from the pillow or the lap, and the fluſhing of the cheeks, I once conſidered as affording indubitable marks of the diſeaſe; but in a child which I ſometime ſince attended with Dr. Aſh, the pulſe was uniformly about 85, (except during the firſt week, before we had the care of the patient.) The child never ſhewed any averſion to the light; never had dilated pupils, never ſquinted, never ſcreamed when raiſed from the lap or taken out of the bed, nor did we obſerve any remarkable fluſhing of the cheeks; and the ſleep was quiet, but ſometimes moaning.

Dr. Whytt Robert
Whytt (1714-66).
President of the Royal
College of Physicians
of Edinburgh. His
book *Observations on
the Dropsy in the Brain*
was published in 1768.

Frequent

Frequent vomiting exifted from the firft, but ceafed for feveral days towards the conclufion. One or two worms came away during the illnefs, and it was all along difficult to purge the child. Three days before death, the right fide became flightly paralytic, and the pupil of that eye fomewhat dilated.

After death, about two ounces and a half of water were found in the ventricles of the brain, and the veffels of the dura mater were turgid with blood.

If I am right as to the nature of hydrocephalus, that it is at firft dependant upon inflammation, or congeftion; and that the water in the ventricles is a confequence, and not a caufe of the difeafe; the curative intentions ought to be extremely different in the firft and the laft ftages.

It happens very rarely that I am called to patients at the beginning, but in two inftances wherein I was called at firft, the patients were cured by repeated topical bleedings, vomits, and purges.

Some years ago I mentioned thefe opinions, and the fuccefs of the practice refulting from them, to Dr. Quin, now phyfician at Dublin. That gentleman had lately taken his degree, and had chofen hydrocephalus for the fubject of his thefis in the year 1779. In this very ingenious effay, which he gave me the fame morning, I was much pleafed to find that the author had not only held the fame ideas

two ounces and a half of water See note to p. 97.

Dr. Quin Charles William Quin (born *c*. 1755). Studied first at Trinity College Dublin, then at Edinburgh, graduating MD in 1779 with the dissertation *De Hydrocephalo Interno*. Quin first heard of the use of the foxglove when Stokes lectured at Edinburgh in 1779 (see p. xx), but did not use it systematically until after Withering's *Account* was published. Quin's book *A treatise on the dropsy of the brain . . . [and] on the use and effect of Digitalis purpurea in dropsies* was published in 1790 (see also p. 308).

ideas relative to the nature of the difeafe, but had alfo confirmed them by diffeions.

In the year 1781, another cafe in the firft ftage demanded my attention. The reader is referred back to Cafe LXIX for the particulars.

I have not yet been able to determine whether the Digitalis can or cannot be ufed with advantage in the fecond ftage of the hydrocephalus. In Cafe XXXIII. the fymptoms of death were at hand; in Cafe LXIX. the practice, though fuccefsful, was too complicated, and in Cafe CLI. the medicine was certainly ftopped too foon.

When we confider what enormous quantities of mercury may be ufed in this complaint, without af-feting the falivary glands, it feems probable that other parts may be equally infenfible to the action of their peculiar ftimuli, and therefore that the Di-gitalis ought to be given in much larger dofes in this, than in other difeafes.

ought to be given in much larger doses Withering is right in principle, although in practice doses large enough to be effective would have caused severe toxicity (see note to p. 36).

HYDROTHORAX.

§ 18. UNDER this name I alfo include the dropfy of the pericardium.

The intermitting pulfe, and pain in the arms, fuf-ficiently diftinguifh this difeafe from afthma, and and from anafarcous lungs.

It is very univerfally cured by the Digitalis.

§ 19. I lately

§ 19. I lately met with two cafes which had been confidered and treated as angina pectoris. They both appeared to me to be cafes of hydrothorax. One fubject was a clergyman, whofe ftrength had been fo compleatly exhaufted by the continuance of the difeafe, and the attempts to relieve it, that he did not furvive many days. The other was a lady, whofe time of life made me fufpect effufion. I directed her to take fmall dofes of the pulv. Digitalis, which in eight days removed all her complaints.' This happened fix months ago, and fhe remains perfectly well,

HYDROTHORAX and ANASARCA.

§ 20. THIS combination is very frequent, and, I believe, may always be cured by the Digitalis.

§ 21. Dropfies in the cheft either with or without anafarcous limbs, are much more curable than thofe of the belly. Probably becaufe the abdominal vifcera are more frequently difeafed in the latter than in the former cafes.

I N S A N I T Y.

§ 22. I APPREHEND this difeafe to be more frequently connected with ferous effufion than has been commonly imagined.

§ 23. Where appearances of anafarca point out the true caufe of the complaint, as in cafes XXIV, and XXXIV.

INSANITY It may be that Withering's success (and that of others, e.g. Jones 1787) in treating cases of insanity with digitalis was due to correction of hyponatraemia due to severe cardiac failure, perhaps in conjunction with over-enthusiastic diuretic treatment (e.g. with mercurials).

XXXIV. the happieſt effects may be expected from the Digitalis ; and men of more experience than myſelf in cafes of infanity, will probably employ it fuccefsfully in other lefs obvious circumſtances.

NEPHRITIS CALCULOSA.

§ 24. WE have had fufficient evidence of the efficacy of the Foxglove in removing the Dyfuria and other fymptoms of this difeafe ; but probably it is not in thefe cafes preferable to the tobacco.*

OVARIUM DROPSY.

§ 25. THIS fpecies of encyfted dropfy is not without difficulty diſtinguiſhable from an afcites ; and yet it is neceffary to diſtinguiſh them, becaufe the two difeafes require different treatment and becaufe the probality of a cure is much greater in one than in the other.

§ 26. The ovarium dropfy is generally flow in its progrefs ; for a confiderable time the patient though fomewhat emaciated, does not lofe the appearance of health, and the urine flows in the ufual quantity. It is feldom that the practitioner is called in early enough to diſtinguiſh by the feel on which fide the cyft originated, and the patients do not attend to that circumſtance themfelves. They generally menſtruate

Dr. Fowler The same as at p. 121. His *Medical reports, of the effects of tobacco in the cure of dropsies and dysuries* ... was published in 1785.

* See an original and valuable treatife by Dr. Fowler, entitled, *Medical Reports of the Effects of Tobacco.*

ftruate regularly in the incipient ftate of the difeafe, and it is not until the preffure from the fac becomes very great, that the urinary fecretion diminifhes. In this fpecies of dropfy, the patients, upon being queftioned, acknowledge even from a pretty early date, pains in the upper and inner parts of the thighs, fimilar to thofe which women experience in a ftate of pregnancy. Thefe pains are for a length of time greater in one thigh than in the other, and I believe it will be found that the difeafe originated on that fide.

§ 27. The ovarium dropfy defies the power of medicine. It admits of relief, and fometimes of a cure, by tapping. I fubmit to the confideration of practitioners, how far we may hope to cure this difeafe by a feton or a cauftic. —— In the LXIft cafe the patient was too much reduced, and the difeafe too far advanced to allow of a cure by any method; but it teaches us that a cauftic may be ufed with fafety.

§ 28. When tapping becomes neceffary, I always advife the adoption of the waiftcoat bandage or belt, invented by the late very juftly celebrated Dr. Monro, and defcribed in the firft volume of the Medical Effays. I alfo enjoin my patients to wear this bandage afterwards, from a perfuafion that it retards the return of the difeafe. The proper ufe of bandage, when the diforder firft difcovers itfelf, certainly contributes much to prevent its increafe.

O V A-

seton A thread drawn though the skin in order to cause a discharge (see also footnotes to pp. 21, 40, 65 and 86).

Dr. Monro Alexander Monro, the elder (1697-1767). Professor of Anatomy at Edinburgh from 1720 (see also pp. 244-5). The paper to which Withering refers was entitled *Improvements in performing the Operation of the Paracentesis, or Tapping of the Belly* (Monro 1752). When performing abdominal paracentesis (i.e. removal of fluid from the belly) it was the custom to wrap the belly with a bandage, towel, or roller after inserting the trochar, in order to express the fluid under pressure, and to prevent the collapse which occurs following the rapid removal of ascitic fluid (by preventing pooling of blood in the splanchnic circulation and thus maintaining the intravascular fluid volume). In the case of ovarian dropsy a measure of this kind is being recommended here to prevent reaccumulation of the encysted fluid. Monro invented a belt which could be tightened gradually as the belly slackened and in which there was a window through which the wound could be dressed. The belt is described and illustrated in his paper.

OVARIUM DROPSY with ANASARCA.

§ 29. THE anasarca does not appear until the encysted dropsy is very far advanced. It is then probably caused by weakness and pressure. The Digitalis removes it for a time.

PHTHISIS PULMONALIS.

§ 30. This is a very increasing malady in the present day. It is no longer limited to the middle part of life : children at five years of age die of it, and old people at sixty or seventy. It is not confined to the flat-chested, the fair-skinned, the blue eyed, the light-haired, or the scrophulous : it often attacks people with full chests, brown skins, dark hair and eyes, and those in whose family no scrophulous taint can be traced. It is certainly infectious. The very strict laws still existing in Italy to prevent the infection from consumptive patients, were probably not enacted originally without a sufficient cause. We seem to be approaching to that state which first made such restrictions necessary, and in the further course of time, the disease will probably fall off again, both in virulency and frequency.

§ 31. The younger part of the female sex are liable to a disease very much resembling a true consumption, and from which it is difficult to distinguish it ; but this disease is curable by steel and bitters. A criterion of true phthisis has been sought for in the
state

brown skins A particular kind of brown pigmentation of the skin is associated with Addison's disease, i.e. hypoadrenalism, the commonest cause of which in the eighteenth century would have been tuberculosis.

the disease will probably fall off again The prevalence of tuberculosis has indeed fallen steadily in the U.K. in the last 150 years, and the death rate has fallen at a rate of about 25 deaths per year each year. The fall is thought to be almost completely attributable to improvements in social conditions (McKeown and Lowe 1966).

a disease very much resembling a true consumption Probably iron deficiency anaemia due to excessive menstrual blood loss. It would have responded to 'steel', i.e. iron (see note to p. 12).

ftate of the teeth ; but the exceptions to that rule are numerous. An unufual dilatation of the pupil of the eye, is the moft certain characteriftic.*

§ 32. Sydenham afferts, that the bark did not more certainly cure an intermittent, than riding did a confumption. We muft not deny the truth of an affertion, from fuch authority, but we muft conclude that the difeafe was more eafily curable a century ago than it is at prefent.

§ 33. If the Digitalis is no longer ufeful in confumptive cafes, it muft be that I know not how to manage it, or that the difeafe is more fatal than formerly ; for it would be hard to deny the teftimony cited at page 9. I wifh others would undertake the enquiry.

§ 34. When phthifis is accompanied with anafarca, or when there is reafon to fufpect hydrothorax, the Digitalis will often relieve the fufferings, and prolong the life of the patient.

§ 35. Many

---

* Many years ago I communicated to my friend, Dr. Percival, an account of fome trials of breathing fixed air in confumptive cafes. The refults were publifhed by him in the fecond Vol. of his very ufeful Effays Medical and Experimental, and have fince been copied into other publications. I take this opportunity of acknowledging that I fufpect myfelf to have been miftaken in the nature of the difeafe there mentioned to have been cured. I believe it was a cafe of *Vomica*, and not a true *Phthifis* that was cured. The Vomica is almoft always curable. The fixed air corrects the fmell of the matter, and very fhortly removes the hectic fever. My patients not only infpire it, but I keep large jars of the effervefcing mixture conftantly at work in their chambers.

Sydenham Thomas Sydenham (1674-89). 'The English Hippocrates', the pre-eminent physician of his day. He was the first to describe many diseases, including the tertian ague of malaria, hysteria, and the chorea which bears his name.

intermittent An intermittent fever.

I wish others would undertake the enquiry Others did, notably Dr Thomas Beddoes who wrote (Beddoes 1799) that 'an effectual remedy for consumption appears to have been nearly ascertained; ... there existed, before the two physicians [Nathan Drake and Richard Fowler], who have taught its safe, easy, and effectual employment, such proofs of the antiphthisical powers of the FOX-GLOVE, that one must wonder its use had not, a number of years ago, become general' (see also pp. 310-12).

Dr Percival Thomas Percival (1740-1804). Physician at Manchester. His *Essays Medical and Experimental* appeared between 1767 and 1773.

fixed air Carbon dioxide.

Vomica A lung abscess, due to infection other than tuberculosis.

§ 35. Many years ago, during an attendance upon Mr. B——, of a confumptive family, and himfelf in the laft ftage of a phthifis; after he was fo ill as to be confined to his chamber, his breathing became fo extremely difficult and diftreffing, that he wifhed rather to die than to live, and urged me warmly to devife fome mode to relieve him. Sufpecting ferous effufion to be the caufe of this fymptom, and he being a man of fenfe and refolution, I fully explained my ideas to him, and told him what kind of operation might afford him a chance of relief; for I was then but little acquainted with the Digitalis. He was earneft for the operation to be tried, and with the affiftance of Mr. Parrott, a very refpectable furgeon of this place, I got an opening made between the ribs upon the lower and hinder part of the thorax. About a pint of fluid was immediately difcharged, and his breath became eafy. This fluid coagulated by heat.

Mr. Parrott ?

This fluid coagulated by heat Because it contained, as would be expected, albumin.

After fome days a copious purulent difcharge iffued from the opening, his cough became lefs troublefome, his expectoration lefs copious, his appetite and ftrength returned, he got abroad, and the wound, which became very troublefome, was allowed to heal.

He then undertook a journey to London; whilft there he became worfe: returned home, and died confumptive fome weeks afterwards.

PUER-

P U E R P E R A L   A N A S A R C A.

§ 36. THIS difeafe admits of an eafy and certain cure by the Digitalis.

§ 37. This fpecies of dropfy may originate from other caufes than child birth.   In the beginning of laft *March*, a gentleman at Wolverhampton defired my advice for very large and painful fwelled legs and thighs.   He was a temperate man, not of a dropfi-cal habit, had great pain in his groins, and attri-buted his complaints to a fall from his horfe.   He had taken diuretics, and the ftrongeft draftic pur-gatives with very little benefit.   Confidering the anafarca as caufed by the difeafed inguinal glands, I ordered common poultice and mercurial ointment to the groins, three grains of pulv. fol. Digitalis night and morning, and a cooling diuretic decoction in the day-time.   He foon loft his pain, and the fwellings gradually fubfided.

T H E   E N D.

This disease admits of an easy and certain cure Probaby all Withering's successes in this disease were due to spontaneous resolution, and were nothing to do with the foxglove (see note to p. 19).

diseased inguinal glands Although this patient presented with the same symptoms as in the post-partum cases, and both would have been due to venous obstruction, in this case the obstruction was caused by the lymph nodes pressing on the veins from *without*, while in the post-partum cases it would have been due to clotting *within* the veins. In this case too *lymphatic* obstruction might have occurred from external pressure.

mercurial oint-ment Metallic mercury triturated with lard and suet, also called blue ointment.

G.G.J. and J. Robin-son George, George, John, and James Robinson. George (*c*. 1735–1801) came to London in 1755 where he was apprenticed to John Rivington, and was later assisted, by the loan of money, by Thomas Longman. In partnership with John Roberts he set up as a bookseller and publisher at 25 Pater-noster Row in 1764, and by 1780 he had the largest wholesale trade in London. In 1784 he took his son George and his brother John into the business, and they traded as G.G.J. and J. Robinson from 1785 to 1793. The business survived under a variety of Christian names until 1830. Robinson paid his authors well and that may be why Wither-ing had so many of his books published by his firm (see the biblio-graphy on pp. 265–7). Robinson also published some of Withering's books in conjunction with other London pub-lishers, e.g. Thomas Cadell and Peter Elmsley of The Strand, and Benjamin White of Fleet Street.

Sir TORBERN BERGMAN (1735–84). Professor of Chemistry, Uppsala. Like Withering (see p. 38) he prepared artificial mineral waters.

BOOKS,

Printed for G. G. J. and J. ROBINSON, Bookfellers, Paternofter-Row, London.

AN ACCOUNT OF THE

Scarlet Fever and Sore Throat,

Or, SCARLATINA ANGINOSA;

Particularly as it appeared at BIRMINGHAM in the Year 1778.

By WILLIAM WITHERING, M. D.

Price 1s. 6d.

Alfo, Price 2s. 6d.

Outlines of MINERALOGY,

Tranflated from the original of Sir TORBERN BERGMAN; with NOTES,

By WILLIAM WITHERING, M. D.

Member of the Royal Medical Society at Edinburgh.

———————

In the Spring of the Year 1786, will be publifhed, by the fame Author, a New Edition of the

BOTANICAL ARRANGEMENT.

With very great Additions; in Three Vols. large Octavo.

AN
ACCOUNT OF THE
FOXGLOVE
AND ITS MEDICAL USES
1785-1985

J. K. ARONSON MA DPhil MB FRCP

Clinical Reader in Clinical Pharmacology (Wellcome Lecturer),
University of Oxford
Honorary Consultant in Clinical Pharmacology to the
Oxfordshire Health Authority

PART I

INTRODUCTION

CHAPTER 1

THE FOXGLOVE AS FLOWER AND HERB

When William Withering published his *An Account of the Foxglove* in 1785, he was referring to the purple foxglove, which grows wild in Great Britain and in many other countries, both in Continental Europe and elsewhere. The picture of the foxglove in the frontispiece to this volume is taken from the plate included in the *Account* (see also p. xxi). After the Preface Withering gives an account of the botany of the foxglove (pp. xi–xiv), and I am inclined to follow his example.

THE BOTANY OF FOXGLOVES

The purple foxglove is one of several foxgloves belonging to the genus *Digitalis*, which in turn belongs to the order of Scrophulariaceae. Modern taxonomy recognizes at least eleven species, four of which have two or more subspecies, and one other of uncertain status (Heywood 1972). The main species are: *Digitalis dubia, ferruginea, grandiflora, laevigata, lanata, leucophaea, lutea, obscura, parviflora, purpurea*, and *thapsi* (compare Boerhaave's list of eleven species given in the note on p. xi).

The purple foxglove, *Digitalis purpurea*, is a biennial, or rarely perennial, plant, which usually flowers between July and September in its second year. It had three subspecies: *purpurea, mariana*, and *heywoodii*. It is a tall plant, between 3 and 6 feet high, with leaves varying in length between 6 and 12 inches. Its flowers are bell-like, and purple, pale pink, or white, the exact colour being genetically determined. The flowers are usually spotted red or yellow, and have short cilia on the outside and a few long hairs on the inside. It is pollinated by bees and is commonly found in open spaces (e.g. burnt areas) in woods, etc., and on heaths and mountain rocks, at heights of up to about 3000 feet. It prefers a light, dry, acid soil. For more details see Heywood (1972).

TERMINOLOGY

Before any further discussion I shall define the terms I shall use in describing the *Digitalis* plants and the drugs derived from them.

There are numerous plants which contain active principles with chemical structures and pharmacological actions similar to those of the active principles found in *Digitalis* plants. The general term for these substances is 'cardiac glycosides', because their main site of action is the heart, and because they contain as part of their structures glucose-like moieties. There are many such naturally-occurring substances, the incomplete list given by Gibbs (1974) extending to 26 pages. A few examples are listed in Table 1.1 with an indication of some of their natural sources.

Strictly speaking, the term 'digitalis' should be used only to refer to those cardiac glycosides which are obtained from plants of the *Digitalis* genus. However, it is common for the term to be used in reference to *any* cardiac glycoside used in clinical practice, even those which do not originate from a *Digitalis* plant (e.g. ouabain). Since this loose nomenclature can give rise to confusion I shall adopt the following usages in this account:

Digitalis = a member or members of the plant genus.
Digitalis or digitalis glycoside = any drug derived from a *Digitalis* plant.
Glycoside or cardiac glycoside = any drug with an action similar to that of digitalis, but derived from any source (including *Digitalis* plants).

Table 1.1 Some naturally-occurring cardiac glycosides and some of their plant sources.

Cardiac glycoside	Source
Adonitoxin	*Adonis vernalis*[1] (false hellebore)
Antiarin	*Antiaris toxicaria*[2] (the upas tree)
Convallatoxin	*Convallaria majalis*[3] (lily of the valley)
Cymarin	*Apogynum cannabinum*[4]; *Strophanthus kombé*[4]
Deslanoside*	*Digitalis lanata*[5] (woolly foxglove)
Digitoxin*	*Digitalis purpurea*[5] (purple foxglove)
Digoxin*	*Digitalis lanata*[5]
Hellebrin	*Helleborus niger*[1] (hellebore)
Helveticoside (erysimin)	*Erysimum helveticum*[6]
Lanatoside C*	*Digitalis lanata*[5]
Neriantin	*Nerium oleander*[4] (oleander)
Oleandrin	*Nerium oleander*[4]
Ouabain (strophanthin-G)*	*Strophanthus gratus*[4]; *Acokanthera schimperi*[4]; *Acokanthera ouabaio*[4]
Periplocin	*Periploca graeca*[7]; *Strophanthus preussii*[4]
Peruvoside*	*Thevetia nereifolia*[1]
Proscillaridin*	*Urginea (Scilla) maritima*[3] (squill)
Sarveroside	*Strophanthus sarmentosus*[4]
Strophanthin-K	*Strophanthus kombé*[4]
Tanghinin	*Tanghinia venenifera*[4]
Thevetin	*Thevetia nereifolia*[1]

* These glycosides are in clinical use.

Orders: [1] Ranunculaceae; [2] Moraceae; [3] Liliaceae; [4] Apocyanaceae; [5] Scrophulariaceae; [6] Cruciferae; [7] Asclepiadaceae.

NAMING THE FLOWER

The term 'Scrophulariaceae' was applied to the large order of plants to which the *Digitalis* genus belongs because it was thought that some of them were useful for the treatment of scrofula, a form of tuberculosis. 'Scrofula' derived from the Latin word for swelling of the lymph nodes, *scrofulae*, the diminutive form of the word for pigs (*scrofae*), which were supposed to be susceptible to such an illness.

The term 'Digitalis', the adjectival form of the Latin word for a finger, *digitus*, was first applied to the foxglove by the Tübingen botanist Leonhardt Fuchs (1501-66) in his herbal, *De historia stirpium* ... (Fuchs 1542). The text was written in Latin, interspersed with the German names for the plants, and the entry '*De Digitali*', describing the *Digitalis purpurea* and the *Digitalis lutea*, forms the penultimate chapter (cap. CCCXLII). Fuchs wrote:

> *Appellavimus autem digitalem, alludentes ad germanicam nomenclaturam* fingerhut/*sic enim Germani hanc stirpem nominant, a florum similitudine* ...
> [We have called it Digitalis, in allusion to the German name 'thimble', so-called by the Germans because the flowers resemble one ...]

The origin of the word 'foxglove' is not so clear. The *Oxford English Dictionary* gives 'foxes glove' from the Old English *foxes glófa*, but the editor, James Murray, and his colleague Henry Bradley, who was responsible for the letter *F*, were unable to explain the association with the fox. A more romantic suggestion is that the word derives from 'folks' glove', that is 'fairies' glove'.

There is no help from foreign languages in differentiating between these two possibilities. Most foreign words for the plant derive either from the Latin *digitalis*, for example *digitale* (Italian) and *digital* (Spanish), or from native words meaning 'thimble', 'thimble-flower', or 'thimble-weed', for example *dedalera* (Spanish), *sormustinkukka* (Finnish), *gyüszürvirág* (Hungarian), and

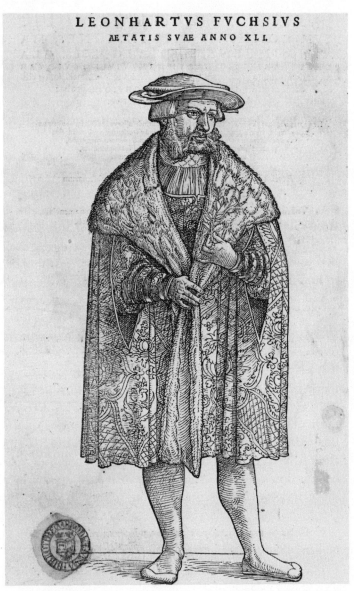

LEONHARTVS FVCHSIVS
ÆTATIS SVÆ ANNO XLI.

Leonhardt Fuchs, from the woodcut forming the frontispiece to his *De Historia Stirpium* ... (1542). Reproduced by the kind permission of the Curators of the Bodleian Library, Oxford.

naprstnik (Czechoslovakian). In two languages only do the words used refer to foxes or fairies: in Norwegian the word is *revebjelle* (fox bell), while in old Welsh it is either *menygellyllon* (elves' gloves) or *menyg y llwynog* (foxes' gloves). In modern Welsh the term *bysedd y cwn* (dogs' fingers) is found.

The Norwegian term strongly suggests that the true derivation is from the word 'fox', since it has nothing etymologically to do with the English word, and that is supported by two of the Welsh forms. The third Welsh form, invoking elves, may simply have come about by translation from a corrupt English form, although that could also be argued about the 'fox' forms. In their *Dictionary of English plant-names* Britten and Holland (1886) suggest that the derivation is more likely to be from 'folks' glove', and they quote in support of this the numerous common terms for the foxglove which invoke fairies (see below). However, they neglect to point out that there are as many which invoke dogs or foxes. It is not necessary, however, to discount completely the more romantic origin, since the two different possibilities meet in the old legend that bad fairies put foxglove flowers on foxes' feet to muffle their footsteps at night.

Not only is there doubt about the origin of the involvement of the fox, but some doubt has also been cast on the obvious explanation that the word 'glove' refers to the shape of the flower. An alternative suggestion is that the word comes from 'foxes-glew', literally 'foxes' music', 'in allusion to an ancient musical instrument composed of bells, pendent from an arched support' (Prior 1863). The Anglo-Saxon word *gléow* meant to play an instrument.

Common names for the foxglove abound (Britten and Holland 1886), and can be grouped according to origin:

> from the colour of the flower—bloody finger, bloody man's finger, bluidy bells;
> from the shape of the flower—

    (i) bluidy bells, dead men's bells, dead men's bellows, fairy bells;

   (ii) bloody finger, bloody man's finger, dog-fingers, fairy fingers, finger flower, finger-root, fox-fingers, lady's purple fingers;

  (iii) fairy glove, lady's glove;

  (iv) fairy thimbles, lady's thimble, witches' thimble;

   (v) dog's-lugs;

  (vi) fairy cap;

 (vii) dragon's mouth, lion's mouth, tiger's mouth, snap-dragon, snaps. (All these terms are more commonly applied to the snapdragon, and derive from the fanciful notion that the shape of the lips of the flower resembles those of the animals.)

from the height of the flower—fox-tree, king's ellwand (an ell-wand being a yardstick).

from those to whom they 'belong'—cottagers (so-called in Ireland 'because they belong to the poor people'), rabbit's flower.

from the habit of children of inflating the flowers like balloons and making them pop (also used in reference to a variety of other flowers)—flop poppy, green pops, pop-dock, pop-glove, poppers, poppy.

for other reasons, which I have been unable to unravel—blob, cowslip or cowslop, dock, docken, flap-dock, flobby-dock, goose flops, lusmore, Scotch mercury (perhaps because it is also another name for the snapdragon), snoxums, wild mercury.

The origin of the term 'lady' in some of these common names is hinted at in the common French name *gants de Notre-Dame*, i.e. 'Our Lady's gloves' (also *doigts de la Vierge*, 'Virgin's fingers'). The connection with the Virgin Mary may have been that the plant was considered to be a 'herb of grace', that is a herb with great healing properties (see Chapter 2).

In its turn the word 'foxglove' has been used to describe plants which are not foxgloves at all, but which have been confused with foxgloves, e.g. *Verbascum thapsus* (foxglove or ladies' foxglove) (see note to p. xi), *Campanula trachelium* (blue or white foxglove), Phytolacca decandra (West Indian foxglove or pokeweed), and various species of *Gerardia* (false foxgloves).

THE FOXGLOVE IN LITERATURE

Despite being a common wild flower the foxglove has received scant attention from poets, playwrights, and novelists. Shakespeare, for example, does not mention it at all, and the 'long purples' or 'dead men's fingers' mentioned in *Hamlet* (IV. vii. 173), which some have thought to be foxgloves, are a different plant altogether, probably early purple orchids, *Orchis mascula*. Walter de la Mare (1960) suggested that Shakespeare may never have seen a foxglove when a child because

> it appears that foxgloves are to be found near Stratford, but only by the elect, so to speak, and in occasional clumps, There were foxgloves at Lapworth, for example, in the summer of [1927]. But none now grows on the bank that Oberon knew, with its thyme, oxlip, violet, musk rose and eglantine; and in South Warwickshire what foxgloves there are tend to disappear . . . How else can we explain [the foxglove's] absence, say, from *A Midsummer Night's Dream*—its natural earthly paradise.

Poets who *have*, at least in passing, mentioned the foxglove include Wordsworth, Keats, Tennyson, and Scott:

> . . . bees that soar for bloom
> High as the highest Peak of Furness-fells
> Will murmur by the hour in foxglove bells.
> (Wordsworth 1807, 'Nuns fret not at their
>   convent's narrow room'.)

. . . let me thy vigils keep
'Mongst bough pavilioned where the deer's swift leap
Startles the wild bee from the fox-glove bell.
(Keats 1817, 'O Solitude! if I must with thee dwell'.)

Bring orchis bring the foxglove spire
    The little speedwell's darling blue
    Deep tulips clash'd with fiery dew
Laburnums, dropping-wells of fire
(Tennyson 1850, *In Memoriam A.H.H.*, lxxxiii.)

Foxglove and nightshade, side by side,
Symbols of punishment and pride.
Grouped their dark lines with every stain
Their weather-beaten ways retain
(Scott 1810, *The Lady of the Lake*, Canto I. xii.)

Scott was asked about the origin of the symbolism he uses here,
and his explanation is to be found in a letter he wrote to Lionel
Thomas Bergner, on 20 October 1812:

> I incline to think that I have confused the nightshade with
> hemlock, used, you know, for the execution of criminals, and
> so far therefore an emblem of punishment; and that the fox-
> glove from its determined erect figure and decisive colour,
> might be no bad emblem of pride.

However, these words do not ring true, and I suspect that Scott
chose those particular flowers for the sonority of their names,
rather than for any symbolic reason.

I have found no poem, however, completely devoted to the
foxglove, in the way, for example, that Shelley devoted his *The
Sensitive Plant* (1820) ostensibly to the mimosa.

Erasmus Darwin, a poet in aspiration only, wrote a long poem in two parts, entitled *The Botanic Garden*. Although it cannot be counted as literature I shall quote a few lines here, because of Darwin's importance in the story of digitalis (see Chapter 4). These lines give the flavour of the poem perfectly. After having described 'pale dropsy', Darwin describes its treatment. Dropsy is compared to Tantalus with 'parch'd tongue' and 'hollow eye':

> Divine HYGEIA, from the bending sky
> Descending, listens to his piercing cry;
> Assumes bright DIGITALIS' dress and air; . . .
> O'er him she waves her serpent-wreathed wand,
> Cheers with her voice, and raises with her hand,
> Warms with rekindling bloom his visage wan,
> And charms the shapeless monster into man.

> (*The Botanic Garden*, Part II, Canto II)

While I am quoting bad poetry, I cannot resist the lines written in around 1820 by Miss Sarah Hoare, whose mother was a friend of Mrs Schimmelpenninck (see p. 288). These lines merit inclusion since the version given here was quoted in the third volume of the 7th edition of Withering's *Botany*, published in 1830, and have been attributed by some to him, despite the clear attribution in the volume to 'S.H.'. They are taken from a poem called *The pleasures of botanical pursuits*, quoted in full in *An introduction to botany* by Priscilla Wakefield (1823). [A slightly different version is given by Feil (1966).]

> The Foxglove's leaves, with caution giv'n,
> Another proof of favouring Heav'n
>   Will happily display;
> The rapid pulse it can abate;
> The hectic flush can moderate;
> And blest by Him whose will is fate,
>   May give a lengthen'd day.

Note the word 'hectic', suggesting the use of digitalis in treating tuberculosis (see above and Chapters 5 and 6).

I am spared here from quoting the dreadful lines inscribed on William Withering's monument in Edgbaston, since they contain no reference to the foxglove. A photograph of the memorial is included in Peck and Wilkinson's biography of Withering (1950).

The references to the foxglove to be found in novels are more interesting. The first of which I am aware is in the first and second chapters of George Eliot's novel *Silas Marner*:

> Marner had cured Sally Oates, and made her sleep like a baby, when her heart had been beating enough to burst her body, for two months and more, while she had been under her doctor's care . . . he had inherited from his mother some acquaintance with medicinal herbs and their preparation—a little store of wisdom she had imparted to him as a solid bequest—but of late years he had had doubts about the lawfulness of applying this knowledge, believing that herbs could have no efficacy without prayer, and that prayer might suffice without herbs; so that the inherited delight he had in wandering in the fields in search of foxglove and dandelion and coltsfoot, began to wear to him the character of a temptation . . . One day, taking a pair of shoes to be mended, he saw the cobbler's wife seated by the fire, suffering from the terrible symptoms of heart-disease and dropsy which he had witnessed as the precursors of his mother's death. He felt a rush of pity at the mingled sight and remembrance, and, recalling the relief his mother had found from a simple preparation of the foxglove, he promised Sally Oates to bring her something that would ease her, since the doctor did her no good.

Silas Marner was set in around 1810, but was written in 1861, when knowledge of the usefulness of digitalis in heart disease was widespread among medical men at least. However, George Eliot was from Warwickshire, and Withering noted (p. 9) that 'a person in the neighbourhood of Warwick' possessed 'a famous family receipt for the dropsy, in which Foxglove is the active medicine'. I do not know what the source of George Eliot's knowledge was.

A novel called *Precious Bane* was published in 1924. It was by Mary Webb, whose novels were later brilliantly parodied by Stella Gibbons in *Cold Comfort Farm* (1932), and was set in a fictitious village in Shropshire, the home of the woman whose receipt Withering was shown in 1775 (see p. 2). In *Precious Bane* the foxglove is used by the narrator's brother, Gideon, to poison their mother when it appears that she will live for many years bedridden and a burden on the family:

> 'Seems to be in a fever all the while. Heart's likely to burst sometimes. I suppose a dose of foxglove ud put her right, maybe?'
> 'Ah. Foxglove'll lower the pulse as quick as anything.' ... I looked up, and there was Tivvy, coming running in a great courant, all distraught. 'Come quick, Prue!' she said. 'Her's took very bad. The tea didna agree. He says, give her it strong, he says, for it'll do more good the like of that'n. So I did. And she said it was a bitter brew. But she drank it. And in a while she went ever so quiet, and I couldna hear her breathe. And then she gave a guggle and whispers—
> 'Go for Prue.'
> I was only just in time to kiss Mother, who was all shrunken down in her pillows. She whispered—
> 'A bitter brew!' and smiled, and caught her breath, and was gone.

A more famous murder with digitalis is that of General Fentiman, described by Dorothy Sayers in *The Unpleasantness at the Bellona Cub* (1921). Lubbock, the pathologist, carries out a post-mortem examination of the exhumed body of the General, and writes to Lord Peter Wimsey:

I tested the viscera for poison and discovered traces of a powerful dose of digitalin, swallowed not very long previous to
decease. As you know, with a subject whose heart was already
in a weak state, the result of such a dose could not but be fatal.
The symptoms would be a slowing-down of the heart's action
and collapse—practically indistinguishable from a violent
heart attack.

Later we hear that 'the dose given was enormous: nearly two
grains'. In a contemporary pharmacopoeia (Squire 1916) four
different formulations of digitalin, of varying strengths, are listed:
digitalin amorphous (Homolle), dose 1/100 to 1/40 grain; digitalin crystallized (Nativelle), dose 1/240 to 1/100 grain; digitalin
German, dose 1/20 to 1/4 grain; digitalinum verum, dose 1/270
grain every 2 or 3 hours. Whichever of these the General was
given, even the least potent, it would almost certainly have been
enough to kill him, since he had a 'weak heart' and was already
taking a normal maintenance dose of digitalin.

Also of interest, as a reflection of current beliefs, at least as
interpreted by Sayers on the basis of the medical information
available to her, is the conversation between Inspector Parker and
Fentiman's doctor, Dr Penberthy:

'Is digitalin a thing one takes for heart disease?'

'Yes; in certain forms of heart disease, digitalin is a very valuable stimulant.'

'Stimulant? I thought it was a depressant.'

'It acts as a stimulant at first; in later stages it depresses the
heart's action.'

'Oh, I see ... It first speeds up the heart and then slows it
down.'

'Not exactly. It strengthens the heart's action by retarding the
beat, so that the cavities can be more completely emptied and the
pressure is relieved.'

The medical literature Sayers quoted in the book, and which can be taken as being some of her sources of information were the ' "Materia Medica", "Pharmacopoeia" Dixon Mann, Taylor, Glaister, and other of those writers who had so kindly and helpfully published their conclusions on toxicology'.

THE CARDIAC GLYCOSIDES IN *DIGITALIS* PLANTS

Of all the *Digitalis* plants the most important from the medical point of view are the *Digitalis lanata*, and the *Digitalis purpurea*, from which the principal cardiac glycosides in clinical use today are extracted. Because the cardiac glycosides cannot yet be synthesized, they are prepared by growing *Digitalis* plants, harvesting their leaves, and extracting their active principles.

The following are examples of the glycosides to be found in the leaves of the two *Digitalis* species (Cowley and Rowson 1963):

> *Digitalis purpurea* —digitalinum verum, digitoxin, gitoxin, purpurea glycosides (desacetyldigilanides) A and B, and strospeside.
> *Digitalis lanata* —acetyldigoxin, desacetyl-lanatoside C (deslanoside), digitoxin, digoxin, gitaloxin, lanatosides A and D, purpurea glycoside A, and strospeside.

It is not surprising, considering this bewildering array of compounds, that unpurified extracts of these plants should be so variable in their effects, since each of these different glycosides has pharmacological characteristics which differ from those of its neighbour, in terms of both its pharmacokinetic properties (i.e. the way in which it is absorbed, distributed around the body tissues, and eliminated from the body) and the potency of its pharmacodynamic properties on the tissues (i.e. what it does when it gets to the site of action). It is only because the majority of the glycosides in these plants are present in relatively small quantities that there is not even more variability from formulation to formulation of unpurified preparations.

The two digitalis glycosides in most common clinical use are digitoxin (extracted from *Digitalis purpurea*) and digoxin (extracted from *Digitalis lanata*). William Withering used *Digitalis purpurea*, and although other foxgloves were later also used elsewhere the purple foxglove was the principal source of digitalis glycosides throughout most of the world until the identification and isolation, during this century, of digoxin (Smith 1930).

THE PHARMACOLOGY OF DIGITOXIN AND ITS INFLUENCE ON WITHERING'S METHODS OF TREATMENT WITH THE FOXGLOVE

In order that the general reader may be able to understand the implications of the pharmacology of the purple foxglove in relation to the historical account which follows, I shall outline some of the important facts in regard to digitoxin, and show how they may have influenced the ways in which Withering used the drug.

Digitoxin is quickly and well absorbed after being taken orally. One would therefore expect its initial effects to be seen quite soon after its first administration (say within an hour or two). However, matters are complicated by the fact that during repetitive therapy there is accumulation of the drug in the body. This phenomenon is illustrated schematically in Fig. 1.1. (solid line). Following the administration of a single dose of the drug the amount in the body rises rapidly as the drug is absorbed, and then falls as it begins to be distributed to the tissues and eliminated from the body. This decay is not a simple process and can be likened to the decay of a radio-active isotope, in that it is characterized by a 'half-time'. In other words the amount of drug in the body is reduced by a half within a given time, that time being the same no matter what amount of drug is in the body. For digitoxin this half-time is very long, of the order of seven days, so that it will take seven days before half of the drug is removed, another seven days before half of what is left is removed, and so on. If, therefore, another dose of the drug is given before there has been much decay of the first dose (Fig. 1.1), the amount of drug in the body will accumulate, and this process continues until a so-called steady state is reached, at which time the same amount of drug is leaving the body during a single dosage interval as the dose that is being given. The steady state does not occur until about five half-times, or in the case of digitoxin about 5 weeks, no matter what the frequency of dosing. Of course, it was common practice to give doses of the purple foxglove at frequent intervals. Withering, for example, describes dosage regimens such as two grains two hourly (e.g. Case XLV, p. 44).

The consequences of giving repeated doses of digitoxin every four hours are illustrated in Fig. 1.1 (dotted line), for comparison

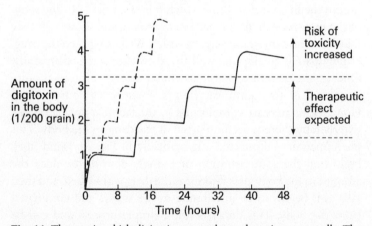

Fig. 1.1. The way in which digitoxin accumulates when given repeatedly. The graphs show the time course of the amount of digitoxin in the body at a dose of 1/200 grain, given either twice daily (solid line) or four-hourly (dotted line), both over a period of two days. Accumulation to much higher amounts would occur for up to about five *weeks* if these doses were continued.

with twice daily dosage (solid line), and it will be immediately seen that dangerous accumulation would quickly occur were the drug to be continued in the same dose at the same dosage interval. After some experience, Withering recognized (p. 186) that it was important to avoid giving the drug too frequently:

> . . . it was moreover of consequence not to repeat the doses too quickly, but to allow sufficient time for the effects of each to take place, as it was found very possible to pour in an injurious quantity of the medicine, before any of the signals for forbearance appeared.

This explains why Withering, in around 1782, reduced the frequency of dosing from two- or four-hourly to once or twice a day, and also why he used the foxglove for a few days only at a time. It explains why others, continuing treatment for longer, frequently caused their patients to become ill because of digitalis toxicity. And it explains why toxicity, once established, took so long to wear off, since it would take a week for only half the drug to be removed from the body (see, for example, the cases at pp. 72-3 and 134-8). Of course, if one were to use a much *smaller* dose of purple foxglove, given say once a day, then one could achieve the same therapeutic effect eventually with a much lower risk of toxicity, and the dose could then be continued indefinitely. However, if one did that one would have to persist for three to four weeks before producing the optimum therapeutic effect, a delay which would be unacceptable in most cases.

The ideal compromise, then, would be to give a large dose to start with (a loading dose), in order to boost the amount of drug in the body rapidly, and then to give a much smaller dose at longish intervals in order to make good the losses from the body, and thus maintain body stores at a relatively constant level (a maintenance dose). In fact Withering never adopted this strategy, and indeed there seemed no need for him to do so, since in cases where his treatment was successful his patients generally remained in remission, either completely or at least for several

weeks or months thereafter. This contrasts sharply with the
modern practice, recently questioned, of giving digitalis therapy
indefinitely (discussed in Chapter 8).

The half-time of a drug is dependent partly on the rate at
which it is eliminated from the body and partly on the extent to
which it is bound by the tissues and therefore kept away from the
sites of elimination. In the case of digitoxin a major factor retarding its elimination is the fact that it is highly bound by proteins
both in the tissues and in the blood. Both of these factors can vary
quite a lot from individual to individual, but it is not possible to
say to what extent such variability would have influenced
Withering's therapy. In addition, since the elimination of digitoxin from the body is mostly by its being converted in the liver
to inactive compounds, one would expect some variability to
have occurred by virtue of different degrees of liver function in
his patients. Again, however, it is not possible to determine
whether or not this influenced his therapy, since we cannot judge
from his reports the extent of impairment of liver function in an
individual case. Nonetheless, in his patients with ascites he did
not experience higher rates of toxicity amongst heavy drinkers
compared with those more abstemious, and it may be either that
liver function did not influence his results very much, or that he
compensated empirically by altering dosages appropriately.

MODE OF ACTION OF DIGITALIS

Although the way in which digitalis produces its beneficial effects
at a molecular level has not been fully established, it seems likely
that it acts by inhibiting the normal transport of sodium and potassium across cell membranes. This alters the electrical activity of
fibres in the heart and results in two principal effects. The first of
these is a slowing of the heart rate, particularly in cases where the
heart rate is increased, and especially so in the form of fast arrhyth-

mia known as atrial fibrillation, in which the atria of the heart beat very rapidly and incoherently, so that their impulses are only irregularly transmitted to the ventricles, which, as a result, beat quickly, irregularly, and with varying strength from beat to beat. It is this arrhythmia which Withering and his correspondents are describing when they talk about a fast, irregular pulse or an 'intermitting' pulse (e.g. Case XX, p. 25, and Case CXXIX, p. 85). Curiously, although Withering discussed the effect of digitalis on the pulse he mentioned the pulse in only 17 of his 163 cases, in contrast to his correspondents, who mentioned it significantly more frequently (in 15 cases of 53). In only 10 of the total 32 can we be reasonably sure that the description is of atrial fibrillation.

The second effect of digitalis on the heart, probably also mediated by its effects on sodium and potassium transport, but via an intermediate effect on the disposition of calcium within the cardiac cells, is to increase its ability to contract. It is this effect which is primarily responsible for the therapeutic efficacy of digitalis in heart failure. Although digitalis does have a small direct effect on the kidney, causing a diuresis, that effect is negligible when compared with the diuretic effect which results from increased contractility of the heart.

Digitalis also causes increased contractility of the smooth muscle of blood vessels, perhaps by a similar mechanism to that whereby it increases the contractility of the heart, although that is much more debatable (Aronson 1984). This effect does not seem to have much consequence during the treatment of heart failure, but it caused a great deal of interest in the late nineteenth century (see Chapter 6), and has more recently become of interest because of the notion that hypertension might be due to an endogenous substance acting rather like digitalis.

Digitalis has several effects on the nervous system, the clinical relevance of all of which is not clear, but some of which are responsible for the common manifestations of toxicity.

DIGITALIS TOXICITY

Digitalis has a low 'therapeutic ratio'. In other words toxicity can easily occur with a very small increase in dose above that which produces a satisfactory therapeutic response. The signs and symptoms of digitalis toxicity are of two types—cardiac and non-cardiac.

The *non-cardiac* effects are: anorexia, nausea, and vomiting (due to an effect on the vomiting centres in the brain); diarrhoea (cause unknown, but perhaps due to a direct effect on the bowel); drowsiness, dizziness, confusion, and, in severe cases, dementia (all due to direct effects on the brain); colour vision abnormalities (usually the patient complains that objects look yellow, so-called 'xanthopsia'—a direct effect on the retina). Sweating, which Withering describes (see p. 184), has been described only once to my knowledge in modern times (see Aronson 1981).

The *cardiac* effects of digitalis toxicity are of two types: abnormal rhythms of the heart, usually manifesting as extra beats, and a block of the normal conduction of impulses from the atria to the ventricles (heart block). It is the latter that Withering is describing when he says that the patient's pulse dropped to around 40 beats per minute, which is the rate at which the ventricles beat when the natural pacemaker of the heart is no longer in control.

All of these effects are described by Withering at various points in his *Account* and are summarized by him on pp. 184-5. However, as he put it: '. . . these sufferings are not at all necessary; they are the effects of our inexperience . . .'.

CHAPTER 2

USES OF THE FOXGLOVE
BEFORE WITHERING

The foxglove and its pharmacological cousins, particularly the squill (*Scilla* see Table 1.1), was used for medical purposes for hundreds, or even thousands of years before Withering.

Squill was used by the ancient Egyptians (Turkel 1931) and is recommended in the Syriac *Book of medicines* (Budge 1913):

> . . . for the stomach, and for shortness of breath, and for pain in the sides, and for those who do not digest their food, and for eructations that leave behind a bitter (or, sour) taste, and for pain in the liver and spleen . . .

> Wine of squills . . . is good for an evil condition of the liver and stomach, and for those who collect water.

This suggests that the Syrians may have used squills for oedematous states. The advice on dosages is extraordinarily perceptive:

> Administer to the patient a spoonful at first and add to the dose gradually until it becometh five spoonfuls. Then diminish the dose until it become one spoonful only.

The advice here is to give a loading dose (albeit in divided doses rather than as a single initial dose), followed by a maintenance dose, and in this respect it coincides with the habits of today (see pp. 227-30).

Squill was reintroduced into clinical practice by van Swieten in the mid-eighteenth century (van Swieten 1764), and was used extensively in the treatment of dropsies by physicians, including Withering, the extent of whose use of it can be judged from the number of times it is mentioned in his *Account* (see the index on p. 386). That squill should be effective in heart failure is not surprising, since it contains several cardiac glycosides, including proscillaridin, which is in use in purified form in some countries today.

The earliest mention that I have been able to find of the use in medicine of foxgloves as such is in the Bury St Edmunds herbal *Herbarium Apuleius Platonicus* (*c.* 1120), in which it is stated that its alternative name is Apollinaris, because of the legend that Apollo discovered it and gave it to Aesculapius. It is not clear, however, precisely what it was used for. There may be earlier references still, since Fuchs (1542) says, '*Nam, ut testatur Galenus libro iiii. de simp. med. facul. cap. xvii . . .*', which may be a reference to a plant known as ephemerum, which was known to Dioscorides. However, there is no conclusive evidence that ephemerum and foxglove are the same plants, and Gerard wrote (1597) that '[according to the ancients, the foxgloves] are of no use, neither have they any place amongst medicines'.

The foxglove was known to the family of Welsh physicians, the Myddvai, who practised between the thirteenth and eighteenth centuries, and it is mentioned among the 900 or so drugs included in their pharmacopoeia (McKenzie 1927). Brooks (1933) wrote that among American Indians 'foxglove . . . was widely employed in the districts where it grows', but he does not specify when or for what purpose. However, they are unlikely to have used foxgloves before Withering's day, since the foxglove was probably not native to America (see Hall Jackson's letter to Withering on p. 296), and there may be confusion here with another plant used for its purgative properties, *Euonymus atropurpureus* or 'wahoo'.

USE OF THE FOXGLOVE
IN TUBERCULOSIS

In the Middle Ages the foxglove seems to have been used as a cure-all and was regarded as a 'herb of grace', that is, a herb with extensive healing properties. However, all the references to the medical uses of the foxglove from the sixteenth century onwards suggest that it was used most commonly for tuberculosis.

There is clear evidence of its use in the form of tuberculosis called scrofula, since that is mentioned as a specific indication by Parkinson (1640), Culpeper (1653), and Salmon (1710). For example, Salmon wrote that it was:

'an extraordinary good wound-herb, prevalent against the King's Evil, and may be used instead of gentian.'

Parkinson's comments and other references to its use in scrofula are given by Withering (pp. xvii–xviii).

However, the foxglove was also used as a salve for wounds of all kinds, of which scrofula may have simply been one example. Martin Martin, a physician who travelled in Scotland, published his diary in 1695, recommending foxglove for external use (Hamilton 1981); Quincy (1742) referred to its reputed 'vulnerary' properties (i.e. its ability to heal wounds and ulcers), and Culpeper wrote:

The herb is frequently and familiarly used by the Italians to heal any fresh or green wound, the leaves being but bruised and bound thereon; and the juice thereof is also used in old sores, to cleanse, dry, and heal them . . . an ointment of it is one of the best remedies for scabby head that is.

The reference to the Italians may derive from the medieval Italian proverb *aralda tutte le piaghe salda* (the foxglove salves all sores). Other references to its use in treating wounds from Lobel and Hulse are given by Withering (see p. xviii).

There is also evidence that the foxglove was used for *pulmonary* tuberculosis, although some of the wording used in old herbals is not definitive. For example Fuchs wrote:

> *Nam . . . amari sapores abstergunt, expurgant, et quae in venis est crassitiem incidunt. Quamobre menses etiam quae amara sunt movere possunt, et ex thorace et pulmone pus educere.*
> [For [these flowers] drain bitter humours, purge, and cut into whatever is thick in the veins. For this reason they can cause even bitter menses to flow, and draw pus out of the chest and lungs.]

Gerard, too, recommended the foxglove to 'cut and consume the thick toughness of grosse and slimie flegme, and naughty humours', and Parkinson wrote that it should be used 'whensoever there is need of a rarefying or extenuating of tough flegme or viscous humours troubling the chest'. Salmon was more specific, writing:

> It is a specific which transcends all other vegetable medicaments for the cure of consumptions; cleaning and healing after an admirable manner ulcers of the lungs . . . It cures a phthisick or ulceration of the lungs, when all other medicines have failed, and the sick been esteemed past cure. It opens the breast and lungs, frees them from tough phlegm, cleans the ulcer, and heals it, where all other remedies act without effect. I have known it do wonders, and speak here from a long experience. Persons in deep consumptions, and given over by all physicians, have, by the use of this syrup, or rob, been strangely recovered, and so perfectly restored as to grow fat again.

(Withering quotes the relevant passages from Gerard and Parkinson on pp. xviii-xix).

It may have been that the persistence with which it was used in the treatment of tuberculosis in the late eighteenth century and throughout the nineteenth century (see pp. 309-12 and 320-22) was in part bolstered by the memory of these old recommendations, which were frequently cited.

USE OF THE FOXGLOVE
IN EPILEPSY

The other main indication for its use before Withering was epilepsy, and here too we see the possible influence of the old writers on both Withering and his contemporaries, who used it for that indication (see, for example, p. 312). It was recommended by Parkinson and Culpeper (for the 'falling sickness') and by Salmon, who wrote that 'two handfuls of the herb taken with polypody helps the epilepsy', this being a straight quote from Parkinson (see p. xvi). Parkinson's indication of the precise dosage leaves something to be desired, but I find that two handfuls of the fresh leaves of the purple foxglove could weigh at least 150 grains, and perhaps as much as 1000 grains! Thus, the dose that Parkinson was recommending was enormous.

That digitalis had adverse effects on the brain was known to the common folk, as is demonstrated by what William Withering Junior wrote in the seventh edition of his father's *Botany*, published in 1830:

> 'Women of the poorer class in Derbyshire, drink large draughts of Foxglove tea, as a cheap means of obtaining the *pleasures*, or the forgetfulness, of *intoxication*!'

There was not, however, unanimous agreement about the foxglove's therapeutic usefulness. For example, Boerhaave made scathing comments about its value (quoted in the note at p. xiv), and Ray criticized Parkinson's recommendation that it be used in epilepsy:

Medicamentum hoc robustioribus tantum convenit, siquidem violenter admodum purgat, et vomitiones immanes excitat.

[This drug is suitable only for the stronger type of patient, since it purges powerfully and causes violent vomiting.]

Ray was suggesting that a drug with such severe effects would be more likely to precipitate fits than to prevent them. Again, Quincy, mentioning its reputation as a 'vulnerary and emetic', at the same time denied that it had any value in the 'present practice'.

The effects of the foxglove as an emetic and purgative were well known, and it was presumably used as such from time to time, although there were many safer alternatives. Parkinson commented that it 'purge[s] the body both upwards and downwards', although his terms are ambiguous, since he goes on to refer to 'tough flegme, and clammy humours' (see pp. xviii-xix). Dodoens and Lewis referred directly to its emetic effects (quoted on p. xiv), and both Ray and Haller (see pp. xiv and xv) mentioned its emetic and purgative powers. Culpeper wrote that '[it is] of a gentle cleansing nature, and withal very friendly to nature', perhaps also referring to its purgative properties.

USE OF THE FOXGLOVE
IN DROPSIES

The question of whether the foxglove was used by physicians and apothecaries for the treatment of dropsies before Withering cannot be answered, although I think it likely that it was not.

Perhaps the 'bitter humours' referred to by Fuchs in the extract from his De historia stirpium . . . quoted on p. 236 were dropsical, but I doubt it. Fuchs would almost certainly have recognized foxgloves as being emetic and purgative, and it is those actions to which he was surely referring. Others ambiguously wrote that the foxglove had beneficial effects on 'naughty humours' (Gerard), 'clammy humours' (Parkinson), and 'choleric humours' (James 1745), but these are Aristotelian/Hippocratic references, invoking the idea that imbalances in the four humours of the body, the phlegm, blood, choler, and black bile, could cause ill-ness, and that the treatment of disease should aim at redressing the balance. Nowhere is dropsy mentioned as a specific indica-tion for the foxglove.

Whatever the opinion of these old authors (and it must be remembered that they not infrequently plagiarized their pre-decessors' texts, sometimes without even rewording, and often without crediting the original), there is good evidence that the foxglove was not used extensively, except perhaps for scrofula and wounds, during the eighteenth century. For example, in his *Medicinal Dictionary*, James (1745) wrote of the *Digitalis purpurea* that it 'is rarely used inwardly, being strongly emetic'.

Nonetheless, it is clear that the foxglove *was* current as a folk remedy for dropsies in Withering's time, since that was how he and others learnt about it (see pp. 2, 3, and 109), and Withering cited other instances (see pp. 9–10).

One other physician came to try it before Withering in the treatment of dropsy in the 1760s, as recorded by Lettsom in his report to the Medical Society of London in 1788 (Lettsom 1789) (the italics here are mine):

> A physician of distinguished eminence informs me, that from the successful exhibition of it, in a case of dropsy, *about 22 years ago*, he was induced to give it repeatedly to the patients of the hospital, to which he was then physician, but without one instance of success; and although he continues high in his profession, the late encomiums [i.e. the recent praises the drug has received] have never drawn him to repeat his experiments.

['The successful exhibition of it, in a case of dropsy' was very likely by a layman.]

In typical eighteenth century style Lettsom does not say who the physician was, and there are no clues to his identity. Whoever he was he may have been unlucky in his choice of cases, or in the doses or formulation that he used, since, had he proved successful at that time, it might have been his name that we would have been commemorating today. For we must remember, when judging Withering's contribution, that he had been in a similar position when he first tried the foxglove in dropsies (see pp. 2-3); having learnt about its use by an old woman, he found it to be a powerful diuretic, but initially used doses which he later realized were too high, and all but stopped using it. At that time he simply commented in his *Botany* (see pp. 250-4) that the *Digitalis purpurea* 'merits more attention than modern practice bestows upon it'. Only when the report of *another* layman's use of the drug came to his ears (pp. 3 and 109) did he start again.

The extent of the influence of lay opinion on medical practice in the eighteenth century was considerable (Jewson 1974) and there have also been examples in recent times of the influence of the general public on medical discoveries, the best known being the diagnosis of Lyme disease (Harris 1983). How long would we have had to have waited for digitalis had it not been for 'an old woman of Shropshire' and 'a carpenter at Oxon'?

PART II

WILLIAM
WITHERING
OF
BIRMINGHAM

CHAPTER 3

WILLIAM WITHERING
OF BIRMINGHAM

William Withering was born on 17 March 1741, in the town of Wellington in Shropshire. He was the second child of Edmund Witherings [*sic*] and Sarah Hector, and had an elder sister, Mary, and a younger sister, Sarah. Virtually nothing is known of his boyhood beyond the fact that he was educated in the classics by the Reverend Henry Wood of Ercall. However, he grew up at a time of great social change in Britain, when dissension and non-conformism were flourishing in both theology and science, and when communications in the country were rapidly improving, with the building of new roads and canals. Coming as he did from a well-educated and well-to-do family, Withering would have doubtless grown up exposed to the stimulation of controversial opinion current at the time, and may even have met some of the intellectual luminaries of his day at the house of his uncle, Dr Brooke Hector, in Lichfield.

Withering's father was a successful apothecary, and there were several physicians on his mother's side of the family—his grandfather was George Hector, who delivered Samuel Johnson, according to Johnson's own account in his autobiography of his first eleven years (Johnson 1805); his uncle, Brooke Hector, was a well-known physician at Lichfield; and another uncle, George, and a cousin, Edmund, were surgeons. It is no surprise, therefore, that Withering's father wanted him to train as a physician. The process began, according to Withering's son, William Withering the Younger, in his memoir of his father (Withering 1822), by his being apprenticed to 'an experienced and deeply interested practitioner', who is not identified, but who was probably his uncle,

Brooke Hector. In 1762, at the age of 21, after four years of this apprenticeship, Withering was sent to study medicine at Edinburgh University.

Edinburgh was at that time one of the major centres of medical teaching in the British Isles, and boasted several eminent physicians and scientists. Many of the men mentioned in Withering's *Account* either studied at Edinburgh or had some important connection with Edinburgh University during their careers.

Withering's training included anatomy, chemistry, materia medica, and medicine, both theoretical and clinical. Anatomy was taught in classes of about 200 students by the then Associate Professor of Anatomy, Alexander Monro secundus (1733-1817), who was in the process of succeeding the then Professor of Anatomy, his father Alexander Monro primus (1697-1767), and who was to be succeeded in turn by his son, Alexander Monro tertius (1773-1859). Domination of a subject by a family in this way (for the 126 years from 1720 to 1846 in the case of the Monros) was not unusual in Edinburgh at that time, other dynasties including those of the Hamiltons and the Duncans. Chemistry, actually clinical chemistry and pharmacology, was taught at that time first by William Cullen (1710-90), one of the founders of the medical school at Glasgow and one-time Professor of Medicine there, and then in 1766 by Cullen's successor and pupil, Joseph Black (1728-99), the discoverer of fixed air (carbon dioxide) and of the principles of latent heat and specific heat. Cullen subsequently lectured on clinical medicine when he became Professor of the Institutes of Medicine in succession to Robert Whytt, the first physician to the King of Scotland. The Professor of Medicine was John Rutherford (1695-1799), and he was succeeded in 1766 by John Gregory (1724-73), later physician to the King of Scotland; he was succeeded in turn by Cullen in 1773. The Professor of Botany was John Hope who acceded to the Regius chair in 1761 and made great improvements to the physician's botanical garden and arranged its plants according to the Linnaean system.

It was the custom of the day to appoint, on behalf of each student, a tutor to take a special interest in the progress of that student. The tutor was expected to act not only as a teacher but as a moral guide and mentor, and tutors frequently entertained their students at their houses, as did Withering's tutor, a Dr Hay, about whom little is known, but who seems to have made Withering most welcome and to have contributed much to the young man's comfort and enjoyment while in the city.

Withering graduated MD in 1766 with a dissertation entitled *De Angina Gangraenosa*, dedicated to the Reverend Wood and to his uncle, Brooke Hector. The signatures on his diploma, dated 31 July (Osler Bequest 1928), are those of Alexander Monro (secundus), John Hope, Thomas Young, Alexander Monro (primus), William Cullen, and John Gregory. Of all his teachers Withering was likely to have been most influenced by Cullen and Black. Cullen was such an excellent lecturer that in 1771 his lectures were printed and published by a local publisher without his consent. He later came to an agreement with the publisher and sanctioned the publication. He is said to have been 'distinguished for his clearness of perception and sound reasoning and judgment rather than for epoch-making originality' (Bettany 1888), qualities which Withering would undoutedly have admired. Black, although a researcher of great insight and originality, gave up his research to devote himself full time to teaching after his appointment at Edinburgh in 1766. John Robison in his preface to Black's lectures, published in 1803, wrote:

'His personal appearance and manner were those of a gentleman, and peculiarly pleasing. His voice in lecturing was low but fine; and his articulation so distinct that he was perfectly well heard by an audience consisting of several hundreds. His discourse was so plain and perspicuous, his illustrations by experiment so apposite, that his sentiments on any subject never could be mistaken, even by the most illiterate; and his instructions were so clear of all hypothesis or conjecture, that the hearer rested on his conclusions with a confidence scarcely exceeded in matters of his own experience'.

The last comment on hypothesis and conjecture rings curiously similar to Withering's advice in a letter to Lady Catherine Wright, written at a later date (see note to p. xiii).

Withering would also have been influenced to some extent by Alexander Monro secundus, who was said to have been the finest of the three Monros, and John Gregory, since both were fine lecturers with simple, direct styles of presentation. Of Monro, Benjamin Rush is quoted (Wright-St Clair 1964) as having written that

'in anatomy he is superior perhaps to most men in Europe, he speaks with great propriety, and as he commits all his lectures to memory, he embellishes them when speaking with all the graces of elocution. He is a gentleman of great politeness and humanity, and much admired by every one that knows him'.

In contrast John Hope, while a good scientist, was not an inspiring lecturer, and Withering failed to show any interest in botany at that time (see p. 250).

After his graduation Withering made a tour of France, visiting Paris, but cut short his visit when his companion, a Mr Townshend, died following a wound which became infected and gangrenous. He returned at Christmas in 1766 and started to look around for a suitable position, chosing to practise first in Stafford on the death there of a Dr Buchanan, whose place he took. He helped to found the Stafford Infirmary and was one of its first two physicians, with Dr Archibald Campbell. One of Withering's first patients at Stafford in 1767 was Helena Cookes, the then 17-

year-old daughter of the Town Clerk, and Withering married her on 12 September 1772, after she had come of age.

Withering would probably have been content at Stafford had his wage not been so relatively low, averaging about £100 per annum, and he kept an eye open for more lucrative appointments elsewhere. His apportunity came in 1775, when he received a letter from Erasmus Darwin, who was a much respected physician in and around Lichfield, and the grandfather of Charles Robert Darwin (quoted by Roddis 1936).

Lichfield, February 25th, '75.

Dear Doctor

I am at this moment returned from a melancholy scene, the death of a friend who was most dear to me, Dr. Small, of Birmingham, whose strength of reasoning, quickness of invention, learning in the discoveries of other men, and integrity of heart (which is worth them all), had no equal. Mr Boulton suffers an inconceivable loss from the doctor's mechanical as well as medical abilities.

A person at Birmingham desired I would acquaint you with Dr. Small's death as soon as I could, but would not permit his name to be mentioned, lest he might disoblige some whom he did not wish to disoblige. It was said that Dr. Smith, who has been there a few months, had not chance at all of succeeding in that place from his defect in hearing. Now it occurred to me that if you should choose that situation your philosophical taste would give you the friendship of Mr. Boulton, which would operate all that for you which it did for Dr. Small. I saw by Dr. Small's papers that he had gained about 500 pounds a year at an average taking the whole time he had been at Birmingham, and above 600 pounds on the last years. Now as this was chiefly in the town, without the expense and fatigue of travelling and horsekeeping, and without being troubled and visiting the people, for he lived quite a recluse studious life, it appears to me a very eligible situation. Add to this that he had increased his fortune by some other circumstance of manufacture or schemes which such a town affords. If you should think that prospect worth your going to see Mr. Boulton at Soho to inquire further into, I will take care to leave at home a proper letter for you to him if I should not see you.

I was very fortunate in recommending Dr. Bates to Aylesbury, and Dr. Wright to Newark, but think in my own mind this of the internal business of Birmingham to be, all put together, the most eligible of any country situation, but I think no one who has not some philosophical acquirements as well as medical is likely to succeed in it.

I shall not mention having wrote this letter to you but I shall be glad of a line in answer, and please to put private on the internal cover.

Adieu,

E. Darwin.

To Dr. Withering.

Private.

The Mr Boulton referred to here was Matthew Boulton, a wealthy industrialist, who had a large factory in Soho, just to the north of Birmingham. He was also a Fellow of the Royal Society, and a founder member, with Darwin, Small, and Josiah Wedgwood, of the Lunar Society (Schofield 1963). He was an influential member of the committee of the Birmingham General Hospital.

Darwin's letter raises at least two questions: how did Darwin know, or know of Withering? and who was the anonymous recommender? If they had not yet met, Darwin could only have known of Withering's 'philosophical taste' from his sound but unimpressive paper on the type of soil known as marle, published in the *Philosophical Transactions* of 1773 (see p. 265). However, Darwin's letter is couched in such a way that suggests that he did know Withering personally, and it is likely that they met at the house of Brooke Hector in Lichfield, where Withering spent his holidays while studying at Edinburgh. Withering's anonymous benefactor may have been John Ash, an eminent Birmingham physician, and Small's close associate. This view is to some extent supported by a letter which Ash wrote to Withering on 2 March 1775, when it appeared that Withering would not be appointed to the vacant position (quoted in Peck and Wilkinson 1950).

> Sir,
>
> I should have been happy to have seen you at Birmingham to have had an opportunity of a free conversation with you on the subject of your settling here. All I wish for is an agreeable sensible man with whom I could live on the best of terms of a friendship such as my late dear friend, Dr. Small. A Dr. Merriott, from Shrewsbury is arrived. I am informed, but I have not seen him yet. I can't take any conspicuous part on such an occasion, but believe me to be your most sincere friend and honourable senior,
>
> John Ash.

Whatever happened to Dr Merriott, or the other contenders for the position, Withering was eventually appointed and moved on his own to Birmingham in May 1775, leaving his wife and daughter with his cousins in Tettenhall for the time being. To begin with he took lodgings at No. 10 The Square, with a Mr Wheeley, but he later moved to 9 Temple Row, which had been Small's residence, next door to John Ash, and brought his family. Later still, in 1786, he leased Edgbaston Hall, where he lived almost until his death, using No. 15 The Square as a town house.

Withering flourished in Birmingham and within a year he was

earning twice as much as he had at Stafford. He travelled extensively by horse-drawn carriage (over 6,000 miles in 1785, by his
own calculations) and his practice grew so rapidly that it was said
to be the largest outside of London. His income soon exceeded
£1,000 per annum, although, however large this may seem, it did
not rival the income of the most successful London physicians,
some of whom made in excess of £5,000 per annum. Withering's
income was undoubtedly restrained by his habit of treating poor
patients free (two or three thousand such each year) both in and
around Birmingham, where he held a daily clinic for the poor,
and in Stafford, which he visited regularly to attend his patients at
the Infirmary until the appointment of his successor, Dr Thomas
Fowler (see p. 121).

From 1776 onwards Withering was to suffer repeatedly from
fever and a chest complaint, and following the episode alluded to
in the *Account* (see p. 73) he correctly diagnosed tuberculosis. In
subsequent years this undoubtedly limited his activities. In 1790
he suffered a further attack of pleurisy, and in 1792 and 1793 he
took trips to Portugal to escape the English winter, staying at
Cintra near Estoril. However his health worsened gradually over
the next 6 years and in 1799, because he thought it bad for his
health to live at Edgbaston, he sold his house and bought a house
called Fairhill, on the high ground outside the city. Fairhill had
been the property of Joseph Priestley, but had been badly
damaged in the Birmingham riots of 1791. Withering renamed
the house The Larches and moved into it on 28 September. He
died eight days later on 6 October 1799, aged 58, and was
entombed in Edgbaston Old Church on 10 October.

WITHERING THE BOTANIST

As I have noted above, Withering was not excited to an interest in
botany by his studies under John Hope, the Professor of Botany at
Edinburgh. Indeed it seems to have been quite the reverse, for in a
letter to his parents he wrote:

WILLIAM WITHERING 251

The Botanical Professor gives annually a gold medal to such of his pupils as are most industrious in that branch of science. An incitement of this kind is often productive of the greatest emulation in young minds, though, I confess, it will hardly have charm enough to banish the disagreeable ideas I have formed of the study of botany.

We do not know how or why Withering subsequently became interested in botany, although it is characteristic of him that, having become interested in the subject, he made himself a master of it. Only two other possible influences can be adduced. One of his intimate friends while at Edinburgh and later was Richard Pulteney (1730-1801) who was subsequently to publish the first English biography of Linnaeus in 1781 and *The Historical and Biographical Sketches of the Progress of Botany in England* in 1790. It is not clear to what extent Pulteney influenced Withering, but when he met his future wife, Helena Cookes, in 1775, Withering started to scour the countryside around Birmingham for plants for her to sketch, and their flourishing relationship doubtless encouraged Withering in his botanical interests. To what extent his wife subsequently maintained his motivation is also not clear, but by 1776 Withering's knowledge of botany was sufficient for him to publish what in subsequent editions became the standard work in its field for many years to come, *The Botanical Arrangements of all the Vegetables naturally growing in Gt. Britain*. Withering's studies continued and in 1787 he published the second edition of his botany in two volumes, entitled *A Botanical Arrangement of British Plants* .... A third volume, produced in collaboration with his friend Jonathan Stokes, appeared in 1792. For reasons which are not entirely clear (Peck and Wilkinson 1950; Schofield 1963), Withering and Stokes fell out subsequently and Withering produced the third edition on his own; it appeared in four volumes in 1796, under the title *An Arrangement of British Plants*.

Withering's *Botany* was the first to delineate systematically in English the flora of Great Britain using the Linnaean system of classification. His contribution was widely recognized, to the extent that he was elected a Fellow of the Linnean [*sic*] Society in 1789 and had a genus named after him, the *Witheringia solanacea*, by the French botanist L'Héritier de Brutelle. Withering's obituarist, J Crane, wrote of it (Crane 1799) that while the first edition

> could be considered as little more than a mere translation from Linnaeus of such *genera* and species of plants as are indigenous in Great Britain; and in which Ray's Synopsis Methodica Stirpium Britannicum, and Hudson's Flora Anglica, could not fail to afford him great assistance;

in the two other editions

> this Arrangement has been so much improved and enlarged, as to have become, in a great measure, an original work; and certainly as a national Flora, it must be allowed to be the most elaborate and complete performance that any country can boast of.

Following Withering's death a further four editions of the botany appeared under the editorship of his son and entitled *A Systematic Arrangement of British Plants*. It continued to appear after his death under the editorship of William Macgillivray, and achieved great popularity, seeing 14 editions in all, the last appearing in 1877, 101 years after the first edition, although by that time it was said that it was 'very good; but long since superceded' (Allibone 1877).

In the painting of Withering made in 1792 by the Swedish artist Carl Frederik von Breda, Withering is shown holding a foxglove and glancing past a copy of the second volume of the second edition of his *Botany*, which is propped open on the table beside him at the entry on digitalis, article 816 on p. 654. The entry repeats the statement made in the first edition, that 'a dram

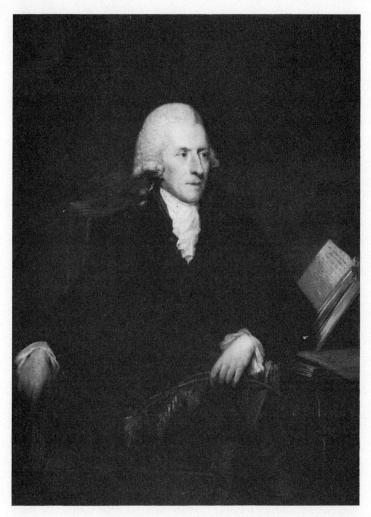

William Withering, by Carl Frederik von Breda (1792). Reproduced by permission of the Swedish National Museum, Stockholm.

of it taken internally excites violent vomiting. It is certainly a very active medicine and merits more attention than modern practice bestows upon it.' It adds 'for an account of its medical properties see Withering on the Foxglove, *Med. trans*. iii and *London Medical Journal*'. I shall discuss these sources later (see p. 280), since a study of them yields a fascinating story in regard to the first publications of accounts of the action of digitalis in dropsies.

WITHERING'S OTHER SCIENTIFIC ACTIVITIES

In the days of the Enlightenment, the so-called Age of Reason, it was common for men of an academic bent to take an interest in divers scientific matters, and Withering's interests went beyond medicine and botany. He took an avid interest in metallurgy and chemistry, and was an active member of the Lunar Society of Birmingham (Schofield 1963).

The Lunar Society was one of many similar associations of men interested in exchanging ideas and sharing friendship, and of all such associations it was said to be the most illustrious. It was called the Lunar Society from the habit of its members of meeting on the Monday nearest the full moon of each month, so that they might have the benefit of a moonlit night for travelling. It grew out of the association of Erasmus Darwin, Matthew Boulton, William Small, and Josiah Wedgwood, and first met in around 1765. However, the term 'Lunar Society' does not seem to have been used formally until about 1776, and it has been suggested (Schofield 1963) that the term 'Lunar Circle' be used for the group which met before that time, since they did not yet consider themselves to be a properly formed Society. In addition to their monthly meetings they met each other frequently, since they mostly lived in or around Birmingham, and corresponded frequently with each other too. The members of the circle were given to discussing a wide variety of scientific matters, and exchanged ideas and details of experiments they had carried out. On one occasion, for example, Darwin wrote to Boulton outlining his scheme for a 'fiery Chariot' based on his, admittedly imperfect, understanding of the workings of the steam engine. On other occasions they discussed the development of canals, the nature of electricity and magnetism, and the constitution of mineral ores. Indeed, there was little of current scientific interest that did not at some time or other come under the scrutiny of the members of the Lunar Society, who also included James Watt, R Lovell Edgeworth, the Samuel Galtons secundus and tertius, and Samuel Parr.

When Withering came to Birmingham in 1775 he took Small's place not only in the Birmingham General Hospital, but also as Boulton's physician, and subsequently in the Lunar Society, although he did not remain on such good terms with its members as Small had been, falling out as he did at least with Darwin and with Stokes, who joined the Society in 1779.

The list of Withering's publications (see pp. 265-7) demonstrates his wide scientific interests, which included, in addition to botany, medicine, and materia medica, soil analysis, mineral analysis, and chemistry. Indeed, his interest in chemistry was at one point so overwhelming that he wrote, in 1776, 'Botany now no longer presides at my board,—her season is past,—and chymistry overspreads the table' (quoted in Withering 1822). He was not, however, as widely accomplished as some of the other members of the Lunar Society, not having the wild inventive mind of Darwin, nor, by the evidence of his publications, the mechanical, mathematical, or astronomical interests of Small. However, in his memoir of his father, which is admittedly clearly inaccurate in parts, his son writes that his father's 'mechanical talents were exercised in the construction of philosophical apparatus, particularly in the improvement of electrical machines', and that 'he took some pains to ascertain how far the prevalent opinion of the weather being influenced by the lunar phases was consistent with facts'. Furthermore, it is known that he took an interest in the archaeology of Stonehenge from the letters his son included in his father's *Miscellaneous Tracts* (Withering 1822).

In 1784 Withering published his *Experiments and Observations on the Terra Ponderosa*, a paper in which he distinguished barium carbonate (terra ponderosa aerata) from barium sulphate (terra ponderosa vitriolata, or barytes). In making this distinction Withering invented the procedure which subsequently became the standard test for sulphates, using the property of terra ponderosa salita (i.e. barium chloride) to form the insoluble precipitate, barium sulphate. In his honour barium carbonate was later called Witherite by the German geologist Abraham Gottlob Werner (Hoffman 1789).

Withering was expert at the analysis of mineral waters, and studied many English waters, including those of St Erasmus's Well near Ingestre in Staffordshire, the Salt Marsh Water in the same part of the country, and Rowton Well in Sutton Park Warwickshire. His son wrote (Withering 1822) that he 'compounded in exact imitation the waters of Spa, Pyrmont, and Seltzer', and Withering himself wrote that he had analysed the Nevil Holt water, between Market Harborough and Uppingham 'which I can destroy and re-produce at pleasure'. Withering's analytical skill was acknowledged by Joseph Priestley, who wrote, in a paper on the 'principle of acidity, the composition of water, and phlogiston' (Priestley 1788):

> Dr. Withering was so obliging as to examine some of these liquors for me (for, not being much accustomed to these analyses, I had requested him to undertake it).

Consequently, when Withering visited Portugal in 1793 he was asked by the Portuguese government to undertake an analysis of the waters at Caldas da Rainha to the north of Lisbon. He completed his analysis satisfactorily, published the findings in Portuguese and English in 1795, and was honoured by being elected a Foreign Corresponding Member of the Portuguese Academy of Science.

In contrast to these successes Withering contributed little to the controversy surrounding phlogiston. What his precise attitudes to the theory were is not known. It seems that most, if not all the members of the Lunar Society, Priestley predominant amongst them, were in favour of the theory, but Withering is said to have delivered a humorous poem to the Society in 1796 entitled *The Life and Death of Phlogiston*. No copy of this poem exists, and it is not known whether Withering was being satirical or ironic, or truly expressing his own feelings about the theory.

WITHERING'S CHARACTER

It is an attribute of some biographers that they uncritically adulate the subjects of their biography. This is unfortunately true both of William Withering Junior in his 1822 memoir of his father, and of Peck and Wilkinson in their 1950 biography. The former can be excused (and indeed in his preface asks to be excused) on the grounds of filial devotion, but Peck and Wilkinson go to too great lengths to paint their hero in glowing terms, presumably having been overawed by his undoubted clinical expertise, scientific abilities, and important discoveries. Schofield, in his dispassionate and scholarly account of the Lunar Society of Birmingham (1963), is more realistic and recognizes Withering's faults as well as his virtues.

What sort of man was Withering? His son writes that 'during his earlier years [he] benefited by the counsels and instructions of his parents, who lost no opportunity of imbuing his mind with just moral sentiments and the genuine principles of religion', and this we can believe, for throughout his dealings with others Withering shows himself to be of high moral rectitude, although

at times he must have seemed to others to be somewhat sancti-
monious. He was not endowed, as I have mentioned above, with
great imagination, and we can again believe his son when he
writes that 'his juvenile course corresponded with each progres-
sive period of life; more distinguished for steady sense and correct
judgement than for the flights of fancy or the eccentricities of
genius.'

Although they contain much of scientific interest Withering's
letters are tedious in their composition, and particularly so when
they deal with domestic matters. From reading them one cannot
imagine that he was the most entertaining of companions, and
Withering realized this himself, as can be judged from a letter he
wrote to the Rev. Scholefield from Lisbon on 11 November 1792,
dealing with the sea voyage to Portugal:

> Some of the party at times diverted themselves by drawing [Dr.
> James Graham] out into conversation, but on these occasions I
> retired, finding my presence spoiled the sport.

James Graham was an eccentric quack who was on his way to
Portugal in the hope of giving unsolicited help to the sick Portuguese queen. Withering writes that Graham was 'either mad or
hypocritically religious', so that Withering's sport-spoiling was
unlikely to have been due to his having defended Graham against
the bear-baiting indulged in by his fellow travellers.

It is true that in his youth Withering seems to have had many
interests outside of medicine and science. He was a keen musician
and his son claimed that he 'excelled on the German [i.e. trans-
verse] flute, and was likewise a proficient on the harpsichord: he
well understood the science of music, and wanted only leisure, to
have become a fine performer on several instruments'. He is also
said to have tried the bagpipes when in Scotland. He was not
averse to sport and indulged in field activities in England and golf
in Scotland, although he probably did not take the latter seri-

ously, since at that time it involved very crude equipment and demanded a great deal of persistence to become expert. He became a Mason in Edinburgh, but there is no evidence that he persisted with Freemasonry on his return to England, where it was not held in such high regard as in Scotland, and in any case he seems to have joined only because 'to be associated with that fraternity had become a general recommendation'. He wrote poetry in the Ossianic style, and even in the composition of verse his depth of seriousness can be judged from his son's remarks: 'Nor did he unfrequently attempt the lighter kinds of poetry' but 'they displayed more the art of the scholar than the fire of the *poeta nascitur*'. Nor was he unromantic; his son wrote that while he was at Edinburgh 'the attractive *coteries* of what may there, with peculiar propriety, be termed the *fair sex*, whose *naïveté*, wit, and beauty could not but prove alluring', and that 'Horace, Tasso, the poems of Miss Carter, and Young's Night Thoughts, were also sharers of his walks'. However, it is hard to believe that Withering could have been able to devote much time to these pursuits; the work at Edinburgh was hard and he spent many a night in his room writing out full versions of his lecture notes for careful study; later, when he set up practice in Stafford he would have been thoroughly occupied, not only in his work, but also in his 'hobbies', i.e. researching his *Botany* and doing chemical and mineralogical experiments, not to mention giving private tuition to Miss Helena Cookes, to indulge spare-time activities. As Crane (1799) put it:

[he] devoted those hours which remained after the business of the day was over to philosophical and scientific pursuits.

Withering was a shy man and 'little qualified, either by constitution of body or turn of mind, for genial and social intercourse with the world . . . With his family and among his friends he was chearful and communicative; but with the world at large, and even in his professional character he was shy and reserved' (Crane 1799). However, although he was shy, Withering was also arrogant, or perhaps it would be more accurate to say self-satisfied (to use his own word). That that is so is amply illustrated by his dealings with his colleagues, in which he could be most irascible in cases where dispute occurred, and in which he thought himself to be in the right. The first occasion on which this happened was in the dispute with Erasmus Darwin, outlined in Chapter 4 (pp. 280-7), and he came into dispute with the Darwin family again in 1788 over the affair of Mrs Houlston, which is thoroughly documented by Peck and Wilkinson (1950). In brief, Withering was asked by an apothecary, Mr Cartwright, to attend Mrs Houlston in Wellington, which he did, travelling 26 miles to do so. Withering discovered that Dr Robert Darwin, Erasmus's third son, had attended her the day before and, disagreeing with Darwin's diagnosis, changed the prescription from port and quinine to calomel. Mrs Houlston became seriously ill and when Withering could not attend her he asked Darwin to do so. Withering attended her again on 8 October, and she seems to have made a slow recovery thereafter. However, shortly afterwards Withering was accused by Darwin of 'un-genteel medical behaviour' in the case, and Darwin claimed that Withering had slandered him by casting doubt on his (Darwin's) diagnosis. It is not possible to say from the subsequent exchange of letters, which are equally vituperative on both sides, which of them, if either, was in the right in this case. Young Darwin may have been incited by his father to attack Withering, and indeed the subsequent publication of their correspondence, at whose instigation it is not known, suggests that the Darwins may have felt there was some gain to be had from their publication, at Withering's expense. Withering for his part was exceptionally ungracious in his handling of the affair, and his insistence on the correctness of his behaviour in the matter seems only to have

WILLIAM WITHERING 261

inflamed the dispute. A more judicious approach than that which
he adopted might have allowed the matter to die down much
more quietly. In illustration of his attitude take the letter he sent
to Robert Darwin on 30 November 1788:

> Possessed, therefore, as I am of self-satisfaction, of the good
> opinion of the world at large, and of medical men in particular,
> your enmity or your friendship, your good or your bad
> opinion, are to me equally insignificant.

In fairness to Withering it must be stated that he did not seek
controversy at any time, but whether right or not in this case, and
Withering was the much more experienced of the two, Robert
Darwin being only 22 at the time, Withering's handling of the
affair betrays his arrogance and self-satisfaction, whether justi-
fied or not. It may be that his later dispute with Jonathan Stokes
was also exacerbated by his own intransigence and pride.

On another occasion Withering showed himself unable to
contain himself. When his *Botany* was unfavourably reviewed by
an anonymous reviewer in the *Monthly Review* of June 1785
Withering wrote to the editor, Griffiths, to complain on several
counts. Fortunately, the editor's response was placatory and ends
'I shall be glad to receive yr treatise on the *Foxglove*, and I make no
doubt but it will be candidly and properly treated in our Journal'.
It was (Anon. 1785d) (see p. 293).

No doubt some of this arrogance was due to Withering's
desire for accuracy, about which he was most punctilious, an
impression which is supported by Mrs Schimmelpenninck's
description of him in her autobiography (see p. 290). For example,
when Erasmus Darwin heard that he was preparing his *Botany*
for publication he wrote to Withering, not unreasonably,
suggesting that 'The Title of your Book should be easily remember'd, and easily distinguished from Lee etc. as "The Scientific
Herbal," "Linnean Herbal," "English Botany," "Botanologie

anglica in which the science of Botany is reduced to English," etc.'. Withering ignored Darwin's suggestions, choosing instead a much more cumbersome, albeit accurate, title, occupying 137 words in 24 lines on the title-page.

Withering's desire for strict accuracy is reflected in his introductory remarks in the *Account* (see p. v), in which he makes it clear that he would not have written the book at all had it not been for what he saw to be the widespread misuse of the foxglove as a therapeutic agent. Even so, and this may simply be false modesty, he appears to feel that his experience is still insufficient for the task: 'I am at length compelled to take up the pen, *however unqualified I may feel myself for the task*', and again, '... it is better the world should derive some instruction, *however imperfect*, from my experience ...' (my italics).

It is a curious thought that we might never have had Withering's *Account* to enjoy had it not been for the misunderstanding and inadequate practice of others.

A CHRONOLOGY OF
WITHERING'S LIFE

1708	Sarah Hector born, 18 November
1712	Edmund Witherings born, 30 December
1739	Withering's elder sister, Mary, born, 1 September
1741	Withering born, 17 March (his gravestone at Edgbaston says 28 March), Wellington, Shropshire Baptized, 13 April.
1750	Withering's younger sister, Sarah, born, 12 February
1758	Apprenticed to an unknown physician (?Brooke Hector)
1762	Goes to Edinburgh to study medicine
1766	Graduates from Edinburgh, MD. Dissertation *De Angina Gangraenosa* Tours France with Mr Townshend
1767	Starts to practise in Stafford Meets Miss Helena Cookes
1769	Edmund Witherings dies of contagious fever, buried 7 November
1772	Marries Helena Cookes, 12 September
1775	Moves to Birmingham Joins Lunar Society Withering's first child, Helena born (dies 10 March, 1776)
1776	First edition of the *Botany* published in May First signs of tuberculosis William Withering Junior born
1778	Outbreak of scarlet fever in Birmingham Charlotte Withering born

1779   *An Account of the Scarlet Fever* published
         Appointed honorary physician at the Birmingham
         General Hospital, September

1781   Carriage accident, breaks collar-bone and is concussed

1783   Severely ill with tuberculosis (which he diagnoses)

1784   Discovers Witherite (barium carbonate)

1785   Elected a Fellow of the Royal Society
         Publication of *An Account of the Foxglove*, 8 July

1786   Leases Edgbaston Hall

1787   Second edition of the *Botany* published
         Elected to the London Medical Society
         Witheringia solanacea named after him by L'Héritier de
         Brutelle

1789   Elected a Fellow of the Linnean Society
         Mother dies, 3 July

1791   Birmingham riots, July; Priestley's house ruined

1792   Painted by Carl Frederik von Breda
         Third edition of the *Botany* published
         Resigns as honorary physician from the Birmingham
         General Hospital, June
         Winters in Portugal

1793   Winters in Portugal
         Studies the waters of Caldas da Rainha

1795   Elected Foreign Corresponding Member of the Portu-
         guese Academy of Science

1799   Moves to Fairhill, Priestley's old house, which he
         renames The Larches
         Dies, 6 October
         Entombed in Edgbaston Old Church, 10 October

WITHERING'S PUBLICATIONS

1766   *Dissertatio medica inauguralis, de angina gangraenosa.* Edinburgh, Auld and Smellie. (An English translation has been published in 1953 in the *Journal of the History of Medicine*, **8**, 16-45).

1773   *Experiments upon the different kinds of marle found in Staffordshire. *Phil. Trans.* **63**, 161-2.

1776   *A botanical arrangement of all the vegetables naturally growing in Great Britain.* T. Cadell, P. Elmsley, and G. Robinson, Birmingham.

1779   *An account of the scarlet fever and sore throat or scarlatina anginosa ... particularly as it appeared in Birmingham in 1778.* T. Cadell, London.

1782   *An analysis of two mineral substances, viz. the Rowley rag-stone and the toad-stone. *Phil. Trans.* **72**, 327-36.

1783   *Outlines of mineralogy.* T. Cadell, G. Robinson, J. Balfour, and C. Elliott, London (Translation of Torbern Bergman's *Sciagraphia regni mineralis*.)

1784   *Experiments and observations on the terra ponderosa. *Phil. Trans.* **74**, 293-311.

1785   *An account of the foxglove and some of its medical uses: with practical remarks on the dropsy, and some other diseases.* G. G. J. and J. Robinson, London.

1786   *A letter on the arsenical solution. In *Medical reports of the effects of arsenic in the cure of agues, remitting fevers, and periodic headaches.* (T. Fowler). J. Johnson and W. Brown, London. pp. 113-31.

1787-92 *A botanical arrangement of British plants*, 2nd edn. M. Swinney, Birmingham (Vols. 1 and 2, 1787; vol. 3, 1792).

1788   *A letter to Joseph Priestley, L.L.D. on the principle of acidity, the decomposition of water. *Phil. Trans.* **78**, 319-30.

1790   *An account of some extraordinary effects of lightning. *Phil. Trans.* **80**, 293-5.

1793   *An account of the scarlet fever and sore throat, or scarlatina anginosa; particularly as it appeared at Birmingham in the year 1778, 2nd edition, to which are now prefixed, some remarks on the nature and cure of the ulcerated sore throat*. G.G. and J. Robinson, London.

1794   *A new method for preserving fungi, ascertained by chymical experiments. *Trans. Linnean Soc.* **2**, 263-6

1794   A letter on pulmonary consumption and other letters. In *Letters from Dr. Withering, Dr Ewart, Dr Thornton, and Dr Briggs together with some other papers supplementary to two publications on asthma, consumption, fever, and other diseases*. (ed. T. Beddoes) Bristol.

1795   *Analyse chimica da aqua das Caldas da Rainha. A chemical analysis of the water of Caldas da Rainha*. Lisbon. (Portuguese and English)

1796   Observations on the pneumatic medicine. *Ann. Med.* **1**, 392-3.

1796   An arrangement of British plants, 3rd edn. M Swinney, Birmingham.

1799   *An account of a convenient method of inhaling the vapour of volatile substances. *Ann. Med.* **3**, 447-51.

William Withering Junior published his *Miscellaneous Tracts* in
1822, in two volumes, containing his own Memoir of his father,
some miscellaneous correspondence (including that with James
Morris on the subject of Stonehenge), and other minor items,
followed by those of the publications asterisked above.

Many of Withering's unpublished letters are held in the Royal
Society of Medicine and the Birmingham Reference Library.

CHAPTER 4

WITHERING'S DISCOVERY AND USE OF THE FOXGLOVE

During one of his journeys in 1775, perhaps when visiting his patients at Stafford, Withering was shown a 'receipt' for the treatment of the dropsy and was asked his opinion on it. As he later wrote in his *Account* (see p. 2):

> I was told that it had long been kept a secret by an old woman in Shropshire, who had sometimes made cures after the more regular practitioners had failed. I was informed also, that the effects produced were violent vomiting and purging; for the diuretic effects seemed to have been overlooked. This medicine was composed of twenty or more different herbs; but it was not difficult for one conversant in these subjects, to perceive, that the active herb could be no other than the Foxglove.

There is no evidence that Withering ever met the old woman of Shropshire, who has come to be known as Mrs Hutton, and neither is there any clue as to who brought her recipe to his attention. The ease with which Withering picked out the active principle of the recipe from among twenty or so herbs seems astounding, but, as I have discussed in my note to p. 2, may have been based on the obvious worthlessness of most, if not all of the other ingredients, and perhaps on the analogy with the actions of the squill, which he knew to be effective in dropsy, and which he knew shared certain other properties with the foxglove, namely its ability to cause nausea, vomiting, and purging.

True to his character (see pp. 257-62), Withering was at first cautious. He started to give the foxglove to the poor patients he treated free in Birmingham and found that it succeeded in only a few. Of these cases Withering reported only one (p. 11), a case with a successful outcome, and in the first edition of his *Botany* he restricted himself to saying that the *Digitalis purpurea* 'merits more attention than modern practice bestows upon it' (see pp. 253-4).

In 1776 Withering heard from his friend Dr John Ash of the case of Dr Cawley. Ash had presumably heard of the case from Dr William Vivian, Cawley's physician, a fellow of Corpus Christi College, Oxford, and Regius Professor of Medicine at the Radcliffe Infirmary. Dr Ralph Cawley, the President of Brazen Nose (now Brasenose) College (see p. 3), had been treated for dropsy by Vivian and physicians from London, but without success. As his brother, Robert Cawley, later informed Withering in his letter dated 31 May 1785 (see p. 109), Ralph Cawley had been told of 'a carpenter at Oxon that had been cured of a hydrops pectoris by the foxglove root', and had dosed himself with such a preparation with success sufficient to prolong his life, his brother thought, for the space of a year. From the account of the prescription Cawley had used Withering deduced that he might have taken twelve times the usually effective dose, and he expressed surprise that Cawley had survived so long. However, the content of glycosides in foxgloves varies through the year, and the root has the lowest content of all, so that Cawley's method may have been, albeit by good luck alone, correct (see p. 111).

It was Ash's description of the case when Cawley was still alive that prompted Withering to take up the use of the plant more vigorously than he had before, and again his knowledge of botany seems to have proved useful. He knew that the amounts of active principles, both in different parts of a biennial plant and at different times of the year, would be variable. He therefore decided to use only one part of the plant, namely the leaves, and to gather them always at the same time of the year, namely when the plant was about to flower, in order to ensure some degree of uniformity of dosage. He started by using a *decoction* of the dried leaves but became dissatisfied with that formulation, because he found firstly, that great accuracy of dosing was required for a satisfactory therapeutic effect without toxicity and secondly, that the reproducibility of extraction of the active principles from the plant by preparing a decoction was poor. As he put it (p. 4), 'I suspected that this degree of accuracy was not reconcileable with the use of a *decoction*, as it depended not only upon the care of those who had the preparation of it, but [also since] its active properties might be impaired by long boiling'. He consequently experimented with an *infusion*, and later still, presumably hoping to improve his methods even further, and looking for greater accuracy in dosing, tried a formulation of *dried powdered leaf*.

ANALYSIS OF WITHERING'S RESULTS

To what extent did Withering's strategy of changing his formulations of the foxglove pay off? In an attempt to answer this and other questions about Withering's use of the foxglove, I have analysed the 162 cases he treated during the ten years from 1775 to 1784. The results are shown in the several Figures which follow, some of which can be compared with the similar previous analysis of Estes and White (1965).

In Fig. 4.1 is shown the age and sex distribution of the patients Withering treated. Their average age was around 46 years. This is a much lower average figure than one would expect today, since about 90 per cent of patients being treated with digitalis nowadays are over 60 years of age. However, this difference reflects the difference in life expectancy between the eighteenth and the twentieth centuries, the average life expectancy at the end of the eighteenth century being around 40 years of age (see note to

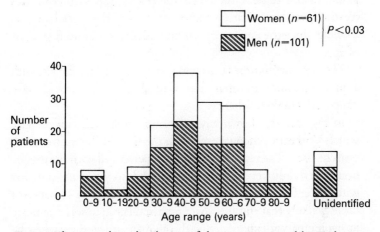

Fig. 4.1. The age and sex distribution of the 162 cases treated by Withering (1775-84).

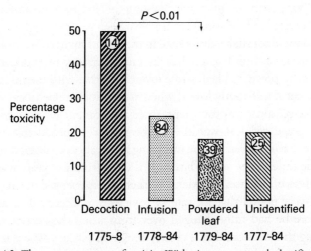

Fig. 4.2. The percentage rates of toxicity Withering encountered, classified by the different formulations of digitalis he used. The numbers in each bar refer to the numbers of cases treated with the relevant formulation. 'P' refers to the statistical comparison between groups (chi-square test).

p. 64). In this respect, therefore, the population Withering was treating was not entirely representative of the population as a whole, since the average age of his patients was around 46 years of age.

The sex distribution of his patients was unequal (Fig. 4.1) with a preponderance of men, but I think that that could have happened simply by chance.

In Fig. 4.2 are shown my estimates of the rates of toxicity which Withering encountered with the three different formulations he used. The rate of toxicity he experienced with the decoction is certainly very high, being around 50 per cent, and that with the infusion much lower, around 25 per cent. However, I think it likely that this improvement in technique was due more to his increasing experience with the drug at the time when he was changing formulations, rather than to the change in formulation itself, for four reasons. Firstly, I do not think it likely that the variability in glycoside content of the two formulations (decoction and infusion) would have been great enough to have accounted for such a difference in the rate of toxicity. Secondly, it can be seen from Fig. 4.2 that the rate of toxicity he experienced with the powdered leaf, while lower than that with the infusion, was not significantly lower, whereas in this case one *would* have expected some improvement, since the content of glycoside in the powdered leaf would have been more reproducible from time to time, given that he was using leaves always gathered at the same time of the year. Thirdly, it is clear from my year-by-year analysis of the rates of toxicity Withering experienced during this ten-year period that his rate of toxicity was already decreasing before he had fully changed over from using the decoction to using the infusion; that is clearly shown in Fig. 4.3, where it can be seen that his toxicity rate declined steadily from 1775/76 to 1779/80, despite the fact that he only started to use the infusion in 1778. Fourthly, there is the matter of Withering's *therapeutic* success with the foxglove, which was the same with all three formulations (see below). All this is not to say that Withering's strategy in changing formulations as he did was unreasonable—far from it—his strategy was sensible and based on sound reasoning. It is simply that the effect this strategy had on his success with the foxglove in terms of avoiding toxicity was probably small by comparison with the effect of his increasing experience with the drug.

Turning to Withering's success in terms of the therapeutic efficacy of the foxglove in cases of dropsy, my analysis is shown in Fig. 4.4. His success rate was very high, being around 65 per cent to 80 per cent, and did not differ greatly from formulation to formulation. However, it is curious that in the 25 cases for which he does not say which formulation he used, his success rate was very poor, being around 20 per cent, significantly lower than his

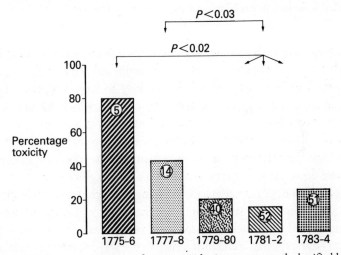

Fig. 4.3. The percentage rates of toxicity Withering encountered, classified by the year of use. The numbers in each bar refer to the numbers of cases treated during the relevant years. 'P' refers to the statistical comparisons between the groups (chi–square test).

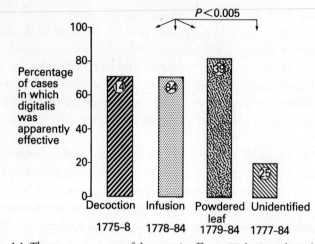

Fig. 4.4. The percentage rates of therapeutic efficacy Withering achieved with the foxglove, classified by the different formulations he used. The numbers in each bar refer to the numbers of cases treated with the relevant formulation. 'P' refers to the statistical comparison between the groups (chi-square test).

success rate with each of the three formulations, when specified. This is a phenomenon which I find difficult to explain. The difference is so large that it is unlikely to have happened by chance, and I suspect that these are cases in which his lack of success made him keep less than perfect notes, or perhaps cases in which he was in too great a hurry both to keep proper notes and to treat the patients in as careful a manner as he would otherwise have done. As to his success rate with the foxglove over the ten years, that does not seem to have changed much, as shown in Fig. 4.5, and that is not surprising, since the mixture of cases Withering treated was much the same from year to year, and one would not have expected much difference in the way his patients would have responded at different times.

In Table 4.1 are listed the various types of cases which Withering treated, showing my estimates of his rates of efficacy and

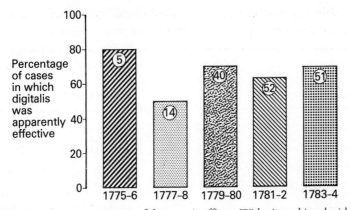

Fig. 4.5. The percentage rates of therapeutic efficacy Withering achieved with the foxglove, classified by the year of use. The numbers in each bar refer to the numbers of cases treated during the relevant years.

toxicity. In making this list I have largely kept to Withering's own terms, which are a mixture of descriptions of syndromes (e.g. anasarca, ascites) and definitive diagnoses (e.g. ovarium dropsy). This is because in the majority of the former it is not possible to give a definitive aetiological label to the cases, although in some cases the diagnosis can be hazarded with a reasonable degree of confidence, for example the case of hypertrophic obstructive cardiomyopathy (p. 66). The difficulty of making accurate diagnoses can be illustrated by considering the problem of ascites in heavy drinkers, which was likely to have been due to alcoholic cirrhosis, but could also have been due, at least in part, to heart failure, which in turn might have been due to alcoholic cardiomyopathy or to some other cardiac disease unrelated to alcohol; alternatively heart failure in those patients could have led to hepatic cirrhosis because of long-standing hepatic venous congestion.

It is clear from Table 4.1 that while Withering's rates of toxicity did not differ greatly from disease to disease, his rates of

Table 4.1. Withering's rates of therapeutic success and toxicity in the different types of condition he treated (162 cases)

Condition	Total	Effective	Toxic
		Number of patients treated	
1. Asthma + dropsy	28	25 (89%)	10 (36%)
2. Dropsy/anasarca	24	19 (79%)	4 (17%)
3. Anasarca + ascites			
(a) Non-drinkers	39	31 (79%)	10 (26%)
(b) Drinkers	31	15 (48%)	9 (29%)
4. Hydrothorax	4	4(100%)	1 (25%)
5. Tuberculosis	15	3 (20%)	1 (7%)
6. Ovarium dropsy	6	0	2 (33%)
7. Others	15	10 (67%)	3 (20%)
(a) Phlegmasia	4	4	1
(b) Hydrocephalus	3	1	0
(c) Renal stone	3	3	1
(d) [Acute renal failure]	2	0	0
(e) Epilepsy/vomiting/lead poisoning (one case each)	3	2	0

Statistical comparisons. The following groups differ significantly from each other in terms of the frequency of therapeutic response (chi-square test; probabilities, P, that there are no differences given in parentheses):

Drinkers versus non-drinkers ($P < 0.01$)
Patients with tuberculosis versus groups 1, 2, and 3(a) ($P < 0.0001$)
Patients with ovarium dropsy versus groups 1, 2, and 3(a) ($P < 0.0001$)

efficacy reflect precisely what one would expect from our current understanding of the actions of digitalis: high success rates in patients with cardiac failure, however it presented (e.g. with asthma, i.e. left ventricular failure, or with anasarca, i.e. oedema), and low success rates in almost all other conditions. His apparently high rate of success in cases of post-puerperal pelvic vein thrombosis (phlegmasia) was almost certainly due to spontaneous resolution of the condition, as presumably it was in cases of renal stone.

It is of interest to note that if one divides those cases of anasarca with ascites into those patients whom Withering says were drinkers and those about whom he says nothing of their drinking habits, the success rates are significantly different. Presumably many of those whom he says were intemperate or 'loose livers' had hepatic cirrhosis, in which cases one would not expect digitalis to be of great value.

Striking for their low rates of efficacy are two conditions, ovarium dropsy (i.e. ovarian cyst) and tuberculosis. The results in ovarium dropsy were so clear cut and the condition so relatively simple to understand that digitalis seems not to have been used again for that indication. However, in the case of tuberculosis, although he did write that it is not useful, Withering was dubious about his lack of success, and he makes it clear, both by his persistent use of it, even after failure in most of the cases in which he tried it, and by his comments towards the end of the *Account* (pp. 204-6), that he thought that digitalis *should* be effective in cases of tuberculosis. That notion was later promulgated by others (see pp. 309-12 and 320-22).

Most of Withering's conclusions about the effects of digitalis in different diseases cannot be faulted, as can be seen from my summary of his conclusions in Table 4.2, and in those cases where they appear to be wrong he can be seen to have had too little experience to be criticized for his judgments.

It can be seen from this analysis, that by the time Withering was ready to publish his *Account* he had amassed a large amount of experience in the use of digitalis in a wide variety of conditions,

Table 4.2. A summary of Withering's conclusions on which conditions would respond to digitalis and which would not (from pp. 193-207)

Description	Qualifications	Conclusions
ANASARCA	Subcutaneous	. . . generally curable
	In . . . the lungs	. . . generally curable
	[With] enlarged viscera	
	(i) without ascites	. . . incurable
	(ii) with ascites	. . . [the] water may be removed by diuretics
	[Severe oedema]	. . . the cure cannot be effected by diuretics
ASCITES	In children	. . . curable
	In adults	. . . generally incurable by medicines
ASCITES and ANASARCA	[Due to] irremediably diseased viscera or [chronic] gout	Incurable
	In every other situation	. . . yields to diuretics and tonics
ASCITES, ANASARCA, and HYDROTHORAX		[Only] the symptoms admit of relief
ASTHMA	Spasmodic	. . . not relieved
	Anasarca of the lungs	. . . generally to be cured by diuretics
	Infarction of the lungs	. . . incurable
ASTHMA and ANASARCA		. . . expect a recovery
ASTHMA and ASCITES		. . . not incurable if the abdominal viscera are found

Table 4.2. (*cont.*)

Description	Qualifications	Conclusions
ASTHMA, ASCITES, and ANASARCA		THE curability will depend upon [various] circumstances
EPILEPSY	[With] effusion	. . . the Digitalis will effect a cure
HYDATID DROPSY		It does not admit of a cure
HYDROCEPHALUS		I have not yet been able to determine whether the Digitalis [is or is not useful]
HYDROTHORAX	[Including] the dropsy of the pericardium	It is very universally cured by the Digitalis
HYDROTHORAX and ANASARCA		. . . may always be cured by the Digitalis
INSANITY	[If due to] anasarca	. . .the happiest effects may be expected from the Digitalis
NEPHRITIS CALCULOSA		. . . the Foxglove [removes] the Dysuria and other symptoms
OVARIUM DROPSY		. . . defies the power of medicine

Table 4.2. *(cont.)*

Description	Qualifications	Conclusions
OVARIUM DROPSY with ANASARCA		The Digitalis removes [the ana sarca] for a time
PHTHISIS PULMONALIS		... the Digitalis is no longer useful in consumptive cases
PUERPERAL ANASARCA		... admits of an easy and certain cure by the Digitalis

and had become expert at its administration. Yet is appears from his own remarks (see pp. v and 8) that others had not learnt how to use the drug satisfactorily, and that it was that which drove him to publish his *Account*. I think that there were at least two other reasons. Firstly, as I have suggested in Chapter 3, Withering, although shy, was also filled with an arrogant sense of his own correctness in those matters in which he was expert. The last sentence of his preface to the *Account* (p. x) suggests that he wanted to demonstrate his expertise for the sake of both his contemporaries and posterity: 'After all, *in spite of opinion, prejudice, or error*, TIME will fix the real value upon this discovery, and determine whether I have imposed upon myself and others, or contributed to the benefit of science and mankind' (my italics). I do not think that Withering was in any doubt about the matter.

PUBLICATIONS ON THE FOXGLOVE ANTEDATING WITHERING'S *ACCOUNT*

The second reason which I believe contributed towards Withering's decision to publish his *Account* relates to the altercation he had with Erasmus Darwin over the case Withering lists as Case IV. For a more detailed account of the facts surrounding that case we must go back to two of the references Withering gave in the second edition of his *Botany* ('*Med. trans.* iii and *London Medical Journal*'), and from the former of those to a publication of 1780. For the history of the 1780 publication we must first consider the life of one Charles Darwin (E. Darwin 1780).

Charles Darwin was born at Lichfield in September 1758, the son of Erasmus Darwin. Had he lived beyond his twentieth year he would also have become the uncle of his more famous namesake. A child of precocious intelligence, Charles was sent to study at Oxford at the age of 16 and matriculated at Christ Church. He remained there for a year, but 'thought the vigour of the mind languished in the pursuit of classical elegance, like Hercules at the distaff, and sigh'd to be removed to the robuster exercises of the medical schools of *Edinburgh*' (E. Darwin 1780). In 1778 'he gained the first medal offered by the Aesculapian Society for a criterion to distinguish matter from mucus', and in the same year 'prepared a thesis for his graduation on the retrograde motions of the lymphatic vessels in some diseases' (these last two quotations are taken from his monument in St Cuthbert's graveyard in Edinburgh, quoted by E. Darwin 1780). Charles was regarded by his contemporaries as a brilliant young man 'by whose genius and industry the art of medicine might have been much improved' (Anon. 1778), but he died in May 1778 of what sounds from its description in the *Medical Commentaries* (Anon. 1778) like acute adrenal haemorrhage secondary to meningococcal septicaemia (Waterhouse-Friderichsen syndrome), possibly following a wound received during dissecting the brain of a child with hydrocephalus.

Two years later Erasmus Darwin published a pamphlet containing Charles's gold medal essay, along with an English translation of his graduation thesis (C. Darwin 1780). At pp. 103-12 there was added 'A note belonging to *page* 65, *and* 68'. The note contains a description of nine cases of dropsy, eight of which were treated with foxglove—two of anasarca of the lung, two of hydrops pericardii, one of hydrops thoracis, and three of ascites—with varied success. The note ends with nine 'Queries' relating to the nature of dropsies, and the possible use of foxglove 'in hydrocephalus internus, in hydrocele, and in white swelling of the joints [i.e. tuberculous arthritis]'. The chapters to which the note refers are entitled 'The phaenomena of dropsies explained' and 'Of cold sweats'. This material constitutes the first published account of the use of digitalis in the treatment of dropsies, ante-dating Withering's *Account* by five years.

On the face of it, it would appear that the young Charles Darwin had seen and treated eight cases of dropsies with digitalis and had written up his results with the possible intention of publishing them later. Indeed, the section starting on p. 65 to which the 'Note' refers deals with the generalities of the treatment of anasarca with emetics, and specifically mention digitalis: 'repeated vomits, and cupreous salts, and small doses of squill, or foxglove, are so efficacious in this disease'.

There is no doubt that Charles could have come to hear of the efficacy of the foxglove in dropsies by the time he wrote his dissertation, at least from his father, if not from his teachers at Edinburgh, since word might not have reached official ears there before Charles heard of it, and perhaps not even until 1779 (see p. xx). However, there is evidence that it was not Charles, but his father, Erasmus, who wrote the appendix to Charles's post-humous publication. Firstly, there is nothing in that appendix which says clearly that it was written by Charles. The intro-ductory paragraph merely says 'The foxglove has been given to dropsical patients in this country with considerable success: the following cases are related with design to ascertain the particular kinds of dropsy, in which this drug is preferable to squill, or other evacuants'. Secondly, in 1785 Erasmus sent to the College of Physicians of London, for publication in its *Medical Transactions*, a paper dated 14 January 1785 and entitled 'An account of the successful use of foxglove in some dropsies, and in the pulmonary consumption'. In that paper Darwin wrote that in the pamphlet of his son's works, published in 1780 'I subjoined about half a dozen cases of dropsies treated successfully by the decoction of *digitalis*', and that he had since treated 'at least a score of other cases, cured by the same method' (Darwin 1785). In the paper he described seven of those in detail, three of dropsies of the thorax and limbs, three of dropsies of the abdomen, and one of (cardiac) asthma. In addition he described the successful use of digitalis in cases of pulmonary consumption, scrophulous ulcers, and melancholia. He advertised the full title of the pamphlet of his son's works twice in the course of the paper, and at the same time (13 January) wrote to his bookseller offering to send him another hundred copies of 'my pamphlet', no doubt anticipating some demand for the publication following the inclusion of his paper in the *Medical Transactions*. Later, in the first edition of his *Zoonomia*, Erasmus again published his son's pamphlet with its appendix and again laid claim to the authorship of the latter. There seems no reason to doubt his claim.

Darwin's motives in all this are not clear, but one must suspect that he acted as he did in order to have it appear that it was he who had introduced the foxglove into clinical practice, perhaps as a spite to Withering. At no time did he mention Withering's name in connection with the foxglove, and indeed in the *Zoonomia* he went so far as to omit a sentence which had been included in the original 1780 pamphlet, and which might have been taken to refer to Withering. In referring to the aetiology of dropsy Charles Darwin had written: '. . . as I have been well informed by a physician of extensive practice and careful observation', a description which fits Withering perfectly. There is no record of Charles's ever having met Withering, although it is likely that they did meet in Lichfield, but whether or not the careful physician to whom Charles referred was Withering, Erasmus's omission of that sentence, and that sentence alone, from his reprint of Charles's original pamphlet casts suspicion on his intentions in reporting this particular medical discovery.

How did Darwin learn about the foxglove? The answer can be found on pp. 12-16 of Withering's *Account* where he relates the case of a Mrs H——, of A——, near N——: 'I have been more particular in the narrative of this case, partly because Dr. Darwin has related it rather imperfectly in the notes to his son's posthumous publication, trusting, I imagine, to memory ...' (see p. 16). Darwin, having failed to relieve this patient's dropsy asked Withering for his advice on 25 July 1776. Withering instructed him in the use of the foxglove, and together they successfully treated her. The woman was identified by Darwin in his unpublished *Commonplace Book* as Mrs Hill of Aston, and Darwin published her case as the first of the nine appended to his son's pamphlet. I shall give here an account of the case in full so that it can be directly compared with Withering's account on pp. 12-16:

Anasarca of the Lungs

1. A LADY, between forty and fifty years of age, had been indisposed sometime, was then seized with cough, and fever, and afterwards expectorated much digested mucus. This expectoration suddenly ceased, and a considerable difficulty of breathing supervened, with a pulse very irregular both in velocity and strength; she was much distressed at first lying down, and at first rising; but *after a minute or two bore either of those attitudes with ease*. She had no pain or numbness in her arms; she had no hectic fever, nor any cold shiverings, and *the urine was in due quantity; and of the natural colour*.

THE difficulty of breathing was twice considerably relieved

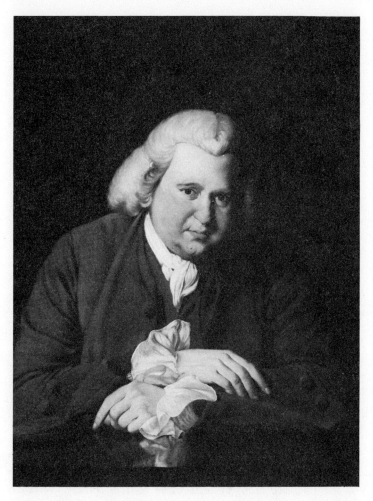

Erasmus Darwin, by Joseph Wright of Derby (1770). Reproduced by permission of the National Portrait Gallery, London.

by small doses of ipecacuanha, which operated upwards and downwards, but recurred in a few days: she was then directed a decoction of foxglove, (digitalis purpurea) prepared by boiling four ounces of the fresh leaves from two pints of water to one pint to which was added two ounces of vinous spirit; she took three large spoonfuls of this mixture every two hours, till she had taken it four times; a continued sickness supervened, with frequent vomiting, and a copious flow of urine: these evacuations continued at intervals for two or three days, and relieved the difficulty of breathing—She had some relapses afterwards, which were again relieved by the repetition of the decoction of foxglove.

Darwin's account of the case is accurate enough when compared with Withering's, albeit incomplete. However, Withering was clearly determined to show that it was he who had taught Darwin about the foxglove, and to do so in a manner which demonstrated Darwin's inability to report a case accurately.

Darwin's 1780 publication was not the only description of the successful use of digitalis in dropsies to antedate Withering's *Account*. In 1781 an editorial note in the *London Medical Journal* stated that 'some experiments have lately been made in the Royal Infirmary at Edinburgh with the *digitalis purpurea*, or *foxglove*, which prove it to be a medicine of considerable efficacy in dropsy' (Anon. 1781). Physicians at Edinburgh had come to learn of the foxglove from at least three sources. Firstly, Jonathan Stokes had delivered a lecture on the subject to the Medical Society of Edinburgh on 20 February 1779, having learnt of it from Withering (see p. xx). Secondly, Charles Darwin would presumably have informed at least his student colleagues, if not necessarily his teachers, of his father's use of the plant. Thirdly, Charles's posthumous pamphlet was reviewed in the *Medical Commentaries*, which were published in Edinburgh under the auspices of the influential physician Andrew Duncan the elder (see p. 8).

In 1785 the editor of the *London Medical Journal* reviewed the reports of their experience with the foxglove that he had received from Dr Karr of Huntingdon, formerly resident at the Edinburgh Royal Infirmary, and Dr Simmons of the Westminster General Dispensary. Dr Karr had been unsuccessful in his efforts, but Dr Simmons, who had heard of its use by 'a very respectable physician at Derby' (probably Darwin, who moved there in 1781), found it of value in certain cases, two of which are described. The editorial is not dated, but it follows an entry dated 23 February, 1785 (Anon. 1785*e*).

Later in the same volume of the *London Medical Journal*, in a letter dated 2 May, 1785, Dr John Warren of Taunton related the successful use of digitalis in four cases of dropsies, quoting Charles Darwin's posthumous pamphlet, evidently believing him to have been the author of its subjoined note (Warren 1785).

Finally, Darwin's paper in the *Medical Transactions* of the College of Physicians of London (Darwin 1785), published in haste in a clear attempt to pre-empt Withering, was followed by a paper by Sir George Baker (Baker 1785c), in which he described the case of a man with anasarca which he had been unable to relieve with quicksilver, squill, salt of wormwood, peruvian bark, lignum quaffiae, oil of juniper berries, a decoction of the tops of broom with salt of tartar, and a powder of broomseeds. He sought the advice of Darwin, who suggested the use of the foxglove, and the patient made a full recovery after a stormy course over the subsequent two months. Baker went on to use the foxglove in other cases, and in his paper describes two such, ending with a short description of the history of the previous medical use of the herb.

Although Darwin's failure to mention Withering in any of his publications was clearly deliberate and reprehensible, the similar failure of the others mentioned above may have been due to their ignorance of Withering's contribution, although competition for publication ran at least as high among medical men of that time as it does today. Sir George Baker, and probably Dr Simmons, learnt of the foxglove through Darwin, and Dr Karr through either Charles Darwin or Jonathan Stokes (although one would have expected the latter to have mentioned Withering in his lecture at Edinburgh). Dr Warren seems to have heard of its use in a fashion similar to Withering and Dr Cawley, as an old wives' recipe. Baker mentions that the case of the 'gentleman at Oxford, who has been reported to have been cured of a dropsy by a decoction of the roots of foxglove, became the subject of medical conversation in London' (presumably through Vivian or Ash), so that knowledge of Dr Cawley's case was another means whereby report may have been spread. However, Baker may also have spoken with Withering about the foxglove for he says that 'a person, who speaks from original experience, has informed me, that the success of this remedy does not depend on its exciting nausea', an observation which was documented by Withering, but which is not to be found in other contemporary accounts

DARWIN'S CHARACTER

It is not perhaps surprising that Withering and Darwin found some excuse for falling out, since they were of vastly different characters, and Withering was the sort of man most likely to annoy Darwin. My assessment of Withering's character is outlined on pp. 257–62, and it contrasts sharply with Darwin's. Although the portrait of him by Joseph Wright of Derby (National Portrait Gallery, London) shows a not unprepossessing man, it seems to have flattered him. Darwin was, in fact, an ugly man, as is clear from the account Mrs Mary Anne Schimmelpenninck (née Galton) gave of him in her Autobiography, in which she reported details of the Lunar Society (Schimmelpenninck 1858):

His figure was vast and massive, his head was almost buried in his shoulders, and he wore a scratch wig, as it was then called, tied up in a little bob-tail behind. A habit of stammering made the closest attention necessary, in order to understand what he said.

She also described his eating habits:

His horror of fermented liquors, and his belief in the advantages both of eating largely, and eating an almost immeasurable abundance of sweet things, was well known to all his friends.

She did not in that passage describe his pock-marked face and rotten teeth. As to her impression of his intellect:

... so far as intelligence was concerned, [one] was not inspired with confidence in beholding him;

but she was wrong, as she quickly admitted. Darwin more than overcame the twin disadvantages of his ugly appearance and stammer by the ebullience of his personality. He had a great imagination and was given to wild flights of ideas, as can be gauged from his letters to Matthew Boulton, proposing the construction of a fiery chariot, or discussing the potential usefulness of the thermometer (both quoted by Schofield 1963). He had an excellent sense of humour and could be corruscatingly witty, so much so as on occasion to offend:

His whole conversation ... was characterised by the merriment and so-called wit which aimed its perpetual shafts against those holy truths which, imperfectly though I yet knew them, afforded me the only comfort in distress which I had ever experienced ... I was struck equally with aversion and indignation at conduct which appeared to me to evince a total want of feeling.

Mrs Schimmelpenninck may, however, have been over-reacting

here since she was only a young girl at the time that this impression was formed. Furthermore, both the Darwins and the Galtons protested at what they saw to be her inaccurate account of Darwin's visits to her sick mother (Schofield 1963). However, her description of Withering merits quotation here, for the contrast it presents:

> He was the personification of that which belongs to a physician and a naturalist; enormous were his organs of proportion and individuality, and great were his powers of active investigation and accurate detail. His features were sharpened by minute and sagacious observation. He was kind, but his great accuracy and caution rendered his manner less open, and it had neither the wide popularity of Mr. Boulton's, nor the attraction of Mr. Watt's true modesty.

Darwin's good-humoured attitude to life is best reflected in a letter he wrote to Matthew Boulton on 5 April 1778:

> I am sorry the infernal divinities who visit mankind with diseases and are therefore at perpetual war with doctors, should have prevented my seeing all your great men at Soho today. Lord! what inventions, what wit, what rhetoric, metaphysical, mechanical and pyrotechnical will be on the wing, bandied like a shuttlecock from one to another of your troop of philosophers! While poor I, I by myself, I imprison'd in a postchaise, am joggled and jostled and bump'd, and bruised, along the King's high-road, to make war upon a stomach-ache or a fever.

Anyone of Darwin's character would have been irritated by Withering's humourless, intense approach, and it seems that he was not alone in his attitude to Withering, who subsequently fell out with other members of the Lunar Society over various matters

(Schofield 1963). Certainly Withering's self-righteousness could only have aggravated his relations with the other 'learned Lunatics', as Darwin liked to call them.

Nevertheless, in the affair of the foxglove Darwin undoubtedly was in the wrong. He and others should have accorded Withering due recognition for his contribution before the publication of the *Account*, and they failed to do so. Darwin ended his paper in the *Medical Transactions* (Darwin 1785) thus:

> [Digitalis] is a newly opened mine, which merits further examination; as it is probably replete with bullion, which only wants polishing to give it lustre; or the stamp of some great name, to make it current amongst the faculty.

Perhaps he thought that his name alone would be enough to give it that currency, but in the event the stamp was applied by Withering, whose studies were subsequently recognized to have been definitive in establishing digitalis as a therapeutically useful drug.

CHAPTER 5

ATTITUDES TO THE USE
OF THE FOXGLOVE
IN WITHERING'S LIFETIME

Withering's *Account* was enthusiastically received as soon as it appeared. The first hint that that would be so came in an item in the same volume of the *Medical Transactions* in which Erasmus Darwin had published his paper on the use of the foxglove in dropsies, and Baker his appendix to Darwin's paper. The item is headed 'Postscript to the appendix to Dr. Darwin's paper on foxglove' (Anon. 1785a), and it had been read at the College of Physicians of London on 6 August, 1785. It reads (the italics are mine):

> Whilst the last pages of this volume were in the press, Dr. Withering, of Birmingham, (who appears to have adopted foxglove from a family receipt, *and to have, for several years, recommended it as a diuretic*) published a numerous collection of cases, in which foxglove has been given, and frequently with good success. To these cases the ingenious author has added some instructions respecting the use of this plant, which claim our attention: for a substance, possessing so extraordinary and peculiar a power over the motion of the heart, if administered by the hand of ignorance and inexperience, is, in its effect, much more likely to be a poison than a remedy.

Although this notice certainly emphasized the prior publications of Darwin and Baker, it made it clear to the casual reader that Withering had had a long experience of the foxglove, and can only have been taken as an encouraging advertisement for the book.

Reviews in the learned journals of the time were complimentary. The reviewer in the *London Medical Journal* (Anon. 1785b) outlined the contents of the book and concluded:

... we cannot conclude the present account of it without expressing our approbation of the great prudence and caution the author uniformly inculcates in the use of this new remedy. That his solicitude to see it administered in small doses, and according to the rules he had laid down, is well founded, we are convinced, from two instances of its virulent effects, when given in large doses, which have lately come to our knowledge.

The reviewer in the *Medical Commentaries* (Anon. 1785c) concluded his review:

... we apprehend that every candid reader who bestows an attentive perusal on this treatise, will allow that the author is not only justly entitled to a high degree of praise for many ingenious observations, but that he cannot be too much applauded for the attention he had bestowed in the collection and preservation of useful facts, and in freely communicating these to the public for the information of others.

Most satisfactorily, from Withering's point of view, the reviewer in the *Monthly Review*, the journal which had printed what Withering considered to have been an unfair review of his *Botany*, compared him to 'the father of physic' and wrote (Anon. 1785d):

We have frequently received great satisfaction from the perusal of the works of this learned physician, and it is with pleasure that we sit down to consider his present publication ... [Although] in this volume there is not wanting evidence of its dangerous operations on the action of the heart ... it must, at the same time, be allowed that in the skilful hands of Dr. Withering [the fox-glove] has been rendered instrumental in the cure of the dropsy, after every other means, tried by able physicians, had failed of procuring relief ... we must beg leave to refer the reader to the work at large; from every part of which he may promise himself instruction . . . We think the public under great obligation to Dr. Withering for the labour he has bestowed on the subject of this book.

Withering soon started to receive the approbation of his colleagues. Cullen, for example (see p. 244), is reported as having said that the *Account* was a book which 'should be in the hands of every pratitioner of physic'. Withering also received letters praising the book (Osler Bequest 1928)—from Jean Hyacinth de Magellan, FRS, 11 August 1785:

I just now (before breakfast) finished reading your [?] present on the foxglove, which I received yesterday from your kind generosity, and for which I return you my most warm thanks, both in my name, and in that of the public at large. Oh! should every practitioner apply all his attentions to observe with so judicious a criterion the phenomena of the various disease which occur in his dayly practice, and to the effect of the medicines applied, what a good large stock of practical knowledge, the only usefull in life, should we possess to avert the summary assault, of pain and torture, to which our weak frame is exposed during the short period of our existence——! I'll send by the first opportunity, this yr publication abroad to various persons of my acquaintance, who may derive considerable advantage from its lecture, and chiefly to a Professor of Medicine of Coimbra, to Madrid, Paris, St Petersburg and Italy both to Milan and Florence: for which purpose I have already got from Robinson *6* copies . . .

. . . and from Andrew Duncan the elder, 5 September, 1785:

I am this day favoured with yours of the 1st of August accompanied with some copies of your very valuable treatise on the Foxglove . . . I have no doubt that I shall receive much satisfaction

from the perusal of it . . . I shall soon probably have opportuni-
ties of giving the Digitalis more trials than I have hitherto done.

Magellan sent a copy to B. P. van Lilyveld in the Hague, and
subsequently received a letter of thanks, dated 14 March, 1786:

> I am to return you my thanks for sending me Dr. Withering's
> account of the Foxglove. As a man labouring from time to time
> under a very disagreeable complaint, I perused the Book with a
> great deal of attention, and, I must say, with equal satisfaction;
> tho' not being myself of the Faculty, I may not be reckoned to
> be a Judge; but clearness and perspicuity will strike a sort of
> persuasion into the minds of even the most ignorant.

Although van Lilyveld's letter was complimentary to Withering
the compliment turned out to have been left-handed, since the
description of his case subsequently given in the letter makes it
clear that he was suffering from *bronchial*, not cardiac, asthma, a
condition which Withering expressly stated was not amenable to
treatment with digitalis (see p. 195). However, not being medi-
cally qualified, van Lilyveld could hardly have been expected to
have distinguished the two conditions, and when Magellan forwarded van Lilyveld's letter to Withering, Withering wrote to
van Lilyveld, giving his advice on the treatment of 'spasmodic
asthma', and not embarrassing van Lilyveld by mentioning the
foxglove. In return van Lilyveld wrote to Magellan:

> Think . . . what pleasure I must have felt by the perusal of Dr.
> Withering's letter upon my subject . . . since the Doctor's ideas,
> reflexions and prescriptions coincide so perfectly with my
> own observations and with the whole tenor of my conduct,
> since several years past.

Copies of the *Account* also found their way to America, and on

9 February, 1786 Hall Jackson (1739-97), a physician at Portsmouth, New Hampshire, wrote to Withering:

> Your inestimable treatise or account of the Foxglove and its medical uses: with practical remarks on dropsy and other diseases, has found its way to this remote part of the globe. It must greatly add to the satisfaction that daily arises in your mind, on seeing so many distressed fellow-mortals relieved by your personal advice, and administrations, to reflect that thousands at the most distant ends of the earth, are wishing to offer their tribute of gratitude for your indefatigable endeavours for the good of mankind . . .

> I have taken your treatise in my pocket for six weeks, I have shown it with the incomparable, accurate, and elegant drawing, to all my acquaintance within twenty miles, but no one can recollect of ever seeing any of its kind in America; I am persuaded, however, that it would arrive to sufficient maturity in this country, by attentive cultivation as our natural productions in general are much the same as those of England; . . .

> I have the honour of being acquainted with John Lane Esquire, merchant in London, to him I have sent for a small invoice of medicines; I have directed a small quantity of *Fol. Digitalis purp. siccat.*, also some of the powder, and seeds, but I greatly fear they have not as yet become articles of the shops, in London; could, I be so fortunate as to obtain (to the care of Mr. Lane) thro' your influence, and direction, a small quantity of the genuine seed, the plant should be most attentively cultivated, most carefully prepared, and as opportunities will not be wanting to administer it, the most accurate observations and remarks, on its operation, and effects, shall be noted, and if you will permit me the honor, shall be communicated to you, for

any further satisfaction, or remarks, you may wish to make on this truly valuable discovery . . .

PS I have directed to be sent me two or three sets of your account of the Foxglove for the purpose of dispersing them.

Withering replied to Jackson after a delay of eight months (his letter is given in full by Estes 1979):

Your letter of Febr. 9th arrived here in due time, and the seed of the digitalis purpurea which accompanies this, will shew that I have not been inattentive to your request. I send much more than will be necessary for your own use, in the hope that you will distribute it into other provinces . . .

I am more and more convinced that the digitalis, under a judicious management, is one of the mildest and safest medicines we have, as well as one of the most efficacious. It is I believe *never* necessary to create nausea or any other disturbance in the system. I never now use more than 1 drachm fol. sicc. to one pound of infusion, and in substance rarely 3 grains in 24 hours. An Account of your tryals with this medicine will be highly grateful to me, and fully recompense any trouble you have given me . . .

Digitalis has cured 2 other cases of insanity in this neighbourhood and 3 cases of haemoptoe. The latter were of the kind attended with a quick bounding pulse, and I directed the medicine from [the] quality I knew it possessed of abating the action of the heart.

Thus was digitalis introduced into America by Hall Jackson, under the influence of Withering. A comprehensive and lucid account of that introduction, and of the practice of medicine in eighteenth century America, has been given by Estes (1979).

THE USE OF DIGITALIS IN DROPSIES BY WITHERING'S CONTEMPORARIES

The pattern of use of digitalis by Withering's contemporaries was not dissimilar from the pattern of use one might expect to see within a newly-introduced drug today. Some of them followed his instructions carefully and proved successful as a result. Others tried the drug, but failed to adhere to the principles he had outlined, and as a result several of their patients suffered digitalis intoxication, in some cases severe enough to prove fatal. In consequence others were discouraged from using the drug at all. Furthermore, several physicians started to use digitalis for the treatment of conditions which we now recognize to be unsuitable for its use, thus setting the pattern for the next hundred or so years. In the rest of this chapter I shall give some examples of these different ways in which digitalis was used.

THE PROPER USE AND THE MISUSE OF DIGITALIS

The physician who was foremost among those who used digitalis properly was John Ferriar (1761-1815). Ferriar studied at Edinburgh and graduated MD there in 1781 with a dissertation entitled *De Variola*. He then practised in Stockton-on-Tees, but in 1785 moved to Manchester where he did a great deal to improve public hygiene. His *Medical histories and reflections* was published in three volumes in 1792, 1795, and 1798, and in the first volume he gave an account of his use of the foxglove in 23 patients with dropsies.

In 1799 Ferriar published a monograph on his experience with the foxglove, and this *Essay on the medical properties of the Digitalis purpurea or foxglove* (Ferriar 1799) was later incorporated into the second edition of his *Medical histories and reflections*. In it he reviewed his experience with the drug and was greatly impressed with its effect on the pulse:

The effect of the foxglove, in retarding the velocity of the pulse, as a direct sedative, was too striking to be long over-looked; and when its application, to diminish morbid irrita-tion in the vascular system, was once pointed out, the consequences of the idea were easily comprehended ... [It is] capable of reducing the pulse, without danger, from 120 in a minute to 75 or 80, at the will of the practitioner ... The diu-retic power of Digitalis, does not appear to me a constant and essential quality of the plant; the power of reducing the pulse is its true characteristic.

He also recognized its direct effect on the heart:

I have had occasion to mention, formerly, the utility of Digi-talis in palpitations of the heart. As the direct action of the medicine, in these cases, it is strongly indicated, and is indeed eminently serviceable.

Because Ferriar laid more emphasis on the effects of digitalis on the pulse rather than on its diuretic effects, while Withering rather stressed its action as a diuretic, some have suggested that Ferriar was the first to recognize that the main action of digitalis was on the heart. However, I believe that he was no nearer the truth of the matter than Withering, for two reasons. Firstly, Withering mentioned the heart three times in his *Account* (pp. 26, 81, and 192), and clearly stated (p. 192) that digitalis had 'a power over the motion of the heart', reasoning (p. 81) from its effect on the pulse. This effect was termed 'extraordinary and peculiar' in the *Medical Transactions* of 1785 (see p. 291). Secondly, although Ferriar recognized that digitalis had a direct effect on the heart, as is shown by the extract immediately above, he clearly thought that it also acted on the arteries: 'it lessens the frequency and quickness of arterial contraction', and elsewhere 'the action of the arterial system is retarded'. Certainly, neither Withering nor Ferriar recognized that the *diuretic* action of digitalis was the direct outcome of an action on the heart, although Ferriar may have recognized that the diuretic effect was linked to the effect on the *pulse*:

> I have seen all the syptoms of general dropsy, attended with a fluttering, feeble pulse, removed by small doses of Digitalis, in the course of a week; and in one remarkable case . . . the vigour and steadiness of the pulse encreased, exactly in proportion as the water was withdrawn from the cellular membrane.

It is not clear, however, from this passage whether he thought the diuretic effect was secondary to the effect on the pulse, or vice versa. He did think, however, that other properties of digitalis were linked to its effects on the pulse:

> I hoped, by diminishing the velocity of the pulse, to lessen one cause of irritation to the lungs . . . [and] that by its continued exhibition, after haemoptysis, it may be possible to procure the cicatrization of the ruptured vessels, and thus prevent the formation of ulcers.

It was on this basis that he and others recommended it in tuberculosis, and others later still for the treatment of fever (see p. 318).

Ferriar's use of the drug was exemplary. In contrast to many others of the time he almost always used the powdered leaf, since he confirmed Withering's demonstration of its greater reliability when compared with the infusion and the decoction. He used low dosages to begin with, increasing the dosage if there was no response and in the absence of toxicity. He gave short courses only, usually for no more than three weeks, although in some cases for up to three months. He would examine the patient hour by hour during the early stages of treatment, watching for the first signs of a slowing pulse or of nausea, when he would withhold therapy.

Although the cases Ferriar chose to treat were of a kind which, on the basis of Withering's *Account*, would have been expected to have responded, his success rate was not as good as Withering's. Of the 23 patients he reported in 1792, nine were cured and two were relieved. Of the others four died and nine were not relieved by the digitalis. Furthermore, three of the nine who responded had 'leucophlegmatia', which would have resolved spontaneously (see note to p. 19). However, in only three cases was there any evidence of digitalis intoxication, and in those cases Ferriar deliberately risked toxicity, increasing the dose in the hope of producing a therapeutic effect.

In contrast to John Ferriar consider John Coakley Lettsom (1744-1815). Lettsom was born of a Quaker family in the Virgin Islands, but came to England at the age of six. In 1761 he was apprenticed to Abraham Sutcliff, a surgeon-apothecary at Settle in Yorkshire, and in 1766 went to study at St Thomas' Hospital in London, and later to the Edinburgh medical school in 1768. He graduated MD at Leyden in 1769 with a dissertation entitled *Observationes ad vires Theae pertinentes*. He returned to London where, although not a great physician, he became eminent in various societies, and was notable as having been one of the founders, in 1773, of the Medical Society of London, to which he donated a house in Bolt Court, Fleet Street, a substantial number of books, and an annual gold medal (the Fothergillian medal) which was awarded for the best medical essay submitted for consideration.

Lettsom first heard of the use of the foxglove in about 1778, but 'its failure in two instances discouraged me from prosecuting further experience at that time' (Lettsom 1789). However, following the publication of Withering's *Account* he was encouraged to try again, and in 1788 presented a report to the Medical Society of London of his use of digitalis in eight cases of dropsy (Lettsom 1789). In all eight patients digitalis toxicity occurred and was frequently severe. A therapeutic effect was achieved in no more than three cases. Lettsom published his report because '[the cases] were such, as has been already observed, as afforded a prospect of successful issue, though the result did not confirm it'. He expressed his surprise that, in his hands, the digitalis had been both ineffective and toxic, and made it clear that he did not doubt the integrity of those who had reported it to be effective and safe:

> As I gave it in the manner prescribed by Dr. Withering, I am at a loss to explain the different results of our experiments. In the cases wherein I have tried it, little or no advantage was procured, while his trials were almost as uniformly successful, and many of them appear to have been much more unpromising. The accuracy of his observations, the candour with which they are published, and above all, the known respectability of his character, place him above the reach of suspicion. I have not only had the correspondence of Dr. Withering himself, but other respectable physicians in the country, have favoured me with accounts of its success, in instances where no improper bias whatever could influence their relations. Future experiment therefore must decide from what unknown causes such different effects have arisen.

Why did Lettsom have such disastrous results? The answer is simple. He did *not*, despite his protestations to the contrary, use the foxglove 'in the manner prescribed by Dr. Withering'.

Firstly, he used it in inappropriate cases. His first case, for example, was one of ascites in a 30-year-old man, without cough or dyspnoea, and there were two other similar cases; Withering had written that uncomplicated ascites was 'in adults generally incurable by medicines' (p. 194).

Secondly, Lettsom used the wrong dosages. It cannot be said from his prescriptions whether or not the *individual* doses he used were too large or not, since he did not specify the source of his supply of the drug, nor at what time of year the leaves were picked, nor the manner of preparation of the formulations he used. However, he undoubtedly gave his patients too much digitalis and in excessively long courses. In one case he ordered the decoction of the foxglove 'to be taken every eight hours, encreasing it as the stomach would admit'. When clear evidence of toxicity occurred he would persist with treatment, sometimes even increasing the dose. For example, of one case in which a therapeutic response occurred, Lettsom wrote:

> I was extremely happy at the prospect I now had, of seeing one successful case from the use of this vegetable, and though he complained of great vertigo, and almost a total loss of vision, with immense prostration of strength, I encouraged him to persevere.

The full folly of Lettsom's methods is illustrated in one incredible passage (the italics are mine):

> In the exhibition of the digitalis purpurea, the first effect I have observed, is rendering the pulse slower than in the natural state of the patient, thus persons whose usual standard may be 70, have had the pulsations reduced to 56, or even less in a minute; this has occurred within 24 hours after the use of this vegetable; but if the same dose be continued, in a day or two the pulse acquires its usual quickness, or even exceeds it, but at the same time it generally becomes depressed, and a languor is diffused over the whole system; the extremities, the hands particularly, acquire a moist clamminess, and feel cold to the touch. *If the dose be encreased till nausea or sickness is excited* , the strength of the patient is still more weakened, and the slowness of the pulse returns as at the first exhibition of the medicine; the sickness resembles sea-sickness accompanied with a confused aching and heaviness of the head. The patient at this period

remarks that he perceives flashes of fire frequently pass across his eyes, and sometimes balls of fire in the room. *An encrease of the dose after this* produces vomiting, and sometimes purging also: he complains of increased headach, or rather of confusion and giddiness; instead of flashes of light, almost all objects he views appear brilliant, and his friends who visit him seem to be surounded with a blaze of fire; his memory is imperfect, and upon attempting to walk, he reels and staggers like a person intoxicated. The dose that brings on these effects, gradually produce confused vision, and at length almost total blindness, which I have known to continue in some instances upwards of a month after the medicine has been omitted. During this time he complains in a particular manner of a throbbing pain in the balls of the eyes, and a sense of fulness and enlargement of them, as if the globes had become too big for the sockets, and were grown out of their natural scite. In two cases that I heard of, the limbs, particularly the lower extremities, were seized with tremors; and from some cause or other both these patients died suddenly, in a manner most resembling apoplexy.

In slight mitigation of Lettsom it must be said that some, but by no means all, of the toxicity his patients experienced may have been due to self-administration of the foxglove, over and above Lettsom's own prescription, as was later related by Sherwen (1800):

In the year 1795, Mr. Martin, a respectable publican, was taking the powder of digitalis in the form of pills, by the prescription of Dr. Lettsom:—while I was attending its administration with all proper caution, I was one day struck with the appearance of a large bowl filled with the leaves of Digitalis infused in boiling water, by his bedside. Upon inquiry, I was informed that a passenger in one of the stage coaches, which had stopped at his door, had told him that foxglove tea was an infallible cure for the dropsy. I believe I need not add, that I rescued this patient from premature dissolution. [In another case] I suspected that this plant had been used; but the fact was most resolutely denied. I have, however, since learned that he really fell a sacrifice to the unguarded use of fox-glove tea, recommended by a person unacquainted with its nature, and ignorant of physic.

In 1787 Lettsom, although he had not met Withering, wrote to him, expressing his 'esteem for his learning, and the useful application of it' and inviting him to become a member of the Medical Society of London. Withering accepted. Later that year Lettsom wrote again to say that Withering had been elected and that his diploma would be forwarded to him on 1 January 1788. In the same letter Lettsom added:

Our second volume [of the *Memoirs* of the Society] will be put into the hands of our Council and Committee for preparation for the press before the end of this year, and I wish we had some communication of thine to increase its value. I am happy at any time to communicate a memoir from thy pen.

Admittedly Lettsom had not followed Withering's precepts on the correct use of digitalis. Admittedly he had published his report of eight improperly treated cases saying that his mode of treatment had been that recommended by Withering. One cannot, therefore, fault Withering for having taken some offence, as indeed he did. However, there is no reason to believe that Lettsom had not acted in good faith, truly believing that his manner of using the foxglove was as Withering had proposed. Furthermore, he had written in complimentary terms to Withering and, although he did not know him, had invited him to become a member of his select society. True to character, Withering's self-righteous self-satisfaction would not allow him to reply to Lettsom in any other than an uncompromising fashion, albeit dressed up with some typical eighteenth century complimentary frills:

Please accept my thanks for your offer of inserting anything new which I might have to say respecting the Digitalis; but I really have nothing new to observe, nor have I anything to retract of what I have said before. Under my own management, under that of the medical practitioners of this part of England, and I may add, also in the hands of some worthy and respectable clergymen in village situations, it continued to be the most certain, and the least offensive diuretic we know; in such cases, and in such constitutions as I have advised its exhibition. I have also the satisfaction to find, by letters from some of the most eminent physicians in different parts of England, that it is equally useful and safe in their hands. But I complain of the treatment this medicine has had in London. Its ill success there cannot be altogether owing to difference of constitutions. Dr. Lettsom has related his unsuccessful attempts with a degree of courage and candour which do the highest honour to his integrity; but no one can compare his choice of patients with my declarations of the fit and unfit, or the doses he prescribed with the perseverance he enjoined, with my doses, rules and cautions, without being astonished that he could suppose he had been given this medicine 'in the manner prescribed by me'. I am fully satisfied, that, had I prescribed it in such cases, such forms, such doses and such repetitions as he has done, the effects would in my hands have been equally useless, and equally deleterious. I must, therefore, suppose that he had forgotten what I had written, without being conscious that his memory had deceived him. Had it been otherwise, after perusing the case I had published at pages 20 and 151 etc. of my Account etc., he would hardly have thought it necessary to have published more instances of what I had stigmatised as bad practice; or to have sought for further proofs, than an active medicine might be employed so as to prove a deleterious poison.

Stripped of its frills this is a most insulting letter, particularly in the way that Withering suggests that Lettsom could not practice medicine as well as any village clergyman. I do not know what Lettsom's response, if any, was, but he seems to have taken heed, for in 1794, when the second volume of the *Memoirs of the Medical Society* was republished in a second edition he added a four-page note to his original article, in which he wrote (Lettsom 1794):

> The cautions contained in the preceding account have been of use, in guarding against temerity, on one hand, and encouraging, on the other prudent experiment. That this medicine is a powerful diuretic was suggested, and further enquiry has confirmed, as well as its dangerous sedative powers; but under the direction of medical skill, I consider it as one of the most powerful diuretics in medicine, and efficacious remedies in ascites and dropsical affections, as far as diuretics can act as curative remedies ... I consider it, therefore, under skilful attention, a valuable addition to our Materia Medica.

These two instances, those of Ferriar and Lettsom, represent the extremes of the ways in which other physicians continued to use digitalis. On the one hand we have clear reports of at least two other physicians who used the drug properly and to some good purpose, namely Charles William Quin (Quin 1790) (see note to p. 199) and Hall Jackson (see Estes 1979). However, although they both used the drug wisely, and achieved rates of toxicity below 20 per cent, Quin's success rate was considerably lower than that of Withering, being around 45 per cent (i.e. comparable to Lettsom's). We can only assume that he was not using the drug optimally, and was undertreating his patients in fear of causing toxicity. Of all these physicians only Hall Jackson achieved a success rate comparable to that of Withering, and his rate of toxicity was even lower than Withering's, being around 9 per cent, although his figure is based on a very small sample (11 patients) (Estes, 1979).

On the other hand we have evidence that some doctors mis-used the drug, although perhaps not to the same extent as Lett-som. For example, in a letter to Lettsom read to the Medical Society of London on 26 October, 1789, William Currie wrote (Currie 1790):

> My own observations of the effects of [Digitalis purpurea] in hydropic affections correspond intirely with yours:—and there is reason to fear, that the general and indiscriminate use of that vegetable, in consequence of the strong recommendations of some respectable physicians, has in many instances been pro-ductive of the most pernicious effects.

The exact extent of misuse of digitalis is not clear, since there are too few reports of this kind to judge from. However, it is not hard to believe that misuse was widespread, as is suggested by the com-ments of Withering in his *Account* (see p. v) and in his letter to Lett-som, and by those of Currie. The reason is that digitalis is very difficult to use. Even today with our understanding of cardiac phy-siology and pathology, our sophisticated methods of monitoring cardiac function, our knowledge of the pharmacology of the car-diac glycosides, and our ability to measure their plasma concentra-tions and to adjust dosages in order to produce optimal effects with minimal risk of toxicity, reported rates of digitalis toxicity are still relatively high (see Aronson 1983a). This is undoubtedly due to the fact that much of the available knowledge, while available to the ordinary practitioner and specialist, is often not assimilated suffi-ciently well to allow optimal use of the drug. How much more difficult would it have been in Withering's day, when virtually none of this knowledge was available? Even in the most careful hands several problems would have arisen—the difficulty of pre-paring reproducible formulations (a problem which is still with us—see for example, Jounela *et al*. 1975), the variability in purity of different formulations, containing different amounts of different glycosides (see pp. 226-7), the difficulty in judging the correct doses to use when the principles of loading dose, maintenance dose, and accumulation were not recognized, the difficulty in failing to recognize that appropriate dosages would vary enormously from patient to patient, particularly in patients with more variable degrees of impairment of liver function than we see today, the difficulty ... but the list goes on and on. Withering's success, based on his monumentally pedestrian care and patience, in the absence of all this basic understanding, demands more and more of our respect.

THE USE OF THE FOXGLOVE IN DISEASES OTHER THAN DROPSIES

For several reasons digitalis was widely used during Withering's day for the treatment of diseases other than dropsies. Firstly, it was thought that its effects in lowering the pulse rate were by virtue of an action on the arterial system (see pp. 230-1); even then there was no agreement as to what it *did* to the arteries, some believing it to be 'stimulant', others believing it to be 'sedative'. It was therefore used in conditions for which it was thought that an action on the arteries, of whatever kind, would be beneficial. Thus William Currie (Currie 1970):

> The great power the Digitalis possesses of diminishing the irritability of the heart, and of weakening the force of the circulation renders it a probable remedy in active haemorrhages.

Secondly, it was thought that its diuretic effects might, in part at any rate, be due to a stimulatory effect on the lymphatics, allowing the reabsorption of fluid. This was one of the reasons for its use in tuberculosis, since it was thought that such a stimulatory effect would encourage the absorption of tuberculous material from the lung. However, there were other reasons, as the following extracts from Nathan Drake's contribution to Beddoes's *Essay . . . on pulmonary consumption* (Beddoes 1799, see below) show:

> It has lately been maintained . . . that pus is a secreted fluid, the consequence of certain diseased motions of the extremities of the blood-vessels . . .

> . . . by powerfully retarding the action of the arterial system, the secretion of matter might be diminished or suspended . . .

> . . . the pulse generally sinks in consequence of nausea; and as subsequent to the retardation of the action of the heart, absorption frequently occurs, it has been supposed that nausea, a diminution of arterial motion, and absorption, are mutually and necessarily related to each other, and that were the first of these phenomena abstracted, the latter, viz. absorption, would not be produced.

One of the foremost proponents of this use of digitalis was Thomas Beddoes (1760-1808), who is perhaps better known for having established, at Clifton, a 'pneumatic institute' for treating diseases by inhalation, and for having there fostered the career of Humphrey Davy, who discovered nitrous oxide while working in the institute. In a letter to his good friend Davies Gilbert (né Giddy) in 1799 Beddoes wrote:

> You will be shocked when you come to know that if I had had as much information on the treatment of consumption when Mrs. Baines first came hither, as I have now, I'd more than probably have cured her! In cases of tubercle and consumption where ulceration is not extensive I have succeeded and am succeeding wonderfully. The cases of success are as yet but few, for I have but just learned the method, in the discovery of which I have had no share. Two of my correspondents without

communication with one another took up the idea of giving digitalis so as to abate the pulse without producing languor or sickness—and both succeeded. From what I have seen and from their testimony I now go to prescribe for patients in the above circumstances with somewhat of the same confidence as for those affected with ague or syphilis. My experience does not warrant me to expect much in the last stage except by way of relief. I hourly expect my correspondents' papers for insertion in our collection, which they will worthily close, and which will appear in a fortnight, and a very valuable large volume it will make. At present I am led to hope that the ravages of this devouring disease will be greatly checked; and by some little further improvements entirely stopped. The digitalis I find an exceptionally ticklish thing to manage in delicate women. My correspondents say they have carried the dose up to near 100 drops of Darwin's Tincture. I cannot get to 30 in such subjects, and I find 10 sometimes sufficient, and the depression from an overdose is terrible.

This letter is to be found in the Cornwall Records Office in Truro, and was brought to my attention by Paul Weindling.

Giddy received this letter on 6 March, and noted that Mrs Baines had died on 3 March. The publication to which Beddoes referred in his letter was the *Essay on the causes, early signs, and prevention of pulmonary consumption for the use of parents and preceptors* (Beddoes 1799), in which he named the two physicians alluded to in his letter as Dr Nathan Drake and Dr Richard Fowler.

The favourable experience of Beddoes and others was not shared by all, and Dr Lachlan Maclean, an Edinburgh graduate working in Sudbury in Suffolk, wrote (Maclean 1799) that 'my own experience in upwards of twenty cases, will not suffer me to speak in such high terms of it [as Dr Beddoes does]'. Nevertheless, digitalis was used to treat tuberculosis for a century or so after, although it was later restricted to treating the fever of the disease (see p. 318). There seems no doubt from the numerous reports of its efficacy in cases of consumption that digitalis had some effect in those cases, and one has to remember that the diagnostic criteria for the disease were very loose, sometimes based on as little as a single episode of haemoptysis, and lacking bacterial confirmation. Thus many of these cases would not have been tuberculosis at all. Both Withering (see item 31, p. 204) and Maclean realized this, the latter commenting that:

> Many cases of chlorosa [i.e. chronic iron deficiency anaemia] are of this description: there is cough, generally dry; pain of the side, chilliness, succeeded by heat, intense thirst, and sometimes night sweats. Many such, that had been pronounced confirmed phthisis by a noted consumption-doctor, have been restored to health under my care, by means of steel . . .

Thirdly, it was recognized that digitalis had at least two different effects on the brain. First, it was thought that digitalis was able to remove 'a superabundance of fluid, extravasated in the different parts of the brain' (Cox 1790). Second, it was recognized that digitalis had a 'sedative' effect on the brain, and it was thought that this 'debilitating power' was by virtue of its 'peculiar property of reducing the pulse, and of occasioning very great nausea' (Cox 1790), although it was, in fact, due to a direct effect on the brain in extreme intoxication. For these reasons digitalis was used in the treatment of hydrocephalus (see, for example, Withering's *Account*, pp. 197-200), of epilepsy, and of insanity (see, for example, Jones 1787). For example, William Currie (1790) described a case of a patient with manic-depressive psychosis, in an acute manic state, in whom 'the sedative effects of camphire intirely failed, and opium, though given in large doses, seldom procured sleep'. After several weeks, during which a wide variety of treatments was tried he gave digitalis:

It was at first given in a pretty full dose, and repeated so as to produce languor, faintishness, and considerable irregularity of the pulse. Its operation was attended by calmness, which was soon followed by sleep.

One cannot but suspect that by that stage the patient was due for a spontaneous remission.

During the nineteenth century many more inappropriate indications were added to the list of uses of digitalis, and I shall discuss those in Chapter 6.

One cannot blame the eighteenth century physicians for their misunderstanding of the appropriate indications for the use of digitalis, based as they were upon an inadequate understanding of the pathophysiology of the diseases they were treating, any more than we can be blamed today for our blind attempts to find specific treatments for diseases such as multiple sclerosis, or the largely empirical ways in which treatments for cancer are developed, based though they are on an understanding of the effects of the drugs we use on the biochemistry of normal and abnormal cells. However, we *can* blame those of them who clearly misused the drug for not having learned how to use it correctly from the example of their more successful colleagues. As Withering put it in a letter to Jonathan Stokes in 1778 (quoted in the *Account*, p. xix):

I wish it was as easy to write upon the Digitalis—I despair of pleasing myself or instructing others, in a subject so difficult. It is much easier to write upon a disease than upon a remedy. The former is in the hands of nature, and a faithful observer, with an eye of tolerable judgment, cannot fail to delineate a likeness. The latter will ever be subject to the whims, the inaccuracies, and the blunders of mankind.

PART III

ATTITUDES TO THE FOXGLOVE AFTER WITHERING'S DEATH

CHAPTER 6

THE NINETEENTH
CENTURY

As far as digitalis was concerned the nineteenth century was something of a fallow period. All that was known about its pharmacognosy, and what we would today call its clinical pharmacology, was reviewed by George Sigmond in his excessively discursive lectures on materia medica and therapeutics given at the Windmill-Street school of medicine (Sigmond 1837), and nearly 50 years later Edward Tibbits, reviewing the current theories of its mode of action, wrote (Tibbits 1881):

> Much has been written about it since that time, but it is extremely doubtful whether at the present day anything more is known with certainty concerning its action than is [in Dr Sigmond's review] set forth.

This view, however, was not precisely true, since, following the publication of a paper by Blake (1839) on the hypertensive action of digitalis on arteries, there was a slow stream of papers (for references see Cushny 1897) demonstrating its effects on the circulation. Furthermore, it was demonstrated, at the beginning of the second half of the century, that digitalis slowed the heart by an action on the vagus (Traube 1871). However, its effects on the contractility of the myocardium were not recognized until relatively late in the century (see Sansom 1886), and the condition of atrial fibrillation had not yet been described in man. Consequently, although digitalis continued to be used in the treatment of dropsy, its use was not widespread (see p. 322).

However, as a result of misconceptions about the actions of digitalis and a lack of understanding of the pathophysiology of many diseases, digitalis *was* used for a wide variety of other diseases, and numerous references are to be found in Neale's *Medical digest* (Neale 1877) to its use in conditions which cover the alphabet, from adenitis, bronchitis, and chordee, to spermatorrhoea, typhoid, and variola. The seemingly haphazard list of 32 conditions referred to by Neale can be rationalized to some extent by considering the actions which digitalis was thought to have.

Firstly, because digitalis strengthened the pulse when weak and slowed it when fast, it was thought to be of value in conditions in which the pulse was weak and fast, e.g. in acute haemorrhage.

Secondly, it was used in the treatment of any condition accompanied by fever, for several reasons:

(a) Because it slowed the fast pulse associated with a fever.
(b) Partly because it slowed the heart rate and partly because it was thought to reduce the tone of the circulation, some thought that it would reduce the amount of blood flowing through the tissues, thereby reducing inflammation—in this respect it was looked on as an alternative to bloodletting, which was also considered to be 'antiphlogistic' (i.e. anti-inflammatory) (Bence-Jones 1855). An alternative view was that the decrease in temperature was due to an *increase* in blood flow in the peripheral circulation, presumably by removing inflammatory humours (Tibbits 1881).
(c) Some inflammatory conditions resulted in dropsy as a complication, and it was thought to be especially valuable in the dropsy associated with scarlet fever (Graham 1844).
(d) It may have been thought that its diuretic effect would cause the removal of poisons from the blood, that being one reason given for its apparent efficacy in delirium tremens (Murchison 1870).

Thirdly, it was recognized that digitalis had effects on the nervous system, both central and peripheral. For this reason it was used to treat delirium tremens (in which 'there is undoubtedly a great disturbance of the vascular system'), mania, migraine, and epilepsy (Serre 1860; Peacock 1861; Murchison 1870; Wiltshire 1870), and cases of opiate withdrawal (Black 1885). Some attributed its apparently beneficial effect in epilepsy to an increase in cerebral blood flow, thought to be reduced during an epileptic fit because of 'a sudden interruption of the nutritive supply of blood to the brain' (Meryon 1871). It was also thought that its effect in reducing the tone of the arterial system was partly attributable to inhibition of the nerves innervating the arteries (Fennell 1869).

Fourthly, it was thought that its diuretic properties would be of value in removing excess fluid from the brain in cases of hydrocephalus (Peacock 1861; see also pp. 197-200). For this reason it was also used in cases of 'suppression of urine' (i.e. acute renal failure) (Reynolds 1869).

Fifthly, it was used in a variety of urogenital disorders, for different reasons. It was thought to cure menorrhagia and metrorrhagia, either by reducing the activity of the nervous ganglia whereby the uterus was stimulated (Dickenson 1855), or, according to some, because it 'excite[d] strong, regular, and intermittent uterine contractions' (Gourvat 1872). For that reason it was also used as an abortifacient and an anaphrodisiac in women. Similarly, in men, because of its supposed inhibitory effects on peripheral nerves, it was used to 'combat erotic excitement, whether due to excitable temperament, sedentary life, stimulant regimen, or the privation or excess of venereal pleasures, etc.' (Brughmanns 1856). Others thought that its 'antiplastic and lowering action' caused a weakening of sexual powers—'the propensities disappear, the secretion of liquor seminis diminishes by degrees, and may at last vanish altogether' (Gourvat 1872). Gourvat attributed the effect on semen production to its antiphlogistic activity, and others used it to treat spermatorrhoea and excessive nocturnal seminal emissions (Laroche 1854). It was also reportedly 'pre-eminently useful when phymosis or paraphymosis . . ., chordee, epididymitis, or adenitis are either present or feared' (Brughmanns 1856), perhaps, although not statedly so, by a conjunction of reasoning about its effects on the urogenital tract and in inflammatory disorders.

THE USE OF
DIGITALIS IN TUBERCULOSIS

The way in which digitalis was used in the treatment of patients with tuberculosis underwent gradual alteration during the course of the nineteenth century. I have outlined the reasons for its use at the end of the eighteenth century in Chapter 5. In the early part of the nineteenth century its use was continued, under the influence of Thomas Beddoes, Nathan Drake, and Richard Fowler, and the issues of the *Medical and Physical Journal* published in the first few years contain many reports attesting to its value, notably a report by J. Magennis (1801) of 72 cases, in which recovery was reported in 40 and improvement in another 24.

Some, however, were not entirely impressed with the efficacy of digitalis, notably Lachlan Maclean, of Sudbury in Suffolk. He reported, firstly in 1799 (see p. 311) and later in 1810 (Maclean 1799, 1810) that his experience had 'corrected the high expectation he had formed of its efficacy' (Anon. 1810). He did not completely abandon its use however, suggesting that it was best reserved for early cases. 'Those who expect wonders from it, or that it will *in general* cure consumption, will be disappointed' (Maclean 1799).

By the second quarter of the century there was more doubt about the value of digitalis in tuberculosis (Forbes *et al*. 1833):

In phthisis ... some [medical writers] regard it as possessed of powers beyond all other remedies, others considering it to have very little efficacy, while a third class have even condemned it as pernicious ... But, whatever be its effects in phthisis, the medicine has wonderfully fallen in the estimation of the profession since the time of Beddoes.

Reviewing the history of its use in tuberculosis Sigmond (1837) wrote, echoing Maclean:

it is only in the early stages that digitalis can be ranked as a curative agent, but it may in its later moments, be equally important as a palliative. The high character it has obtained, has been from its having been employed before the breaking down of tubercles in the lung ...

All this suggests to me that the successes reported by Beddoes and his colleagues were largely due to the spontaneous resolution of disease in cases which were not tubercular.

There is no evidence of the systematic evaluation of digitalis in cases of tuberculosis during this time, but by the third quarter of the nineteenth century it was definitely out of favour as a curative drug, as is evidenced by the following extracts:

It has been recommended in phthisis, but it is not productive of any permanent benefit in this disease. [Garrod 1875.]

Nobody now believes that digitalis will cure consumption. [Anon. 1872.]

Nonetheless, the idea that it was valuable in the treatment of the *symptoms* of tuberculosis persisted. For example, haemoptysis:

I believe we have a remedy [to treat massive haemoptysis] for the majority of patients, in *digitalis*. [Brinton 1861.]

Digitalis is of value in the treatment of haemorrhage, especially from the lungs. [Garrod 1875, despite his opinion about
its curative value quoted above.]

Indeed, digitalis continued to be recommended for the treatment
of *fever* in tuberculosis for many years, and was recommended for
this purpose in Osler's *Principles and practice of medicine* as late as
the 8th edition (1913), but not in the 9th edition (1920). Osler
died in 1919.

THE USE OF DIGITALIS IN DROPSY

It should not be thought from all this that digitalis was not used
for the treatment of dropsy during the nineteenth century, but, if
one takes as evidence the numbers of publications on its therapeutic indications, there is no doubt that it was used much more
frequently for other indications (for a review of the continental
European practice see Ackerknecht 1962). For example, James
Braithwaite, a practitioner in Leeds, was moved in 1883 to
publish a note in the *Lancet* (Braithwaite 1883), describing the
use of digitalis in dropsy:

> Although the diuretic action of digitalis in cardiac disease with
> dropsy is perfectly well known, it is very rarely indeed pre-
> scribed in this part of the country ...

This observation prompts two questions. Why was it used so
much for other diseases? and why was digitalis not used more in
the treatment of dropsy?

The answer to the first question has several components.
Firstly, there is the consideration that, to use Osler's words, 'one
should treat as many patients as possible with a new drug while it
still has the power to heal'. In other words, new drugs may appear
to have therapeutic effects which in fact they do not have. The
concept of the randomized, double-blind, placebo-controlled

trial had not yet been invented in the nineteenth century, and no one would have considered formally testing the possibility that a drug's apparent therapeutic efficacy was due, not to a real effect, but to some problem of diagnosis or spontaneous resolution of the disease. Secondly, the misconceptions relating to the actions of digitalis led physicians to believe that digitalis would be effective in a variety of diseases, as I have shown earlier in this chapter (pp. 317-20). Ackerknecht (1962) has argued that the empirical observation that digitalis appeared to be effective in a particular disease would have led to rationalizations about its mode of action, based on what was thought about it at the time, and I am sure that there must have been some element of such rationalization in some cases. Take, for example, the case report of its use in encouraging the reduction of an incarcerated inguinal hernia. The author did not say why he used digitalis initially, but having used it, as he supposed successfully, he argued (Simmons 1801):

> Reduction [of a hernia] is chiefly prevented by the inflammatory state of the contents of the herniary sac; which state consists in a increased frequency and vigour of the arterial pulsations ... These augmented dimensions are further extended, by the hindrance given to the return of the venous blood, and by the watery fluids of the intestines distilling into the strangulated cavity ... By the Digitalis the supply by the arteries is stinted, and the muscular resistance obviated by it.

Nevertheless, in some cases there must also have been *a priori* reasoning, for example in extending the use of digitalis as a febrifuge, following its first exhibition as such, to any case of fever.

The answer to the question of why digitalis was used so infrequently in the treatment of dropsy is equally complex. Firstly, it is so difficult to use properly (see pp. 227-32). For example (Stirling 1864):

> I have made a trial of digitalis in several cases of mitral incompetence, but cannot speak favourably of its effects.

Yet we know that digitalis is effective in cases of heart failure secondary to mitral regurgitation.

Secondly, a misconception about its action persisted, the old difficulty of knowing whether it was a cardiac 'sedative' or 'stimulant' (see pp. 299 and 318) still being undecided. For example, Sansom, recommending its use as the treatment of choice in cases of mitral regurgitation, wrote (Sansom 1886):

> There is yet some lingering of the old timidity which, regarding digitalis as a sedative and depressant of the heart, would withhold it when the heart is weak.

Thirdly, it was correctly recognized that there were conditions in which the use of digitalis would exacerbate heart failure rather than improve it, although the precise nature of some such cases would not have been understood (e.g. hypertrophic obstructive cardiomyopathy, previously called subvalvular aortic stenosis). In one case there was a clear-cut evidence of this, in Dominic John Corrigan's description of aortic regurgitation (Corrigan 1832). Corrigan (1802-80) was an eminent Dublin physician who had graduated from Edinburgh in 1825. He was president of the Irish College of Physicians five times, and was made a baronet in 1866. It was said that 'his success was due to his good sense and large practical experience, but he was not a profound physician nor a learned one' (Moore 1887). In his paper on aortic regurgitation Corrigan wrote:

> If the action of the heart be rendered very slow [by digitalis] the pause after each contraction will be long, and consequently the regurgitation of the blood must be considerable ... In every case of this disease in which digitalis has been administered, it has invariably aggravated the patient's sufferings. The oppression has become greater; the action of the heart more laboured; the pulse intermittent, and very often dicrotic, from

the heart's being unable by a single contraction to empty itself ... From this state they only recovered by omitting the *digitalis*, and putting them on stimulants. In no case of this disease did *digitalis* produce the slightest good effect; and in all, the patients while under its exhibition were always worse.

Corrigan's observations were later confirmed by others (see, for example, Thorowgood 1864), and there is no doubt that this kind of observation, coupled with the other considerations outlined above, would have discouraged others from using digitalis more widely. It is curious to think that a piece of work could on the one hand have contributed so much to medical understanding, while on the other hand, albeit unintentionally, diminishing the effective usefulness of one of the few active drugs available to the physicians of the time.

CHAPTER 7

THE TWENTIETH CENTURY
1900 to 1950

The twentieth century can be considered as having started, as far as digitalis is concerned, in the 1890s, with the work of Sir James Mackenzie. Mackenzie (1853-1925) was an Edinburgh graduate who went to Burnley in 1879 to practise as a general practitioner and physician to the Victoria Hospital. In 1907 he moved to London, and was given charge of the heart wards at the Mount Vernon Hospital. In 1915 he was elected FRS and knighted. A personal account of some aspects of his life was recorded in an entertaining but journalistic book by R. McNair Wilson (1926), and Thomas Lewis wrote of him (Lewis 1937) that 'An uncommon faculty of criticism, a deep-rooted distrust of authoritative statement, gave him rare discrimination between the known and the unknown; this associated in unusual degree with originality of mind, a retentive memory, and determined purpose, underlay his success as an investigator'.

Despite a busy clinical career Mackenzie found time to carry out clinical research, and his main interest was in the pulse. With the aid of a Lancashire watchmaker he invented a polygraph with which he studied the movements of the jugular venous pulse, publishing his observations in *The study of the pulse* (1902). He was the first to recognize the condition of 'auricular paralysis', or 'nodal rhythm', his original terms for what came to be called auricular or atrial fibrillation, as a cause of an irregular pulse, and he carried out careful studies of the effect of digitalis in slowing the ventricular rate in atrial fibrillation. This work culminated in a series of publications in the *British Medical Journal* (Mackenzie 1905a, b, c, d, e).

THE ACTIONS OF DIGITALIS AND ITS USE IN ATRIAL FIBRILLATION

Mackenzie distinguished several actions of digitalis. Firstly, he described its effects on 'stimulus conduction (dromotropic effect)', by which he meant the propagation of impulses through the atria. He considered that digitalis did not affect this conduction, except when the rate of conduction was already considerably reduced, probably describing what is now called the 'sick sinus syndrome'. Secondly, he described its inhibitory effects on 'stimulus production (chronotropic effect) and excitability (bathmotropic effect)', by which he meant the origination and propagation of the cardiac impulse. He wrote that he could not tell which of these two effects was responsible for the slowing of the heart rate.

Thirdly, Mackenzie described the effect of digitalis on 'contractility (inotropic effect)'. His remarks on the subject are worth quoting in full, because they illustrate how defective reasoning about the relationship between the pulse rate and the contraction of the myocardium continued to lead investigators to erroneous conclusions:

> Within certain limits, the longer the pause [after a contraction] the more vigorous will be the contraction, and the contraction will also last longer. It is a matter of everyday experience that a heart beating at a certain rate which is normal to the individual results in the circulation being efficiently carried on. An excessive slowing is no more conducive to an efficient circulation than an excessive quickening. The rate most compatible seems to be that which permits the heart muscle just enough time to recover its full power of contraction... The good effect of digitalis on contractility may be due simply to the fact that in slowing the rate ... it gives time for the function of contractility to be restored; ...

Mackenzie also observed cases in which he thought that digitalis had reduced the contractility of the heart;

> I am of the opinion that the cause of the slow action of the heart is due to the digitalis depressing the function of contractility after the manner shown in my last paper. It was there pointed out that when digitalis depressed the contractility, if time were not given for the function to be restored, the contraction was less in force and shorter in duration, and experimental evidence was given to show that the fibres might refuse to contract and so a beat might drop out to be followed by a stronger and longer systole.

Elsewhere he wrote (Mackenzie 1905f):

> In my observations on the effect of digitalis on the human heart, I pointed out that when a function such as conductivity or contractility was depressed, digitalis had a tendency to increase this depression. Notwithstanding this I found that while the digitalis depressed these functions a patient's condition may be distinctly improved, and it seems at first sight very anomalous that benefit should be derived from a drug which manifestly injures certain functions of the muscle fibres.

Mackenzie resolved the apparent paradox by invoking another effect of digitalis, its effect in 'restoring the tonicity', attributing dilatation of the heart to lack of tone in the muscle fibres.

Some of the cases in which Mackenzie was describing an impairment of contractility were cases of digitalis toxicity with coupled ventricular extrasystoles, and he expressed his surprise that the 'depressing influence' of digitalis should, in such cases, be accompanied by 'a certain degree of irritability'.

Mackenzie's attitude to the value of digitalis in dropsy with regular cardiac rhythm, as opposed to atrial fibrillation, is unclear. He also certainly attributed the beneficial effects of digitalis in dropsy to its effect in slowing the heart rate and in his second Oliver-Sharpey lecture on heart failure, given to the Royal College of Physicians, he said (Mackenzie 1911a):

> It seems probable that [drugs of the digitalis group] owe their good effect mainly to the amount of rest procured by the slowing of the heart's rate ... The vast majority of patients in whom digitalis acts with such marvellous effect in slowing the rate and improving the condition are those affected by auricular fibrillation. Hearts with the normal rhythm are seldom so sensitive to the digitalis, and in them there is not the same tendency to slowing of the rate.

However, he did recognize not only that improvement in a patient's condition could occur even when the heart rhythm was regular, but also that it could occur without an effect on the heart rate (Mackenzie 1911b):

> There is no doubt that digitalis relieves distress of breathing and reduces dropsy and it does not necessarily do so by slowing the pulse ... That improvement under such circumstances is not due solely to slowing of the heart's action can be inferred from a case of heart block where there was no effect on the pulse rate, but where the improvement was most marked.

However, he probably thought that the beneficial effect in such cases was due to a direct diuretic effect on the kidneys, since he describes the effects of digitalis on urine flow in the following fashion (Mackenzie 1911b):

> ... it was only in exceptional cases that there was a marked increase in the flow of urine and ... these showed signs of renal inefficiency by the presence of dropsy ... In a patient in whom the normal rhythm was present, the increase in the

flow of urine began after he had taken one or two drachms with no perceptible change in the heart's action.

There is no evidence that he connected the beneficial effect in cases of dropsy with regular cardiac rhythm to a direct effect on the heart.

None of these shortcomings, however, should hide the fact that it was through the agency of Mackenzie that the modern use of digitalis in treating fast atrial fibrillation was established.

Mackenzie wrote (Mackenzie 1905b) that he had gained a clearer insight into the action of digitalis by 'the perusal of Professor Wenckebach's book on *Arrhythmia of the Heart*'. Karel Frederik Wenckebach (1864-1940) was Professor of Medicine at Groningen University in Holland, and later in Vienna. His special interest was in cardiac arrhythmias and their treatment, and it was he who first reported the value of quinine in the treatment of atrial fibrillation (Wenckebach 1914). Wenckebach studied the mode of action of digitalis in slowing the heart in man, and concluded (Wenckebach 1910) that it was at least partly via an effect on the vagus nerve. In this he was following the example of Traube (1851, quoted in Cushny 1897), and Cushny (1897) who had demonstrated such an effect in experimental animals, and his findings were subsequently confirmed by Mackenzie and Cushny (Mackenzie 1911a; Cushny *et al*. 1913).

Wenckebach also discussed those of Mackenzie's cases which suggested that digitalis caused decreased cardiac contractility, and concluded (Wenckebach 1910):

> ... such cases have shown me that only in some cases *perhaps* digitalis diminishes contractility. We may further ask if perhaps in those cases digitalis acts by vagus inhibition ... *Conclusion*.—Digitalis increases the strength of the human heart by acting on the heart muscle. Perhaps large doses, or in appropriate cases even small doses, may have an opposite effect (by acting on the vagus?).

He admitted, however, that in cases similar to those of Mackenzie (i.e. those with coupled ventricular extra beats, often due to digitalis toxicity) 'I never saw any effect of vagus pressure'.

Wenckebach's conclusions on the actions of digitalis are vividly expressed:

> Acting on the vagus, it pulls the reins of the heart; acting on the heart muscle, it is a most useful whip, at the same time providing it with food by bettering the circulation.

However, he did not clearly distinguish those cases in which digitalis might and might not be useful, writing (perhaps not unreasonably):

> Give digitalis a fair trial in every case. If ever I should acquire a reputation for treating heart patients with success, it will be from my giving in this way digitalis in cases where authorities and textbooks forbid it.

He was also later quoted (*Lancet* 1932; ii: 633) as having said:

> I owe my reputation as a cardiologist to the fact that I order digitalis in just those cases which textbooks regard as unsuitable and in doses which physicians describe as dangerous.

Although his involvement was more in regard to animal than human observations, the role played by Arthur Robertson Cushny should not be ignored. Cushny (1866–1926) was a medical graduate of Aberdeen University who subsequently studied pharmacology with Oswald Schmiedeberg in Germany. In 1893 he went to Ann Arbor, in Michigan, to be Professor of Pharmacology, returning to Britain in 1905 to take the chair of pharmacology at University College, London, where he collaborated with Mackenzie (then at Mount Vernon). In 1918 he took the chair of materia medica and pharmacology at Edinburgh, in succession to Sir Thomas Fraser.

Cushny's main research interests were the actions of diuretics on the kidneys, the pharmacological differences between optical isomers, and, following his teacher Schmiedeberg, the actions of digitalis and other cardiac glycosides on the cardiovascular system. He suggested that the condition known as 'delirium cordis' was identical with atrial fibrillation, and was subsequently shown to be correct. He also showed that while the effect of digitalis in slowing the heart rate in sinus rhythm was at least partly attributable to its effects on the vagus, that was not the case in atrial fibrillation. He correctly suggested that it was due to impairment of the conduction of impulses from the atria to the ventricles, although he also suggested that it might be a secondary effect following the 'improved nutrition of the heart from the augmented power of contraction of the heart muscle' (Cushny *et al*. 1913).

Cushny's interest in cardiac glycosides culminated in the publication, in 1925, of *The action and uses in medicine of digitalis and its allies*, a comprehensive review of what was then known about the basic pharmacology, clinical pharmacology, and therapeutic uses of digitalis and other cardiac glycosides. In the book Cushny paid tribute to William Withering by reproducing von Breda's painting as frontispiece. In the preface Cushny expressed his regrets for having had to use the engraving of von Breda's painting by W. Bond, but wrote that he had been unable to find the original (it hangs in the Swedish National Museum in Stockholm).

Lest it be thought that there was no controversy surrounding these discoveries, I must at this point introduce Sir Thomas Lewis. Lewis (1881-1945) graduated BSc (first-class honours) in anatomy and physiology from Cardiff, and then studied medicine at University College Hospital, in London, winning a scholarship and five medals before he graduated in 1905. After taking his MD in 1907 he worked with Starling, and spent most of his subsequent working life in London. He met Mackenzie in 1908 and was encouraged by him to study the electrophysiology of the heart. Lewis's views on digitalis were idiosyncratic for his time (Lewis 1919):

> The principle of [therapy with cardiac glycosides] is that, administered to suitable cases, the heart, by means of [them], obtains rest . . . Those who regard digitalis as a cardiac stimulant mistake its character. *To the heart foxglove is not tonic, but powerfully hypnotic*. It extends the diastoles of the heart; it extends the period of sleep.

In 1921 Mackenzie sent Lewis a paper on digitalis for publication in the journal *Heart* which Lewis edited. The story has been related by McMichael (1981); Lewis rejected the paper, writing to Mackenzie (*Lewis-Mackenzie Correspondence, 1909-25*):

> I have read your letter with close attention. May be I am wrong, may be not, on this matter of digitalis and its action on the vagus. My position is that the pure action through the vagus is not proved; and that it can be contended that the main action in fibrillation is a direct one on the muscle.

Mackenzie replied angrily:

> . . . you might as well put upon the forefront of the journal 'No articles will be accepted which are not in accordance with the (temporary) beliefs of the Editor' . . . As this, I suppose, is to be the end of our collaboration, I can assure you that I will follow with interest your future progress, and no one will rejoice more than I at your successes.

THE USE OF DIGITALIS IN HEART FAILURE WITH NORMAL RHYTHM

It is clear from all this that it was recognized that digitalis was of some value in the treatment of heart failure associated with normal cardiac rhythm, but that its effectiveness in such patients was overshadowed by its dramatic effects in patients with atrial fibrillation. The refinement of the electrocardiogram by Einthoven (1903) after its invention by Waller (1887) quickly led to an increased understanding of the nature of different cardiac arrhythmias. Subsequently Cohn (1915) classified heart failure into four types depending on the presence of regular rhythm or atrial fibrillation, and the presence or absence of peripheral oedema. He further subdivided these types according to whether or not the blood pressure was raised. Others later graded heart failure more carefully according to its severity, and these simple devices helped investigators in their studies of the most appropriate circumstances in which digitalis might be used. However, Cohn was hampered by an inability to measure the contractility of the heart in man, and his initial observations were therefore limited to observing heart rate and rhythm. In doing so he made the observation that digitalis alters the T wave of the electrocardiogram (Cohn 1915).

Subsequently, however, in careful clinical studies, and with the use of new techniques, albeit crude ones, for measuring cardiac output (at first indirectly using re-breathing techniques, but later directly by introducing catheters into the heart) and other indices of cardiac performance, two things became clear. Firstly, that digitalis had beneficial effects in cardiac failure *whether it was associated with regular rhythm or with atrial fibrillation*. Secondly, that digitalis increased the contraction of the heart by a direct effect on the cardiac muscle.

Christian (1919) showed that digitalis and strophanthin had beneficial effects in what he called 'chronic myocarditis', that is primary disease of the heart muscle due to any cause, as opposed to heart failure secondary to valvular disease. He attributed the previous failure of others to demonstrate a beneficial effect in patients with regular rhythm to the use of low dosages, and his words echoed those of Wenckebach quoted above:

It seems that in our books and in our teaching, bad effects from overdosage of digitalis and descriptions of contra-indications to its use have been so emphasized that often the physician actually is afraid to give an adequate dose of digitalis.

Drew Luten (1924) confirmed Christian's findings and extended them to show that there was a poor response to digitalis in patients with aortic valve disease, confirming Corrigan's report (see p. 324). Later on Marvin (1927) found that digitalis was of benefit in heart failure due to what he termed arteriosclerotic disease, a term which embraced both ischaemic and hypertensive heart disease, a finding later confirmed by Paul Wood (1940), and that it was of some benefit in patients with syphilitic heart disease. However, he found it to be of no value in a small series of patients with heart failure secondary to rheumatic valvular damage.

Further advances became possible in the late 1930s and early 1940s with the development of methods for measuring cardiac haemodynamics by invasive and non-invasive techniques, resulting in series of papers from H. J. Stewart and from Sir John McMichael, the former showing that digitalis increased cardiac output and reduced the size of the dilated heart in a manner independent of the cardiac rhythm (Stewart *et al*. 1938a, b), and the latter carefully dissecting out the different effects on cardiac function of digitalis and venesection.

McMichael graduated with honours from Edinburgh in 1927 and gained his MD (Gold Medal) in 1933 for his work on splenic anaemia. Working in the British Postgraduate Medical School in the late 1930s and early 1940s, he published a series of papers on the actions of digitalis and venesection in heart failure with Howarth and Sharpey-Schafer. They confirmed that digoxin, which had been isolated from *Digitalis lanata* by Smith in 1930, caused increased cardiac output in patients with heart failure, even when associated with regular rhythm (McMichael and Sharpey-Schafer 1944). However, they reasoned that that effect was due to a primary action of the drug on venous pressure, and were not able to explain such an action. They subsequently showed that venesection and digoxin had similar effects in reducing right atrial pressure and increasing cardiac output, but that the effects of digitalis were consistently greater, suggesting that they might be, at least in part, due to a direct effect on the heart (Howarth *et al*. 1946). They also showed that, while digitalis was beneficial in patients whose heart failure was due to valvular, hypertensive, or ischaemic heart disease, it was of little value in patients whose heart failure was secondary to chronic lung disease ('cor pulmonale').

It is worthy of note that in the interpretation of these studies McMichael and his colleagues were greatly aided by the understanding of cardiac physiology afforded by the studies of Starling and Frank, relating cardiac output to venous pressure in isolated heart preparations (Frank 1895; Starling 1918). Subsequent studies of the actions of digitalis in heart failure may have added much to our understanding of the different ways in which digitalis acts, but our knowledge of which patients may best respond has been little advanced at the clinical level since the publication of these studies.

CHAPTER 8

THE TWENTIETH CENTURY
from 1950

There are two matters to be dealt with in regard to the clinical use of digitalis in the second half of the twentieth century, remembering that it is too soon to gain a proper historical perspective on the events. Firstly, the development of the discipline of clinical pharmacology and its application to the cardiac glycosides, and secondly, the current attitudes to the use of digitalis and other cardiac glycosides. Much of the following account of the history of the clinical pharmacology of cardiac glycosides is, of necessity, and for the sake of the record, technical. However, I have tried to make the account as simple as possible, giving references to more technical review articles for those who want to pursue the details further. Those who are not interested in the drier facts of clinical pharmacology would be well advised at this point to turn to p. 344 and there pursue the story of current attitudes to the clinical use of cardiac glycosides.

CLINICAL PHARMACOLOGY

The subject we now call clinical pharmacology had its roots in what is still in some parts of the country called materia medica, which is, broadly speaking, the study of the use of drugs in man. The term 'clinical pharmacology' should embrace all aspects of this, having four components (see Grahame-Smith and Aronson 1984):

(i) Pharmaceutical matters—by this I mean those aspects of the formulation of drugs in preparations suitable for their

clinical administration, and which may influence the drug's
clinical use.

(ii) Pharmacokinetics—the delineation of the way in which a
drug is absorbed, distributed around the tissues of the body,
and eliminated. All these factors determine how much
drug gets to its site of action. A terse, technical account of
the history of pharmacokinetics has been written by
Wagner (1981).

(iii) Pharmacodynamics—an understanding of what the drug
is doing at its site of action. This can be appreciated at
different levels—for example, digitalis inhibits the transport
of sodium and potassium ions across cell membranes and
this can be considered to be its effect at a molecular level; in
doing so it causes increased contraction of cardiac muscle
fibres (an effect at the cellular level); this effect is in turn
translated into an increase in cardiac output (an effect at the
level of the whole organ); finally, and in appropriate
circumstances, this effect may cause a diuresis in the patient
with cardiac failure and result in improvement in the
patient's symptoms (an effect at the level of the whole body).

(iv) Drug therapy—an understanding of how to use a drug
properly in the treatment of a disease or illness. This last
synthesizes the preceding three, since it involves an understanding of what formulations to use; of what doses to give,
and of how to alter those doses to suit different patients; of
which patients may best benefit from the use of the drug; of
when to start therapy; and of when to stop.

When one considers the long chain of command linking the
harvesting of the leaf of a plant to the final therapeutic outcome it
is not at all surprising that the three complex matters of pharma-
ceutics, pharmacokinetics, and pharmacodynamics lay numerous
traps along the way for the physician attempting to use digitalis in

the best possible fashion, as we have seen in each of the preceding chapters.

PHARMACEUTICAL PROBLEMS

We have already seen how William Withering's careful studies were the first attempt to discover which formulation of crude digitalis, prepared directly from the plant, was ideal (see Chapter 4). He decided that the powdered leaf was the best of the choices available to him, and digitalis leaf remained the best available formulation until it became possible to isolate and purify cardiac glycosides from their plants in the early part of this century. Since then pure formulations of digoxin, digitoxin, and other cardiac glycosides (See Table 1.1, p. 215) have been used.

However, the very fact that highly purified preparations became available caused pharmaceutical problems, since small variations in the way a pharmaceutical formulation releases its active contents into the body can make large differences in the amount of drug getting to the site of action. The story of the 'digoxin affair' has been recounted by Munro-Faure *et al.* (1974), and can be summarized briefly here. In around 1969 Burroughs Wellcome, the principal manufacturer of digoxin tablets in the world, in some way altered the formulation of Lanoxin® tablets. The total amount of drug in the tablets was not changed, but some of the other constituents ('excipients') were, and the change in formulation meant that the digoxin in the tablets did not dissolve as quickly in the stomach as it should have, and that led to decreased availability of the drug for absorption. In May 1972 the formulation was changed again, but in the meantime it was noticed that the absorption of digoxin from the 1969/72 tablets was lower than it should have been (about half as much). This observation led to intensive research on the correct ways in which digoxin should be formulated, and it was discovered, firstly that there were large differences in the absorption of digoxin from different tablets made by different manufacturers, and secondly that there were differences in the absorption of digoxin from different formulations (e.g. tablets compared with elixir, and elixir compared with encapsulated elixir; see p. 183). Problems of this kind with tabletted formulations have now largely been overcome by the introduction of pharmacopoeial standards (Department of Health and Social Security 1975; *British Pharmacópoeia* 1975).

PHARMACOKINETICS

The first studies on the pharmacokinetics of digitalis were carried out at the beginning of this century, and their results were reviewed by Cushny in 1925. However, they were based on measurements of concentrations of cardiac glycosides in body tissues using methods which were very crude, and while it is surprising that the results obtained at that time reflected quite well what we know about the pharmacokinetics of these drugs from modern studies, it is *not* surprising that they were limited in their scope.

In 1949 Friedman and his colleagues invented a relatively sensitive bio-assay for cardiac glycosides, based on their effects on the duck embryo heart. The techniques were too cumbersome, however, for routine clinical use, as were several subsequent methods (for a review see Aronson 1985).

In the meantime, however, investigators had devised other methods for studying the pharmacokinetics of digitalis. The most ingenious of those were the experiments of Gold and his colleagues. They used their observations on the time course of changes in cardiac function following the administration of digitoxin, both by different routes and in different doses, in order to make inferences about the pharmacokinetics of the drug. For example, they showed that it was possible to establish the strength of an unknown formulation of digitalis by observing the

effects of its administration on the T wave of the electrocardiogram, and by comparing those effects with the effects of
preparations of known strength (Gold *et al*. 1942). They showed
that the effect of an oral dose of digitoxin was the same as that of
an intravenous dose, suggesting that digitoxin was completely
absorbed after oral administration (Gold *et al*. 1944). They
quantified the potency of pure digitoxin compared with digitalis
leaf (Gold *et al*. 1944). They showed that the well-known
phenomenon of the accumulation of digitoxin during long-term
therapy, of which Withering had been aware (see Fig. 1.1 and pp.
227-30) and which was clearly described at the beginning of this
century (see Cushny 1925), could be circumvented by using a
small maintenance dose after the initial phase of treatment with
higher doses was complete (Gold *et al*. 1944)—it was largely this
discovery, which Mackenzie had already made empirically
(Mackenzie 1911b), which led clinicians to start using digitalis in
long-term therapy rather than in short courses as they had done
since the time of Withering (see pp. 227-30).

In reviewing all these achievements, Gold wrote (Gold 1946):

> The term 'clinical study' doesn't rate very high in clinical
> circles. The belief prevails that the search for facts on drug
> action in man directly is of necessity inexact, subject to the
> impressions and prejudices of the observer and not amenable
> to the strict control of the animal experiment. [However,]
> there is a vast area of pharmacologic investigation which may
> be developed with the human subject and which, if the experi-
> ments are suitably designed, may be counted on to yield
> important facts in a manner which complies with the strictest
> demands of scientific evidence.

While Gold's defensive attitude is understandable, in view of the
novelty of the methods he was using, and of the whole subject of
clinical pharmacology (although he would not have called it

that), it was unnecessary—there can be no doubt that his studies formed the foundations on which subsequent studies of the pharmacokinetics, and hence of the clinical use, of digitalis were based.

A second method of studying the pharmacokinetics of digitalis, less ingenious, but, because easier, more fruitful in terms of the sheer volume of information gained, was developed in the 1960s—the administration of cardiac glycosides which were 'labelled' with radioactive isotopes such as tritium (^{3}H) and carbon-14. In studies of this kind [^{14}C]digitoxin was used by Okita and his colleagues, and [^{3}H]digoxin by Doherty and Marcus and their respective colleagues (for a review see Doherty 1968). Most of their findings have since been confirmed by studies in which direct measurements of plasma, urine, and other tissue glycoside concentrations have been made using a variety of techniques, principally radio-immunoassay, which was first developed in the late 1960s (Smith *et al*. 1969), and which has since proved the mainstay of such studies.

In addition to its research applications the ability to measure plasma digitalis concentrations has also led to the introduction of such measurements in the routine care of patients taking digitalis, in order to adjust doses to best suit the patient, to diagnosis toxicity, to monitor compliance, and to help make decisions about long-term treatment. I have reviewed this subject in detail elsewhere. For those interested in the precise details of the pharmacokinetics of digoxin and digitoxin, they can be found in various review articles (see Iisalo 1977; Wettrell and Andersson 1977; Aronson 1980a; Aronson 1983b).

PHARMACODYNAMICS

The elucidation of the pharmacodynamic properties of digitalis has travelled the road outlined in paragraph (iii) on p. 338 in the reverse direction. This is not at all surprising, since it is initially simpler to observe the behaviour of the intact organism, despite its greater complexity, than it is to observe the behaviour of individual parts of the organism. Thus, William Withering knew that digitalis has beneficial effects at the level of the whole body—that is it made his patients better—although he had some difficulty in convincing some of his contemporaries of the fact (see pp. 301-9). Later on, early in this century (see Chapter 7) the effect of digitalis at the level of the whole organ (the heart and other tissues) were demonstrated. It was not until the 1950s, however, that the underlying cellular and molecular mechanisms were discovered.

It was already known that cardiac glycosides, at least in toxic doses, altered the intracellular disposition of potassium (Calhoun and Harrison 1931; Cattell and Goodell 1937; Hagen 1939). The discovery of the mechanism of this effect belonged to Schatzmann (1953) who showed that strophanthin inhibited the movements of sodium and potassium across the membranes of red blood cells, and Glynn later showed that this effect was produced by low concentrations of several different cardiac glycosides (Glynn 1957). This observation was subsequently turned to practical use in the development of a sensitive bio-assay for digitalis, based on the dose-responsiveness of the inhibition by cardiac glycosides of potassium transport into red blood cells (Lowenstein and Corrill 1966; Grahame-Smith and Everest 1969), and in the development of a method for monitoring the cellular effects of digitalis in the body during therapy (Aronson *et al*. 1981).

At about the same time Skou described the enzyme, present in cell membranes, which was responsible for providing most of the energy for transporting sodium and potassium across cell membranes (Skou 1957), the so-called sodium-potassium-linked, magnesium-dependent adenosine triphosphatase (Na/K-ATPase for short), and it was not long before it was shown that cardiac glycosides produced their effects by inhibiting that enzyme. Post (1974) has written a brief, but entertaining account of Skou's discovery, and of his own part in the subsequent elucidation of the effects of cardiac glycosides on the Na/K-ATPase.

Since then an enormous amount of evidence has accumulated suggesting that it is by inhibition of the Na/K-ATPase that cardiac glycosides produce their toxic and therapeutic effects on the heart and probably on the eye, if not on other tissues as well (for a comprehensive review see Schwartz *et al*. 1975). The apparently idiosyncratic view that it may be by *stimulation* of this enzyme that the therapeutic effects of digitalis are produced, at least at low doses (see Noble 1980), has led to the careful unravelling of other interesting properties of digitalis (Hart *et al*. 1983), but it is too soon to be able to assess the clinical relevance of these findings.

CURRENT ATTITUDES TO THE CLINICAL USE OF CARDIAC GLYCOSIDES IN HEART FAILURE

There is no doubt that digitalis remains the treatment of choice for the treatment of uncomplicated fast atrial fibrillation. However, its role in the treatment of heart failure, particularly in patients whose heart rhythm is regular, has recently become controversial for several reasons.

In order to gain some perspective on current attitudes to the clinical use of digitalis in the treatment of heart failure it is first necessary briefly to remind those who have struggled through the preceding pages of this chapter, and to tell for the first time those who chose not to, about the different levels at which digitalis acts in producing its therapeutic effects, from the lowest to the highest level, now adding the context of the clinical problems which heart failure may pose.

At the *molecular* level digitalis inhibits sodium and potassium movements across cell membranes—about that there is no doubt (although if those movements are in some way already abnormal, as in overactivity of the thyroid gland, or in response to abnormalities of potassium balance, then the reponse to digitalis may be altered, and the use of the drug limited). Although there is some doubt about the relevance of this effect on sodium and potassium to the clinical effects of cardiac glycosides, the doubt is small enough to be ignored for the present.

At the *cellular* level digitalis increases the rate of contractility of the cardiac muscle fibres—about that too there is no doubt, although it is recognized that, in some circumstances, this may not happen properly, and that abnormalities caused by chronic lung disease (see p. 336), or by acute impairment of the blood supply to the heart, may reduce the clinical usefulness of digitalis (i.e. in 'cor pulmonale', and immediately following a heart attack or in cardiogenic shock).

At the level of the *whole organ*, digitalis increases the cardiac output (and in addition has other effects on the cardiovascular system which I shall not discuss). Although that too is not open to doubt, it is recognized that in some circumstances the increase in contractility may not cause an increase in cardiac output, notably in the condition called hypertrophic obstructive cardiomyopathy (engagingly abbreviated to HOCM, pronounced 'hocum'), in which the muscle at the outlet of the left ventricle is hypertrophied and obstructs outflow, so that any increase in contractility of the left ventricle, including the hypertrophied section, causes worsening of cardiac function rather than improvement.

 · Finally, at the level of the *whole body*, digitalis, except perhaps in those circumstances mentioned above, generally improves the patient's condition, removing, or at least alleviating, the signs and symptoms of cardiac failure. About this fact too, there can be no doubt—the evidence of many clinical investigators since William Withering attests to it (see Chapter 7). It is also recognized that the circumstances in which digitalis is most likely to be of benefit is where cardiac failure is due to chronic impairment of the blood supply to the heart (chronic ischaemic heart disease), or to disease of the mitral valve, or to hypertension (although there is some controversy about the last indication; see, for example, Hamer 1979).

Despite all this apparent lack of doubt, two issues have recently caused controversy. The first relates to the relative value of digitalis compared with other treatments, the second to the long-term efficacy of digitalis.

DIGITALIS COMPARED WITH OTHER TREATMENTS FOR HEART FAILURE

For many years it has been commonplace to use diuretics for the treatment of heart failure. Mercurials, such as calomel, have been known to be diuretics for at least 400 years (see, for example, Withering's use of them by consulting the index on pp. 381-87 under their various names, e.g. calomel and corrosive mercuric sublimate), and they were widely used during the earlier part of this century. However, mercurials are exceptionally toxic substances, and in many cases digitalis would have been preferred, at least as first choice. Following the introduction of safer diuretics, however, during the 1950s, diuretic therapy for heart failure gradually came to assume first place ahead of digitalis, and in many cases it is true that diuretic therapy is adequate and sufficient treatment.

This change has occurred with only minimal attempts to answer certain questions about the relative usefulness of these two different types of treatments. Firstly, in an uncomplicated case of cardiac failure with regular heart rhythm, is it better to use digitalis or a diuretic? There are only two studies in which an attempt has been made to answer this question, and although the results suggest that there is little difference between digitalis alone or in combination with a diuretic, the studies were too poorly designed to be conclusive (Rader *et al*. 1964; Hutcheon *et al*. 1980). The importance of this question is that it is gradually becoming apparent that diuretics may have adverse effects, especially during long-term therapy, which may be more undesirable than the adverse effects of digitalis. The problem, of course, is that the adverse effects of digitalis can be so difficult to avoid, especially in the elderly, that physicians are less trusting of its safety than they are in general of the safety of diuretics.

Secondly, if diuretics fail to work, or produce only incomplete relief, does the addition of digitalis confer any benefit? Surprisingly, there seems to be no answer to this question at present. There is, it must be said, the not altogether unsurprising finding that if a patient has responded satisfactorily to a diuretic then he will not experience any added symptomatic benefit from digitalis (McHaffie *et al*. 1978). However, I have found no more than anecdotal evidence regarding the benefit of adding digitalis when there has *not* been a complete response to a regimen of diuretics.

The problem has recently become complicated by the introduction of vasodilators to the treatment to cardiac failure, and although I still prefer to add digitalis after diuretics, and have seen several cases of dramatic response to such treatment, I cannot summon up firm proof that my method is better than that of those who omit to use digitalis altogether.

THE LONG-TERM USE OF DIGITALIS

It was Withering's habit to use digitalis in short courses only. Exemplary of this is his account of Case XLIII (pp. 40-43), in which he gave several courses of treatment and observed remission following each course for periods of up to five months. In some cases he seems to have given only one course of treatment with life-long cure, although we cannot be sure either of the causes of heart failure in those cases, or even that they were necessarily cases of cardiac failure, rather than some other condition which would not have recurred after its treatment or spontaneous resolution.

Withering's reason for using only short courses of treatment with digitalis was that the doses he used inevitably resulted in toxicity after only a few days because of accumulation (see Fig. 1.1 and pp. 227-30). It was not until the observations of Gold and his colleagues (see p. 340) that it was possible to gauge how accumulation could be avoided by reducing to a maintenance dose after initial therapy, although Mackenzie had also recognized the possibility of such an approach (Mackenzie 1911b). It then became possible to continue digitalis therapy safely for more than a few days, and it subsequently became commonplace for digitalis therapy to be continued life-long.

This was acceptable in many cases of atrial fibrillation, in which it became apparent that continued therapy was necessary in order to continue to control the ventricular rate, which could be slowed by digitalis, but which would speed up again on its withdrawal. That that was so was recognized by Mackenzie (1911b, and see quote on p. 347), and it was subsequently clearly shown to be so by Rogen (1943), although since then it has been recognized that not all patients with controlled atrial fibrillation continue to need digitalis to maintain the heart rate at a normal level after long-term therapy (Liverpool Therapeutics Group 1978; Johnston and McDevitt 1979), and presumably these are patients in whom a sufficient degree of atrio-ventricular block has occurred to prevent the transmission of more than a normal number of impulses from the atria to the ventricles, even in the absence of digitalis.

However, in patients with heart failure associated with regular rhythm it has recently become clear that long-term digitalis therapy may not be required. In fact that was clearly recognized by Mackenzie (1911b):

> The maintenance of the improvement [in cases with the normal rhythm] is one of the most difficult matters to understand. The improvement in most cases of auricular fibrillation lasted only a few days after the cessation of the drug, and an attempt was made to give the patient just enough of the drug as would maintain the good effect without producing the disagreeable symptoms, and in several cases this was very successfully accomplished. With the normal rhythm, this tendency to relapse after cessation of the drug was not seen.

This phenomenon has been clearly demonstrated in several studies (for a review see Aronson 1980b), and is due to several factors. Firstly there are patients in whom heart failure occurs because of a single precipitating factor which, if properly treated, does not recur, for example anaemia and hyperthyroidism (see Dall 1970). Secondly, following the resolution of cardiac failure it is clear that the heart can, in some cases, function quite well for a variable period of time until whatever mechanisms cause heart failure, and they are not clearly understood, cause the syndrome to develop again. In such cases the withdrawal of digitalis may not necessarily lead to recurrence of heart failure, or if it does it may be possible, at least in the first instance, to treat it with increased doses of diuretics.

If one considers all those patients in whom the initial indication for treatment with digitalis was one which would be expected to persist (e.g. chronic ischaemia), and who subsequently continued to take effective doses of digitalis as long-term therapy, then heart failure will not worsen in about two-thirds of those patients following subsequent withdrawal of digitalis. In another one-fifth, whatever worsening of heart function occurs after withdrawal of digitalis can be treated with increased doses of diuretics. In only about one-tenth of all those patients does long-term digitalis prove necessary to maintain reasonable cardiac function.

These figures are remarkably similar to those quoted by Gold, based on his extensive experience of the clinical use of digitalis (Gold 1941):

> Only about 15 percent of cardiac patients owe to the habitual use of digitalis the fact that they are able to carry on with a reasonable degree of comfort. The reputation of the drug is not enhanced, to say the least, by its use in the remaining 85 percent of the cardiac population.

All these factors—the earlier diagnosis of heart failure and its successful treatment with diuretics, the recognition that in some cases (see p. 345) digitalis is not of great benefit to start with, and the observation that long-term digitalis therapy is not necessary in the majority of cases—has led to the belief that, as I heard someone say recently, 'digitalis doesn't work any more'. This attitude is an ironic reflection of Osler's equally ironic comment on the use of new drugs (quoted on p. 322), and it has two separate components. Firstly, it is felt that digitalis is of little or no benefit from the outset in treating cardiac failure, no matter what the cause, and secondly, it is thought, mistakenly, that digitalis does not continue to exert its pharmacological and therapeutic effects during long-term therapy. I say 'mistakenly' firstly, because, although there is indeed evidence that the effects of digitalis at the molecular level do not necessarily persist during long-term therapy (Aronson *et al*. 1981), this phenomenon does not necessarily apply to all cases; secondly, because there is clear evidence that the haemodynamic effects of digitalis may be lost in some patients following withdrawal of digitalis without worsening of heart failure, suggesting that in those patients digitalis was 'working' (i.e. producing an effect at the level of the whole organ), but was not required for its effects on the whole body; and thirdly, because there are manifestly patients, albeit a small number of them, who *do* need continued long-term treatment with digitalis to remain well.

There is still no alternative to digitalis for the first-line treatment of fast atrial fibrillation in the majority of cases. However, digitalis has yet to find its proper place in the therapy of heart failure in patients whose heart rhythm is regular. Despite much research there is still no adequate alternative in terms of a drug which increases cardiac contractility, but equally it has not been shown that there is a clear need for a drug which acts in such a way in the treatment of established heart failure, in preference, say, to diuretics or vasodilators. There is as yet no clear way of distinguishing those patients in whom long-term therapy with digitalis is required, as opposed to those in whom it is not, and the only way of deciding the issue in an individual is by withholding therapy and going through the tedious process of monitoring events day by day, watching for evidence of worsening of cardiac function. This is a process which many physicians would be unwilling to undertake, preferring rather not to use the drug in the first place. Furthermore, despite the development of new, semi-synthetic cardiac glycosides, based on the structure of either the digitalis glycosides (e.g. beta-methyldigoxin) or other cardiac glycosides (e.g. methyl-proscillaridin), there is still no glycoside available which is both effective and safe, and digitalis toxicity continues to be a problem in routine practice.

As William Withering put it, our methods are still 'far from perfect'.

CHAPTER 9

ENVOI

In writing the two parts of this book I have tried firstly to learn about medical practice in the eighteenth century through current understanding, and secondly to determine what can be learned about modern practice from an understanding of the past.

Of course, Withering's *Account* gives us only one face of eighteenth century medicine, dealing as it does with one relatively well-circumscribed group of diseases, but we can nonetheless take away some information from it in relation to eighteenth-century medicine as a whole.

It is clear that, as far as a therapeutic arsenal was concerned, eighteenth-century physicians were not short of ammunition. It is often written that until very recently only a handful of effective drugs was available to doctors (opiates, digitalis, and quinine being the most important), but that is simply not so. The physicians of the eighteenth and nineteenth centuries had many other powerful drugs at their command, as can be seen by reading the index to the drugs Withering used, on pp. 381-87. They had powerful diuretics, emetics, purgatives, febrifuges, carminatives, analgesics, sedatives, hypnotics, tranquillizers, and anticholinergic drugs; even before the discovery of the value of digitalis in dropsies they had drugs which increased the contractility of the heart, notably squill. Their therapeutic problems arose, I believe, not so much out of a poverty of available drugs, although their pharmacopoeia was admittedly much less replete with effective compounds than ours is, but more from other limitations which did not allow them to use what drugs they had to their best advantage.

Their two major problems were firstly, that their understanding of the pathophysiology of disease was rudimentary, and secondly, that their understanding of the actions of the compounds they were using, based as it was on relatively primitive clinical observations and chemical knowledge, was negligible.

These limitations gave rise to secondary problems. Firstly, they resulted in the introduction into the pharmacopoeia of a large variety of valueless, and indeed sometimes dangerous drugs. For example the early editions of the *Edinburgh Pharmacopoeia*, first published in 1699, contained such preparations as 'cranium hominis violenta morte extincti', 'secundia humanum', and 'stercus humanum', and although it was recognized by the beginning of the nineteenth century that those particular formulations were 'useless and disgusting substances' (see Cowen 1957), nonetheless there remained a large number of other preparations which we would nowadays recognize as being equally useless, if not necessarily equally disgusting.

We should not, however, be too scathing about all of those inclusions. For example, ginseng was introduced into the *Edinburgh Pharmacopoeia* in the same year that digitalis was reintroduced into it (1783) and was removed in 1803—it is now to be found in the current edition of *Martindale's Extra Pharmacopoeia* under the heading 'Supplementary drugs and other substances', where it states that 'ginseng has been claimed to enhance the natural resistance and recuperative power of the body and to have stimulant and sedative activity'. It is not yet clear whether or not ginseng or its active principles will prove to be of therapeutic use.

Secondly, even in the cases of drugs with clear pharmacological effects, it was not known how best those drugs should be used in regard to the choice of the drug most appropriate for the condition being treated, the most appropriate formulation, and the correct dosages, frequency of administration, and duration of treatment. In illustration of this, contrast Withering's methods of administering digitalis with that of Gold and his colleagues (see p. 340) and with what would be the modern approach were digitalis to be newly discovered today.

Over a period of ten years Withering, by careful experiment and clinical observation, came to what were substantially correct conclusions about its use (see pp. 179-92), although he could not have explained those conclusions in terms of the actions of the drug. Over a period of about five years Gold and his colleagues, again by careful clinical observations, supplemented with the use of the electrocardiogram, elucidated the accumulation of digitalis during long-term therapy and propounded the principles of the loading dose and maintenance dose, although Mackenzie before them had come to similar conclusions based on less sophisticated clinical observations. Today the same conclusions would be reached within a few months, by appropriately designed pharmacokinetic studies, outlining the absorption, distribution, and elimination of the drug, by means of appropriate plasma and other tissue concentration measurements, and sophisticated mathematical analysis of the data. Appropriate dosage regimens would be quickly developed for patients of different age groups and for patients with different degrees of renal or hepatic function.

However, all this does not mean that we are able to market drugs any faster. We now have to spend the extra time we have gained by studying other facets of the action of the drug, and in recent years increasing attention has been paid to safety and the avoidance of adverse effects. In this sense we are worse off than in the eighteenth century, because of the introduction of potent, synthetic and semi-synthetic drugs, which are not infrequently as potent in causing adverse effects as they are in producing a therapeutically desirable result. Because of the nature of the adverse effects of drugs we should have to spend at least as much time, perhaps more, in the development and marketing of a drug such

as digitalis today as Withering did in developing his own expertise, and at a much greater cost in the use of people and resources.

It must be recognized that we have exchanged simplicity for
the increased, albeit expensive, production of effective drugs, and
that that in turn means that we have to exchange therapeutic
impotence for increased risks of the adverse effects of therapeutically useful compounds. That this is worthwhile there can
be no doubt. We have today at our disposal many life-saving
drugs, such as antibiotics, insulin, and corticosteroids, and many
drugs which alleviate the discomfort of illness, such as drugs used
for treating peptic ulcer, Parkinson's disease, and asthma. We are
beginning to come to terms with the fact that these benefits carry
with them increased risks, and we are continually looking for
ways in which those risks can be minimized.

While the public cannot expect that powerful new therapies
should be completely free from adverse effects, they can expect
that their doctors should be able to use the drugs at their command in the most efficient ways possible, and in that respect too
we can learn from the example of digitalis. Following the publication of Withering's *Account* it is clear (see the discussion on
pp. 298-309) that there was widespread misuse of the drug, partly
because of a failure to understand the correct principles underlying both the precise choice of cases to be treated and of the
correct dosages to be used, as Withering had outlined.

We can easily find examples of this kind of sequence of events
in modern practice. For example, not infrequently drugs are mar-
keted for specific indications and are then used for purposes
other than those for which they were originally indicated, and for
which their value has not been proven. This happens for several
reasons. Firstly, it may appear logical, even if not proven, that a
drug with particular pharmacological characteristics should be
effective in some condition whose pathophysiology is thought to
relate to those characteristics; for example, the use of cimetidine

to treat acute bleeding from a duodenal ulcer, after it had been shown that it was of value of hastening the healing of a chronic ulcer. Secondly, doctors are subject to a lot of pressure from their patients to prescribe effective drugs, and from pharmaceutical companies to prescribe their latest products. As a result it is not uncommon for a doctor to prescribe, for example, the newest antidepressant drug on the market, because his patient has not found complete satisfaction from the more traditional prescription and is asking for something more effective. Because of the intermittent nature of the complaint, and the difficulty in measuring the response in an individual patient, the new therapy may appear, at least for some time, to be more effective than the old, and that in turn reinforces the doctor's attitude to the new drug.

In case this seems too cynical an attitude to new drugs, which may after all be more effective than older remedies, and which not infrequently prove to be so after careful study, it must be remembered, continuing with the example of antidepressants, that in order to demonstrate formally that a new antidepressant is really better than an established antidepressant one would have to carry out a trial to compare the two drugs in over 1000 patients (see Grahame-Smith and Aronson 1984), and that such trials are virtually never carried out. Thus there are many instances in which one does not know that a new drug is better than an established drug in treating a particular disease or illness in the population as a whole. Even if one did know that there was a statistical difference between the two drugs in a large population of patients, one might never know whether or not the drug had produced its beneficial effects in the individual patient.

In turn it must be remembered that the concept of a controlled clinical trial, which makes it possible formally to compare two drugs, and to make some assessment of their relative merits and demerits, was unknown to the physicians of previous centuries. For example, when John Ferriar published his own experience of the foxglove in treating dropsies he accompanied it with a description of the similar use of cream of tartar (i.e. potassium acid tartrate, which is recognized as having slight diuretic properties), but did not think to make a formal comparison of the two compounds beyond presenting a list of the cases he had treated with the two compounds (Ferriar 1792).

THE VALUE OF TECHNOLOGY

While some of the advances which have allowed us to use existing drugs to better advantage than our predecessors did have been based on purely *theoretical* developments, such as the mathematical concepts necessary for the elucidation of the pharmacokinetics of a drug, or the statistical concepts necessary for the design of a clinical trial, most of the advances have been made because of the advent of new *technology*, although frequently in combination with theoretical concepts. For example, without the ability to measure plasma concentrations of drugs by sophisticated techniques, such as radio-immunoassay, there would be no practical applications for pharmacokinetic theory.

It was this absence of appropriate technology that was the largest factor in limiting the ability of physicians of previous centuries to make the best use of the drugs they had. In the case of digitalis, Withering and his contemporaries were unable to do more than to measure its effects on the rate of the pulse, and the output of urine, and to observe its beneficial effects on the whole patient. They were unable to study the subtle ways in which digitalis affects the action of the heart muscle; they were unable to observe its actions on the conducting tissues of the heart, or on its nervous innervation; they were unable to standardize dosages, and to alter dosages appropriately to suit the individual case other than by trial and error.

When technological advances came they were unfortunately of the wrong sort from the point of view of elucidating the *clinical* value of digitalis. The invention of the haemadynamo-meter allowed Blake (1839) to study the effects of digitalis on the blood pressure, an action which is of little importance in the therapeutic effects of digitalis. Subsequent studies by Traube and Cushny (see Cushny 1897), using a variety of relatively simple instruments, including the myocardiograph, which recorded the relative distance between two points on the surface of the exposed heart, while of great theoretical interest, did little to advance the state of knowledge of the actions of digitalis relevant to its clinical use, beyond the further elucidation of its effects in altering the blood pressure, and the admittedly important finding that digitalis has an action on the vagus nerve. It was not until the invention and refinement of the electrocardiograph at the turn of the century (Waller 1887; Einthoven 1903) and the invention by Mackenzie of his polygraph (see Wilson 1926) that it became possible to elucidate the actions of digitalis in the treatment of atrial fibrillation.

Later on, further technological advances allowed physicians to extend their understanding—ballistocardiography, cardiac catheterization, phonocardiography, echocardiography, chemical methods for measuring digitalis concentrations in body tissues, biochemical methods for measuring the effects of digitalis on body tissues at the cellular level—at these and other stages one can chart developments in our understanding which have in turn led to changes in our use of or attitude to the drug.

It is common to liken scientific knowledge to a wide-open area with frontiers which are continually being pushed back, but I have always found this a curious analogy, at least in relation to medical research, in which we are constantly exploring and re-exploring the *same* areas, using increasingly sensitive tools to do so, rather like a hunter using his machete to explore in greater detail that area of the jungle which he already knows so well. In order to explore his part of the jungle in greater detail he relies on the tool-maker to provide him with sharper and sharper machetes. Some hunters make their own machetes, as Mackenzie invented his polygraph, but more usually they rely on collaboration, harnessing the skills of others. Nowhere has this been better demonstrated in recent years than in the invention of the technique of nuclear magnetic resonance spectroscopy by physicists, its development as an analytical tool by biochemists, and its application to the solution of clinical problems by physicians, each working in collaboration with the others.

Although it is still possible for one man to contribute to clinical science by dint of observation alone (for example, Oliver Sacks's observations on the actions of levodopa in postencephalitic Parkinsonism, recounted in his book *Awakenings*), we are coming to rely increasingly on collaborations of the kind exemplified by nuclear magnetic resonance spectroscopy, between scientists of different disciplines, to advance our understanding.

THE ROLE OF THE INVESTIGATOR

Despite these observations it would be wrong to credit only the inventors of new techniques with the improvements in understanding which has come as a result of their application, and to ignore the contribution of those who have applied them. For example, the probability theory developed by the Reverend Bayes in the eighteenth century has only recently come to be used in the development of the process known as decision analysis, simply because no one previously thought of using it for that purpose.

Thus, although the foxglove had been available for centuries before Withering, and although it was known to have diuretic properties, and although at least one other physician had tried it in the treatment of dropsy and had failed (see p. 239), nonetheless, by the application of simple observation, without the aid of sophisticated technology, Withering was able to delineate its clinical properties. (Incidentally, I find it curious that he did not do the same for squill, which had been recognized for much longer to have similar therapeutic effects in the treatment of dropsy and which contains cardiac glycosides similar to those found in *Digitalis* plants.)

Thus, although it had been known for many years that digitalis slowed the pulse, it took Mackenzie, with the aid of his polygraph, to demonstrate conclusively the relative specificity of its effects in atrial fibrillation.

Thus, although it had been suspected on clinical grounds by Withering and Mackenzie that digitalis accumulated in the body during long-term therapy, it took Gold and his colleagues, with the aid of the electrocardiograph, or simply by counting the pulse in atrial fibrillation, to demonstrate that that was indeed so and to develop dosage regimens to circumvent the problem.

Thus, although Withering and some of his contemporaries had shown that digitalis could relieve dropsy associated with normal cardiac rhythm, although they did not recognize it as such, it took investigators such as Christian, Marvin, Stewart, and McMichael and their colleagues to demonstrate that it could, using simple clinical observations, and with the aid of the latest advances in technology.

In each of these and other cases it can be seen that it was not merely the availability of the appropriate technology, but also the presence of the right-minded investigator which led to the clinical advances we now take for granted in our daily use of digitalis. To take a simple analogy from outside the realms of science, consider the way in which Picasso transformed a bicycle saddle and handlebars into the head and horns of a bull—the application of a simple but revealing idea into a work of art. William Withering, and since him many others involved in the history of digitalis, not only in the clinical story which I have related, but in other areas, such as the elucidation of the chemistry of the cardiac glycosides, were equipped with, to use Peter Medawar's striking phrase, the comparable art of making scientific problems soluble.

THE INTERDEPENDENCY OF BASIC
AND CLINICAL RESEARCH

It was once fashionable to regard 'pure' or 'basic' science as being of the utmost importance, but the pendulum has now swung in the opposite direction, and it is now common to hear scientists and politicians talking rather disparagingly about, to use the modern jargon, 'curiosity' science. The reasons are obvious. There are often no immediately obvious practical applications for scientific experiments which are intended to study basic phenomena, and while practical problems exist, and the resources to study them are limited, there will always be pressure to reduce commitment to basic research.

That this is a dangerous attitude cannot be doubted. The clinical scientists of the Enlightenment amused themselves by their basic experiments in physics and chemistry, mineralogy and botany, mathematics and astronomy. They were glad to be able to employ practical applications for their discoveries, and indeed searched for them, but they were not unduly concerned if they did not find them. They derived their stimulation from the acts of discovery and the intellectual debate involved.

When they surveyed the history of discoveries in cardiology and respiratory medicine, Comroe and Dripps (1976) found that about 41 per cent of the key publications were related to non-clinical basic science, the rest to clinical science. They were able to trace, for example, the development of electrocardiography to several scientific discoveries which at first sight would have seemed to have had no application to clinical practice, starting with the simple observation that amber stores electrostatic charge. They used their findings to argue that more resources should be devoted to basic research, but their analysis could equally well be used to support the argument that resources should be divided roughly equally between clinical and basic research.

Neither basic nor clinical research can exist without the other. Unless basic scientists, exercising their curiosity, make fundamental discoveries, clinical scientists will not have the machetes they need to explore their jungles. Unless the clinicians ask the appropriate questions about the problems they face, the tools provided by the basic scientists will prove to be blunt and useless. Whatever it was that sparked Withering's interest in botany (see pp. 250-4) it was almost certainly nothing to do with a desire to use plants medicinally, but the expertise he gained by his studies of a basic science was undoubtedly of major importance in his later successful clinical use of the foxglove.

BIBLIOGRAPHY

Ackerknecht, E. H. (1962). Aspects of the history of therapeutics. *Bull. Hist. Med.* **36**, 389-419.

Allibone, S. A. (1877). *Dictionary of English literature and British and American authors*. J. B. Lippincott, Philadelphia; Trübner, London.

Alston, C. (1683-1760). *Lectures on the materia medica; containing the natural history of drugs; also directions for the study of the materia medica; and an appendix on the method of prescribing*. (ed. J. Hope). E. & C. Dilly, London.

Anon. (1778). [Obituary of Charles Darwin] *Med. Comm*. **5**, 329-36.

— (1781). [Editorial note] *Lond. Med. J*. **2**, 415-16.

— (1785a). Postscript to the appendix to Dr. Darwin's paper on foxglove. *Med. Trans. Coll. Phys. Lond.* **3**, 448.

— (1785b). [Review of Withering's *Account*] *Lond. Med. J.* **6**, 298-305.

— (1785c). [Review of Withering's *Account*] *Med. Comm.* **10**, 133-46.

— (1785d). [Review of Withering's *Account*] *Month. Rev.* **73**, 369-71.

— (1785e). [Editorial note] *Lond. Med. J.* **6**, 55-60.

— (1810). [Review of Maclean, 1810] *Edin. Med. Surg. J.* **6**, 474-86.

— (1872). [The treatment of phthisis] *Lancet* **i**, 653-4.

Aronson, J. K. (1980a). Clinical pharmacokinetics of digoxin. *Clin. Pharmacokin*. **5**, 137-49.

— (1980b). Cardiac glycosides and drugs used in dysrhythmias. In *Side effects of drugs, annual 4* (ed. M. N. G. Dukes). Excerpta Medica, Amsterdam, pp. 123-6.

— (1981). Cardiac glycosides and drugs used in dysrhythmias. In *Side effects of drugs, annual 5* (ed. M. N. G. Dukes and J. Elis). Excerpta Medica, Amsterdam. p. 177.

— (1983a) Digitalis intoxication. *Clin. Sci*. **64**, 253-8.

— (1983b) Clinical pharmacokinetics of cardiac glycosides in patients with renal dysfunction. *Clin. Pharmacokin*. **8**, 155-78.

— (1984). The role of the Na$^+$, K$^+$-ATPase in the regulation of vascular smooth-muscle contractility, and its relationship to essential hypertension. *Trans. Biochem. Soc*. **12**, 943-5.

— (1985). Digoxin. In *Contemporary issues in biochemistry: therapeutic drug monitoring* (ed. B. Widdop). Churchill Livingstone, Edinburgh.

Aronson, J. K. and Ford, A. R. (1980). The use of colour vision measurement in the diagnosis of digoxin toxicity. *Q. J. Med.* **NS49**, 273-82.

—— —— and Grahame-Smith, D. G. (1981). Techniques for studying the pharmacodynamic effects of cardiac glycosides on patients' own erythrocytes during glycoside therapy. *Klin. Wochenschr.* **59**, 1323-32.

Baker, G. (1772a). Several extraordinary instances of the cure of the dropsy. *Med. Trans. Coll. Phys. Lond.* **2**, 235-58.

—— (1772b). An inquiry concerning the cause of the endemial colic of Derbyshire. *Med. Trans. Coll. Phys. Lond.* **2**, 419-70.

—— (1785a). Farther observations on the poison of lead. *Med. Trans. Coll. Phys. Lond.* **3**, 175-240.

—— (1785b). An appendix to Dr. Baker's inquiry concerning the cause of endemial colic of Derbyshire. *Med. Trans. Coll. Phys. Lond.* **3**, 460-9.

—— (1785c). An appendix to the preceding paper [See Darwin, 1785]. *Med. Trans. Coll. Phys. Lond*, **3**, 287-308.

Bauhinus, J. and Cherterus, J. H. (1650-51). *Historia plantarum universalis, nova et absolutissima, cum consensu et dissensu circa eas*. Ebroduni.

Beddoes, T. (1799). *Essay on the causes, early signs, and prevention of pulmonary consumption for the use of parents and preceptors*. Longman & Rees, London.

Bence-Jones, H. (1855). On digitalis. *Med. T. Gaz.* **NS10**, 381-3.

Bettany, G. T. (1888). William Cullen. In *Dictionary of national biography* (ed. L. Stephen and S. Lee. Smith, Elder & Co., London. vol. 13, pp. 279-82.

Black, J. (1803). *Lectures on the elements of chemistry, delivered in the University of Edinburgh* (ed. J. Robison). Longman & Rees, London; W. Creech, Edinburgh.

Black, J. G. (1885). Case (uterine) illustrating the action of digitalis as a depresso-motor. *Lancet* **i**, 886-7.

Blackall, J. (1813). *Observations on the nature and cure of dropsies, and particularly on the presence of the coagulable part of the blood in dropsical urine; to which is added, an appendix, containing several cases of angina pectoris, with dissections, etc.* Longman, Hurst, Rees, Orme & Brown, London.

Blackwell, E. (1737). *A curious herbal, containing five hundred cuts, of the most useful plants which are now used in the practice of physick. To which is added a short description of the plants; and their common uses in physick*. J. Nourse, London.

—— (1750-73). *Herbarium Blackwellianum emendatum et auctum; id est Elisabethae Blackwell collectio stirpium quae in pharmacopoliis ad medicum usum asservantur quarum descriptio et vires ex anglico idiomate in latinum conversae sistuntur* . . ., Vols. 1-5 (ed. C. J. Trew 1750-65), Vol. 6 (ed. C. G. Ludwig, 1773). J. Fleischmann, Nuremberg.

Blake, J. (1839). Observations on the physiological effects of various agents introduced into the circulation as indicated by the haemodynamometer. *Edin. Med. Surg. J*. 51, 330-45.

Bock, H. (1552). *Hieronymi Tragi, de stirpium maxime vero earum quae in Germania nascuntur commentarii*. V. Rihelius, Argentorati.

Boerhaave, H. (1740). *A treatise on the powers of medicines*. J. Wilcox, London.

Braithwaite, J. (1883). A note on the treatment of cardiac dropsy. *Lancet* ii, 855-6.

Brinton, W. (1861). On the treatment of tubercular haemoptysis. *Lancet* ii, 516-17.

British Pharmacopoeia (1975). Addendum. HMSO, London. p. xix.

Britten, J. and Holland R. (1886). A dictionary of English plant-names. Trübner, London.

Brodman, E. (1945). Two different plates in Withering's *Account of the Foxglove. J. Hist. Med*. 17, 415-17.

Brooks, H. (1933). The medicine of the American Indian. *J. Lab. Clin. Med*. 19, 1-23.

Broughton, A. (1779). *Dissertatio medica, de vermibus intestinorum*. Edinburgh.

Brughmanns, M. (1856). Effects of digitalis on generative organs. *Rév. Méd. Chir.* (quoted in *Med. T. Gaz*. NS13, 120-1).

Budge, E. A. W. (trans.) (1913). *Syrian anatomy, pathology and therapeutics, or the book of medicines*. Oxford University Press, London.

Calhoun, J. A. and Harrison, J. R. (1931). Studies in congestive heart failure. IX. The effect of digitalis on the potassium content of the cardiac muscle of dogs. *J. Clin. Invest*. 10, 139-44.

Cattell, M. and Goodall, H. (1937). On the mechanism of the action of digitalis glucosides on muscle. *Science*. 86, 106-7.

Christian, H. A. (1919). Digitalis therapy: satisfactory effects in cardiac cases with regular pulse-rate. *Am. J. Med. Sci.* **157**, 593-602.

Church, G., Schamroth, L., Schwartz, N., Marriott, H. J. L. (1962). Deliberate digitalis intoxication. A comparison of the effects of four glycoside preparations. *Ann. Intern. med.* **57**, 946-56.

Coade, R. (1755). *Boerhaave's materia medica or the druggists' guide*. London.

Cohen, H. (1955). The evolution of the concept of disease. *Proc. R. Soc. Med.* **48**, 155-60.

Cohn, A. E. (1915). Clinical and electrocardiograhic studies on the action of digitalis. *J. Am. Med. Ass*, **65**, 1527-33.

Comroe, J. H. and Dripps, R. D. (1976). Scientific basis for the support of biomedical science. *Science* **192**, 105-11.

Corrigan, D. J. (1832). On permanent patency of the mouth of the aorta, or inadequacy of the aortic valves. *Edin. Med. Surg. J.* **37**, 225-45.

Cowen, D. L. (1957). The Edinburgh Pharmacopoeia. I. Historical development and significance. *Med. Hist.* **1**, 123-39.

Cowley, P. S. and Rowson, J. M. (1963). Clinical studies of the leaves and inflorescences of *Digitalis purpurea* L. and of related species. *J. Pharm. Pharmac.* **15**, 119-22T.

Cox, J. M. (1790). History of a case of insanity, cured by the use of the Digitalis purpurea. *Med. Comm.* **4** (decade II), 261-70.

Coxhill, W. T. (1946). Brasenose College in the time of Principal Ralph Cawley 1770-1777. *B. Litt. Thesis.* University of Oxford.

Crane, J. (1799). [Withering's obituary] *Gentleman's Magazine* **69(ii)**, 907-8.

Culpeper, N. (1653). *Pharmacopoeia Londinensis; or, the London dispensatory further adorned by the studies and collections of the fellows, not living of the said colledg* ... P. Cole, London.

— (1681). *The complete herbal and English physician enlarged.* G. Sawbridge, London.

Currie, W. (1790). Observations on the Digitalis purpurea, or foxglove. *Mem. Med. Soc. Lond.* **4**, 10-15.

Curtis, W. (1777). *Flora Londinensis: or plates and descriptions of such plants as grow wild in the environs of London: with their places of growth, and times of flowering; their several names according to Linnaeus and other authors; with a particular description of each plant in Latin and English. To which are added, their several uses in medicine, agriculture, rural oeconomy and other arts*. London.

Cushny, A. R. (1897). On the action of substances of the digitalis series on the circulation in mammals. *J. Exp. Med.* **2**, 233-99.

— (1925). *The action and uses in medicine of digitalis and its allies*. Longmans, Green & Co., London.

— Marris, H. E., and Silberberg, M. D. (1913). The action of digitalis in therapeutics. *Heart* **4**, 33-58.

Dall, J. L. C. (1970). Maintenance digoxin in elderly pateints. *Br. Med. J*. **i**, 705-6.

Darwin, C. (1780). *Experiments establishing a criterion between mucaginous and purulent matter and an account of the retrograde motions of the absorbent vessels of animal bodies in some diseases*. J. Jackson, Lichfield.

Darwin, E. (1780). Life of the author. In Darwin, C. (1780). pp. 127-35.

— (1785). An account of the successful use of foxglove in some dropsies, and in the pulmonary consumption. *Med. Trans. Coll. Phys*. **3**, 255-86.

— (1789-91). *The Botanic Garden; a poem in two parts*. (Part II published in Lichfield, 1789; part I published in London (J. Johnson), 1791).

— (1801). The phaenomena of dropsies explained. In *Zoonomia, or the laws of organic life*. 3rd edn. J. Johnson, London. XXIX.5.1-2, pp. 477-92.

de la Mare, W. (1960). *Come hither*. Constable, London.

Department of Health and Social Security (1975). Circular DDL (75)1: Digoxin tablets BP. Circulars DDL (75)2, CPH (75)4: Digoxin tablets BP—reminder.

Dickstein, E. S. and Kunkel, F. W. (1980). Foxglove tea poisoning. *Am. J. Med*. **69**, 167-9.

Dickenson, W. H. (1855). On the action of digitalis upon the uterus. *Med. T. Gaz*. **NS11**, 609.

Dodoens, R. (1554). *Remberti Dodonaei, stirpium historiae pemptades*. Antwerp (*see also* Lyte 1578).

Doherty, J. (1968). The clinical pharmacology of digitalis glycosides. *Am. J. Med. Sci*. **255**, 382-414.

Dover, T. (1732). *The ancient physician's legacy to his country. Being what he has collected himself in forty-nine years practice: or, an account of the several diseases incident to mankind, described in so plain a manner, that any person may know the nature of his own disease*. London.

Drake, N. (1799). [On the cure of consumption] *Med. Phys. J*. **ii**, 417-30.

Dunlop, D. and Alstead, S. (1966). *Textbook of medical treatment*, 10th edn. E & S Livingstone, Edinburgh.

Edinburgh Medical and Physical Dictionary (1807). Bell, Bradflute, Doig & Stevenson, Edinburgh.

Einthoven, W. (1903). Die galvanometrische Registrirung des menschlichen Elektrokardiogramms, zugleich eine Beurtheilung der Anwendung des Capillar-Elektrometers in der Physiologie. *Pflüg. Arch. Ges. Physiol*. **99** , 472-80.

Eliot, G. (1861). *Silas Marner; the weaver of Raveloe*. W. Blackwood & Sons, Edinburgh and London.

Estes, J. W. (1979). *Hall Jackson and the purple foxglove: medical practice in revolutionary America 1760-1820*. University Press of New England, Hanover NH.

— and White, P. D. (1965). William Withering and the purple foxglove. *Sci. Am*. **212(vi)**, 114-19.

Evans, F. J. and Cowley, P. S. (1972). Cardenolides and spirostanols in *Digitalis purpurea* at various stages of development. *Phytochem*. **11**, 2971-5.

Feil, H. (1966). The story of a verse on the foxglove. *Bull. Cleveland Med. Libr*. **14**, 12-14.

Fennell, S. (1869). Digitalis in scarlet fever. *Lancet* **i**, 143.

Ferriar, J. (1781). *Dissertatio medica, de variola*.

— (1792). *Medical histories and reflections*. T. Cadell, London.

— (1799). *An essay on the medical properties of the Digitalis purpurea, or foxglove*. Sowler & Russell, Manchester.

Flora danica (1761-1883). *Icones plantarum sponte nascentium in regnis Daniae et Norvegiae, in ducatibus Slesvici et Holsatiae et in comitatibus Oldenburgi et Delmenhorstiae*. Vols. 1-3 (ed. G. C. Oeder, 1761-70), Vols. 4-5 (ed. Q. F. Muller, 1771-82). C & A Philiberti, Hafnia.

Forbes, J., Tweedie, A., and Conolly, J. (eds) (1833). *The cyclopaedia of medical practice*. Sherwood, Gilbert & Piper, and Baldwin & Cradock; Whitaker, Treacher & Co., London.

Fowler, T. (1785). *Medical reports of the effects of tobacco, principally with regard to its diuretic quality, in the cure of dropsies, and dysuries: together with some observations, on the use of clysters of tobacco, in the treatment of colic*. J. Johnson, London.

—— (1786). *Medical reports of the effects of arsenic, in the cure of agues, remitting fevers, and periodic headaches. Together with a letter from Dr Arnold of Leicester, and another from Dr Withering, describing their experience of the effects of arsenic in the cure of intermittents*. J. Johnson, London.

Frank, O. (1895). Zur Dynamik des Herzmuskels. *Z. Biol*. **14**, 370-437 (translated (1959) by C. B. Chapman, *Am. Heart. J*. **58**, 282-317, 467-78).

Friedman, M. and Bine, R. (1949). Study of rate of disappearance of digitalis glycoside (lanatoside C) from blood of man. *J. Clin. Invest*. **28**, 32-4.

Fuchs, L. (1542). De digitali. In *De historia stirpium commentarii insignes maximis impensis et vigiliis eld borati, adjectis parundem viaris plusquam quingentis imaginibus, numquam antea ad naturae imitationem artificiosus effictis et expressis . . . Basileae, in officina isingriniana*. pp. 892-4.

Furukawa, H., Bilezikian, J. P., and Loeb, J. N. (1980). Kinetics and thermodynamics of ouabain binding by intact turkey erythrocytes. *J. Gen. Physiol*. **76**, 499-516.

Garrod, A. B. (1875). *The essentials of materia medica and therapeutics*, 5th edn. Longmans, Green & Co., London, pp. 331-3.

Gerard, J. (1597). *The herball or generall historie of plantes*. J. Norton, London.

—— (1633). The herball or generall historie of plantes. Revised and enlarged by T. Johnson. Islip, Norton & Whitakers, London.

Gibbons, S. (1932). *Cold comfort farm*. Longmans, Green & Co., London.

Gibbs, R. D. (1974). *Chemotaxonomy of flowering plants*. McGill-Queen's University Press, Montreal and London. Vol. 2, pp. 725-50.

Glynn, I. M. (1957). The action of cardiac glycosides on sodium and potassium movements in human red cells. *J. Physiol*. **136**, 148-73.

Gold, H. (1941). [Quoted by Spector, R. Digitalis therapy in heart failure: a rational approach. *J. Clin. Pharmacol*. **19**, 692-6].

—— (1946). Pharmacologic basis of cardiac therapy. *J. Am. Med. Ass*. **132**, 547-54.

—— Cattell, McK., Otto, H. L., Kwit, N. T., and Kramer, M. L. (1942). A method for the bio-assay of digitalis in humans. *J. Pharmacol. Exp. Ther*. **75**, 196-206.

—— —— Modell, W., Kwit, N. T., Kramer, M. L., and Zahn, W. (1944). Clinical studies on digitoxin (digitaline Nativelle) with further observations on its use in the single average full dose method of digitalization. *J. Pharmacol. Exp. Ther*. **82**, 187-95.

Gourvat, A.-P. (1872). Antiplastic and lowering action of digitalis. *Gaz. Med. Paris* [quoted in *Lancet* **i**, 50].

Graham, T. J. (1844). *Modern domestic medicine*. London, p. 35.

Grahame-Smith, D. G. and Aronson, J. K. (1984). *The Oxford textbook of clinical pharmacology and drug therapy*. Oxford University Press, Oxford.

—— and Everest, M. S. (1969). Measurement of digoxin in plasma and its use in diagnosis of digoxin intoxication. *Br. med. J*. **i**, 286-9.

Hagen, P. S. (1939). The effects of digilanid C in varying dosage upon the potassium and water content of rabbit heart muscle. *J. Pharmacol. Exp. Ther*. **67**, 50-5.

Hale-White, W. (1929). The Withering letters in the possession of the Royal Society of Medicine. *Proc. R. Soc. Med*. **22**, 1087-91 (*see also* Osler Bequest 1928).

von Haller, A. (1768). *Historia stirpium indigenarum helvetiae inchoata*. Berne.

Hamer, J. (1979). The paradox of the lack of efficacy of digitalis in congestive heart failure with sinus rhythm. *Br. J. Clin. Pharmacol*. **8**, 109-13.

Hamilton, D. (1981). *The healers. A history of medicine in Scotland*. Canongate, Edinburgh.

Hamilton, W. (1807). *Observations on the preparations, utility, and administration of the Digitalis purpurea, or foxglove, in dropsy of the chest, consumption, hemorrhage, scarlet fever, measles, etc.; including a sketch of the medical history of the plant, and an account of the opinions of those authors who have written upon it, during the last thirty years*. Longman, London.

Harris, E. D. (1983). Lyme disease—success for academia and the community. *New Engl. J. Med*. **308**, 773-5.

Hart, G., Noble, D., and Shimoni, Y. (1983). The effects of low concentrations of cardiotonic steroids on membrane currents and tension in sheep Purkinje fibres. *J. Physiol*. **334**, 103-31.

Herbarium Apuleius Platonicus (c. 1120) MS Bodley 130.

Heywood, V. H. (1972). Digitalis L. In: T. G. Tutin, V. H. Heywood, N. A. Burges, D. M. Moore, D. H. Valentine, S. M. Walters, and D. A. Well (ed) *Flora Europaea*. Cambridge University Press, Cambridge. Vol. 3, pp. 239-41.

Hill, B. (1970). Medical impostors. *Hist. Med*. **2(ii)**, 7-11.

Hoffman, C. A. S. (1789). Mineralsystem des Herrn Inspektor Werners mit desen Erläbnis heransgegeben. *Bergmännisches. J*. **2**, 369-92.

Home, F. (1783). *Clinical experiments, histories, and dissections*. 3rd edn., corrected. J. Murray & W. Creech, Edinburgh.

Howarth, S., McMichael, J., and Sharpey-Schafer, E. P. (1946). Effects of venesection in low output heart failure. *Clin. Sci*. **6**, 41-50.

— — — (1947). Effects of oxygen, venesection and digitalis in chronic heart failure from disease of the lungs. *Clin. Sci*. **6**, 187-96.

Hudson, W. (1762). *Flora anglica, exhibens plantas per regnum Angliae sponte crescens, distributas secundum systema sexuale* ... London.

Hulme, N. (1765). *Dissertatio medica inauguralis, de scorbuto*. A. Donaldson & J. Reid, Edinburgh.

Hulse, E. (1668). *Disputatio medica inauguralis de hydrope*. J. Elsevier, Leyden.

Hutcheon, D., Nemeth, E., and Quinlan, D. (1980). The role of furosemide alone and in combinaton with digoxin in the relief of symptoms of congestive heart failure. *J. Clin. Pharmacol*. **20**, 59-68.

Iisalo, E. (1977). Clinical pharmacokinetics of digoxin. *Clin. Pharmacokin*, **2**, 1-16.

James, R. (1745). *A medicinal dictionary*. T. Osborne, London.

Jameson, E. (1961). *The natural history of quackery*. Michael Joseph, London.

Jewson, N. D. (1974). Medical knowledge and the patronage system in 18th century England. *Sociology*. **8**, 369-85.

Johnson, S. (1805). *An account of the life of Dr. Samuel Johnson from his birth to his eleventh year, written by himself*. R. Phillips, London.

Johnston, G. D., Kelly, J. G., and McDevitt, D. G. (1978). Do patients take digoxin? *Br. Heart J*. **40**, 1-7.

— McDevitt, D. G. (1979). Is maintenance digoxin necessary in patients with sinus rhythm? *Lancet* **i**, 567-70.

Johnstone, E. (1799). *De febre puerperali*. Balfour & Smellie, Edinburgh.

Jones, W. (1787). An account of two cases of insanity, one of which was cured by the use of the foxglove: also a case of hemoptysis, cured by the same remedy. *Med. Comm*. **1** (decade II), 302-16.

Jounela, A. J., Pentikäinen, P. L., and Sothmann, A. (1975). Effect of particle size on the bioavailability of digoxin. *Europ. J. Clin. Pharmacol*. **8**, 365-70.

Laroche, M. (1854). Case of nocturnal seminal emissions successfully treated by digitaline. *Gaz. Méd. Paris* [quoted in *Med. T. Gaz*. **NS9**, 473-4.]

Lely, A. H. and van Enter, C. H. J. (1970). Large-scale digitoxin intoxication. *Br. Med. J*. **iii**, 737-40.

Lettsom, J. C. (1769). *Dissertatio inauguralis medica, sistens observationes ad vires theae pertinentes*. T. Haak, Leyden.

— (1789). Of the Digitalis purpurea in hydropic diseases. *Mem. Med. Soc. Lond*. **2**, 145-76.

— (1794). Of the Digitalis purpurea in hydropic diseases. *Mem. Med. Soc. Lond*. **2** (2nd edn), 145-76 (as in 1st edn) and 177-80 (added in 2nd edn).

Lewis, T. (1919). On cardinal principles in cardiological practice. *Br. Med. J*. **ii**, 621-5.

— (1937). Sir James Mackenzie. In J. R. H. Weaver (ed.) *Dictionary of national biography* 1922-1930. Oxford University Press, London. pp. 543-4.

— and Mackenzie, J. (1909-1925). *Correspondence*. Wellcome Institute for the History of Medicine, London.

Lewis, W. (1761). *An experimental history of the materia medica, or of the natural and artificial substances made use of in medicine: containing a compendious view of their natural history, an account of their pharmaceutic properties and an estimate of their medicinal powers*. Antwerp.

von Linné, C. (1735). *Caroli Linnaei, systema naturae sive regna tria naturae systematice proposita per classes, ordines, genera, et species*. T. Haak, Leyden.

Liverpool Therapeutics Group (1978) Use of digitalis in general practice. *Br. Med. J*. **iv**, 673-5.

Lonicerus, A. (1551). *Naturalis historiae opus novum*. C. Egenhoffs, Frankfurt.

—— (1564). *Kräuterbuch und künstliche conterfeyunge der bäumen, stauden, hecken, kräuten, getreyde, gewürtzer* ... C. Egenhoffs, Frankfurt.

Lowenstein, J. M. and Corrill, E. M. (1966). An improved method for measuring plasma and tissue concentrations of digitalis glycosides. *J. Lab. Clin. Med*. **67**, 1048-52.

Luten, D. (1924). Clinical studies of digitalis. I. Effects produced by the administration of massive dosage to patients with normal mechanism. *Arch. Int. Med*. **33**, 251-78.

Lyte, H. (1578). *A niewe herball or historie of plants* [translation of Dodoens 1554]. Gerard Devves, London.

McHaffie, D., Purcell, H., Mitchell-Heggs, P., and Guz, A. (1978). The clinical value of digoxin in patients with heart failure in sinus rhythm. *Q. J. Med*. **NS47**, 401-19.

McKenzie, D. (1927). *The infancy of medicine. An enquiry into the influence of folk-lore upon the evolution of scientific medicine*. Macmillan, London.

Mackenzie, J. (1902). *The study of the pulse, arterial, venous, and hepatic, and of the movements of the heart*. Y. J. Pentland, Edinburgh and London.

—— (1905a) New methods of studying affections of the heart. I.—Affections of the function of conductivity. *Br. Med. J*. **i**, 519-22.

—— (1905b). New methods of studying affections of the heart. II.—The action of digitalis on the human heart. *Br. Med. J*. **i**, 587-9.

—— (1905c). New methods of studying affections of the heart. III.—The action of digitalis on the human heart—(continued). *Br. Med. J*. **i**, 702-5.

—— (1905d). New methods of studying affections of the heart. IV.—

374   BIBLIOGRAPHY

5Action of digitalis on the human heart in cases where the inception of
the rhythm of the heart is due to the ventricle. *Br. Med. J.* **i**, 759-62.
— (1905e). New methods of studying affections of the heart. V.—The
inception of the rhythm of the heart by the ventricle. *Br. Med. J.* **i**,
812-15.
— (1905f). A preliminary enquiry into the tonicity of the muscle fibres
of the heart. *Br. Med. J.* **ii**, 1689-91.
— (1911a). the Oliver-Sharpey lectures on heart failure. Lecture II.—
The estimation of heart failure and the significance of symptoms. *Br.
Med. J.* **i**, 858-63.
— (1911b). Digitalis. *Heart* **2**, 273-89.
McKeown, T. and Lowe, C. R. (1966). *Introduction to social medicine.*
Blackwell Scientific Publications, Oxford.
Maclean, L. (1799). [On the Digitalis purpurea] *Med. Phys. J.* **2**, 113-27.
— (1810). *An inquiry into the nature, causes, and cure of hydrothorax; illustrated by interesting cases, and many living examples of the success of the
method recommended.* J. Birkitt, Sudbury.
McMichael, J. (1981). Sir James Mackenzie and atrial fibrillation—a new
perspective. *J. R. Coll. Gen. Pract.* **31**, 402-6.
— and Sharpey-Schafer, E. P. (1944). The action of intravenous digoxin
in man. *Q. J. Med.* **NS13**, 123-35.
Magennis, J. (1801). Observations on the effects of the Digitalis purpurea, in the cure of phthisis pulmonalis. *Med. Phys. J.* **5**, 201-16.
Martindale, W. H., Westcott, W. W. (1932-35). *The extra pharmacopoeia*,
20th edn. Vol. 1 (1932), Vol. 2 (1935). H. K. Lewis, London.
Marvin, H. M. (1927). Digitalis and diuretics in heart failure with regular
rhythm, with especial reference to the importance of etiologic classi-
fication of heart disease. *J. Clin. Invest.* **3**, 521-39.
Masson, D. (ed.) (1889-90). *The collected writings of Thomas de Quincy.*
A. & C Black, Edinburgh.
Meryon, E. (1871). On the functions of the sympathetic nervous system
of nerves, as a physiologic basis for a rational system of therapeutics.
Lancet **2**, 704-6.
Monro, A. (1752). Improvements in performing the operation of the
paracentesis, or tapping of the belly. *Med. Essays* **1**, 173-80.
Moore, N. (1887) Sir Dominic John Corrigan. In *Dictionary of national*

biography (ed. L. Stephen and S. Lee) Smith, Elder & Co., London. Vol. 12, pp. 1177-8.

Morison, R. (1672-99). *Historia plantarum universalis oxoniensis seu herbarum distributio nova, per tabulas cognationis et affinitatis ex libro naturae observata et detecta*. Oxford.

Munro-Faure, A. D., Fowle, A. S. E., Johnson, B. F., and Lader, S. (1974). Recognition of variable bioavailability as an international problem: a review of the earlier studies. *Postgrad. Med. J.* **50** (suppl 6), 14-17.

Murchison, C. (1870). Clinical lectures on medicine. Lecture IV, Part III. Treatment of delirium tremens. *Lancet* **ii**, 596-8.

Murray, J. A. (1776-92). *Apparatus medicaminum tam simplicium quae praeparatorum et compositorum in praxeos adjumentum consideratus*. J. C. Dieterich, Göttingen.

Neale, R. (1877). *The medical digest* 3rd edn. Ledger, Smith & Co., London.

Noble, D. (1980). Mechanism of action of therapeutic levels of cardiac glycosides. *Cardiovasc. Res.* **14**, 495-514.

Office of Population Censuses and Surveys, Occupational Mortality (1978). *The Registrar General's decennial supplement for England and Wales*. 1970-72. HMSO, London.

Osler Bequest (1928) Withering's letters, papers, and graduation diploma, catalogued by Sir William Hale-White. In the possession of the Royal Society of Medicine (unpublished) (see also Hale-White 1929).

Osler, W. (1930). *The principles and practice of medicine* 11th edn. Y. J. Pentland, Edinburgh and London.

Parkinson, J. (1640). *Theatrum botanicum; the theater of plants. Or, an herball of a large extent . . . With the chiefe notes of Dr. Lobel, Dr. Borham, and others inserted therein*. T. Coles, London.

Peacock, J. B. (1861). Notes on the treatment of delirium tremens by large doses of tincture of digitalis. *Med. T. Gaz.* **NS23**, 104-6.

Peck, T. W. and Wilkinson, K. D. (1950). *William Withering of Birmingham*. John Wright & Sons, Bristol; Simpkin Marshall Ltd., London.

Pena, P. and de L'obel, M. (1570). *Stirpium adversaria nova, perfacilis vestigatio, luculentaque accessio ad priscorum, presertim Dioscoridi et recentioru, materiam medicam*. T. Purfoetij, London.

Percival, T. (1767-73). *Essays medical and experimental*. J. Johnson & B. Davenport, London.

Post, R. L. (1974). A reminiscence about sodium, potassium-ATPase. *Ann. N. Y. Acad. Sci.* **242**, 6-11.

Priestley, J. (1788). Additional experiments and observations relating to the principle of acidity, the composition of water, and phlogiston. With letters to him on the subject by Dr. William Withering and James Keir. *Phil. Trans. R. Soc. Lond.* **73**, 313-30.

Prior, R. C. A. (1863). *On the proper names of British plants*. Williams & Norgate, London.

Pulteney, R. (1781). *A general view of the writings of Linnaeus*. T. Payne, London.

—— (1790). *Historical and biographical sketches of the progress of botany in England, from its origin to the introduction of the Linnaean system*. T. Cadell, London.

Quin, C. W. (1779). *Dissertatio medica inauguralis, de hydrocephalo interno*. Balfour & Smellie, Edinburgh.

—— (1790). *A treatise on the dropsy of the brain, illustrated by a variety of cases. To which are added observations on the use and effects of the Digitalis purpurea in dropsies*. J. Murray & W. Jones, London.

Quincy, J. (1742). *Pharmacopoeia officinalis et extemporanea, or a complete English dispensatory in four parts* . . . J. Osborne & T. Longman, London.

Rader, B., Smith, W. W., Berger, A., Eichna, L. W. (1964). Comparison of the hemodynamic effects of mercurial diuretics and digitalis in congestive heart failure. *Circulation* **29**, 328-35.

Ray, J. (1686). *Historia plantarum*. H. Faithorne & J. Kersley, London. Vol. 1, p. 768.

—— (1690). *Synopsis methodica stirpium britannicarum, in qua tum notae generum characteristicae traduntur, tum species singulae breviter describuntur: ducentae quinquaginta plus minus novae species parim suis locis inseruntur, partim in appendice seorsim exhibentur*. S. Smith, London.

Revelle, R. (1972). Introduction. In *Population and social change* (ed. D. V. Glass and R. Revelle). Edward Arnold.

Reynolds, H. D. (1869). Case of suppression of urine cured by the external use of digitalis. *Lancet* ii, 635.

Rivinus, A. Q. (1690-9). *Introductio generalis in rem herbariam*. C. Gunther, Leipzig.

Roddis, L. H. (1936). William Withering and the introduction of digitalis into medical practice. *Ann. Med. Hist.* NS8, 93-112 and 185-201.

Rogen, A. S. (1943). Maintenance treatment with digitalis. *Br. Med. J.* i, 694-5.

Sacks, O. (1973). *Awakenings*. G. Duckworth & Co., London.

Salerne, F. (1748). Observation de botanique. *Hist. Acad. R. Sci.* 1, 84-5.

Salmon, W. (1710). *Botanologia. the English herbal: or, history of plants*. H. Rhodes & J. Taylor, London.

Sansom, A. E. (1886). On some modern remedies in heart disease. *Lancet* i, 535-6.

Sayers, D. (1921). *The unpleasantness at the Bellona Club*. Victor Gollancz, London.

Schatzmann, H.-J. (1953). Herzglykoside als Hemmstoffe für den aktiven Kalium- und Natriumstransport durch die Erythrocytenmembran. *Helv. Physiol. Acta* 11, 346-54.

Schimmelpenninck, M. A. (1858). *Life of Mary Anne Schimmelpenninck* (C. C. Hankin, ed). Vol. 1. Autobiography. Longman, Brown, Green, Longmans & Roberts, London.

Schofield, R. E. (1963). *The Lunar Society of Birmingham. A social history of provincial science and industry in eighteenth-century England*. Clarendon Press, Oxford.

Schwartz, A., Lindenmayer, G. E., and Allen, J. C. (1975). The sodium-potassium adenosine triphosphatase: pharmacological, physiological and biochemical aspects. *Pharmacol. Rev.* 27, 3-134.

Serre, C. (1860). Excerpta minora. Quinine and digitalis. *Med. T. Gaz.* NS20, 840.

Sheiner, L. B., Rosenberg, B., Marathe, V. V., and Peck, C. (1974). Differences in serum digoxin concentrations between outpatients and inpatients: an effect of compliance? *Clin. Pharmacol. Ther.* 15, 239-46.

Sherwen, J. (1800). [On digitalis] *Med. Phys. J.* **3**, 307-11.

Sigmond, G. G. (1837). Lectures on materia medica and therapeutics. Lectures XVIII-XXI. *Lancet* **ii**, 457-62, 529-34, 567-72, 609-11.

Simmons, W. (1801). [On digitalis] *Med. Phys. J.* **6**, 133-5.

Skou, J. C. (1957). The influence of some cations on an adenosine triphosphatase from peripheral nerves. *Biochim. Biophys. Acta* **23**, 394-401.

Smith, S. (1930). Digoxin, a new digitalis glucoside. *J. Chem. Soc.* **i**, 508-10.

Smith, W. D. L. (1956). Malaria and the Thames. *Lancet* **i**, 433-6.

Smith, T. W., Butler, V. P., and Haber, E. (1969). Determination of therapeutic and toxic serum digoxin concentrations by radioimmunoassay. *New Engl. J. Med.* **281**, 1212-16.

— Haber, E., Yeatman, L., and Butler, V. P. (1976). Reversal of advanced digoxin intoxication with Fab fragments of digoxin-specific antibodies. *New Engl. J. Med.* **294**, 797-800.

— Butler, V. P., Haber, E., Fozzard, H., Marcus, F. I., Bremner, F., Schulman, I. C., and Phillips, A. (1983). Treatment of life-threatening digitalis intoxication with digoxin-specific Fab fragments. *New Engl. J. Med.* **307**, 1357-62.

Squire, P. W. (1916). *Squire's companion to the British pharmacopoeia*, 19th edn. J & A Churchill, London.

Starling, E. H. (1918). *The Linacre lecture on the law of the heart. Given at Cambridge, 1915*. Longmans, Green & Co., London.

Stewart, H. J., Crane, N. F., Dietrick, J. E., and Wheeler, C. H. (1938a) Action of digitalis in uncomplicated heart disease. *Arch. Intern. Med.* **62**, 546-68.

— Dietrick, J. E., Crane, N. F., and Wheeler, C. H. (1938b). Action of digitalis in uncomplicated heart disease. *Arch. Intern. Med.* **62**, 569-92.

Stirling, D. H. (1864). Digitalis in cardiac disease. *Med. T. Gaz.* **NS28**, 251-2.

Stokes, J. (1782). *Dissertatio inauguralis, de phlogisticato*. Balfour & Smellie, Edinburgh.

— (1812). *A botanical materia medica; consisting of the generic and specific characters of the plants used in medicine and diet, with synonyms, and references to medical authors*. J. Johnson, London.

Thorowgood, J. C. (1864). Digitalis in cardiac disease. *Med. T. Gaz.* **NS28**, 212.

Tibbits, E. T. (1881). On the modern theory of the action of digitalis. *Lancet* **ii**, 586-7.

Topsell, E. (1607). *The historie of foure-footed beasts . . . collected out of all the volumes of Conradus Gesner, and all other writers to this present day.* W. Iaggard.

de Tournefort, J. P. (1700). *Institutiones rei herbariae.* J. Anisson, Paris.

Traube, L. (1871). Digitalis. *Ges. Beit. Path. Physiol.* **i**, 190 and 252; **ii**, 907.

Turkel, H. L. (1931). *Joachim's translation of the Ebers papyrus, as quoted by 'Scillaren'.* American Druggist.

van Swieten, G. L. B. (1764). *Commentaria in Hermannii Boerhaave aphorismos de cognoscendis et curandis morbis.* J. & H. Verbeek, Leyden.

Wagner, J. G. (1981) History of pharmacokinetics. *Pharmacol. Ther.* **12**, 537-62.

Wakefield, P. (1823). *An introduction to botany* 9th edn. Harvey & Darton; J. Harris & Son; Longman, Hurst, Rees, Orme & Co.; Sherwood & Jones; Baldwin, Craddock & Fry; Simpson & Marshall, London.

Waller (1887). A demonstration on man of the electromotive changes accompanying the heart's beat. *J. Physiol.* **8**, 229-34.

Warren, J. (1785). An account of the great efficacy of the digitalis purpurea in dropsies. *Lond. Med. J.* **6**, 145-58.

Webb, M. (1924). *Precious bane.* Jonathan Cape, London.

Wenckebach, K.-F. (1903). *Die Arhythmie als Ausdruck bestimmter Funktions-storungen des Herzens; eine physiologisch-klinische Studie.* W. Engelman, Leipzig. (Translated (1904) by T. Snowball as *Arrhythmia of the heart. A physiological and clinical study.* William Green & Sons, Edinburgh and London.)

— (1910). Discussion on the effects of digitalis on the human heart. *Br. Med. J.* **ii**, 1600-6.

— (1914). *Die unregelmässige Herztätigkeit und ihre klinische bedeutung.* W. Engelmann, Leipzig.

Wesley, J. (1791). *Primitive physick: or, an easy and natural method of curing most diseases* 23rd edn. London.

Wettrell, G., and Andersson, K.-E. (1977). Clinical pharmacokinetics of digoxin in infants. *Clin. Pharmacokin*. **2**, 17-31.

White, C. (1784). An inquiry into the nature and cause of that swelling in one or both of the lower extremities which sometimes happens to lying-in women. C. Dilly, Warrington.

Whytt, R. (1768). *Observations on the dropsy in the brain*. J. Balfour, Edinburgh.

Wilson, R. McN. (1926). *The beloved physician. Sir James Mackenzie*. John Murray, London.

Wiltshire, A. (1870). Digitalis in delirium tremens. Five cases successfully treated by half-ounce doses of the tincture; with remarks. *Lancet* **ii**, 286-7.

Withering, W. For William Withering's publications see the separate bibliography on pp. 265-7.

Withering, W. Jun. (1822). *The miscellaneous tracts of the late William Withering MD FRS including a memoir of his life, character, and writings*. Longman, Hurst, Rees, Orme & Brown, London.

Wood, P. (1940). The action of digitalis in heart failure with normal rhythm. *Br. Heart J*. **2**, 132-40.

Wright-St. Clair, R. E. (1964). *Doctors Monro: a medical saga*. Wellcome Historical Medical Library, London.

INDEX

TO THE NAMES OF MEDICINES AND PLANTS MENTIONED IN WITHERING'S *ACCOUNT OF THE FOXGLOVE* AND IN THE MARGINAL NOTES

Page numbers in bold print refer to items which are given their own marginal notes. Other page numbers refer to items which are to be found either in Withering's text or within a marginal note.

INDEX

TO THE PROPER NAMES MENTIONED IN WITHERING'S *ACCOUNT OF THE FOXGLOVE* AND IN THE MARGINAL NOTES

Page numbers in bold print refer to items which are given their own marginal notes. Other page numbers refer to items which are to be found either in Withering's text or within a marginal note.

GENERAL INDEX

Note: This index does not include the items contained in the previous two indexes, namely the names of medicines, plants, and people mentioned in William Withering's *An Account of the Foxglove*.